Pier Giorgio Malesani
Massimo Guantieri
Carlo Piazza

GUANTIERIAN HYPNOLOGY
Science and the Art of Hypnosis, according to Gualtiero Guantieri.

Dedicated to Gualtiero Guantieri

Istituto Italiano di Ipnologia Gualtiero Guantieri (già Istituito Italiano Studi di Ipnosi Clinica e Psicoterapia "H. Bernheim" - Scuola di Ricerca e Formazione).

Introduction

*Roots and fruits of Guantierian Hypnological Epistemology,
by Consuelo Candida Casula.*

Consuelo Candida Casula is a specialist in Psychology and Hypnotic Psychotherapy, a teacher at the Italian School of Hypnosis and Ericksonian Psychotherapy, as well as current Past President of the European Society of Hypnosis (E.S.H.) and Member of the Education and Training Committee of the International Society of Hypnosis (I.S.H.). She also taught at the S.P.P.I.E. Bernheim School in Verona.

When I enrolled in the A.M.I.S.I. (Italian Medical Association for the Study of Hypnosis) in 1986, I had already encountered Ericksonian hypnosis through the teachings of Norma and Phill Barretta, whom I met in Milan during a Neurolinguistic Programming course. Their teaching fascinated me to such an extent that, shortly after their acquaintance, I attended my first Ericksonian congress, in Phoenix. There, Barretta introduced me to Jeff Zeig, Michael Yapko, Steve Lanckton and Kay Thompson, who have since become inspirational role models and friends. Perhaps because of my basic training, what I was learning from A.M.I.S.I., about the thought and practice of Gualtiero Guantieri, from the president and teacher Giampiero Mosconi, his friend and colleague, was quite familiar to me. Furthermore, during the years in which I taught at the 'H. Bernheim' School of Psychotherapy in Verona I had the opportunity to come into contact with many of his followers, recognizing the complementarity and continuity between the Ericksonian and Guantierian approaches.

Writing these few lines on how much the thought and practice of Gualtiero Guantieri are still present in my way of conceiving and practicing hypnosis, helps me to make explicit what was previously implicit. In my own practice as a psychotherapist specialised in hypnosis and as a trainer of hypnosis in various schools both in Italy and abroad, Guantieri's teaching is an integral part, along with the voices of other masters I have met throughout my life.
With both patients and students, I emphasise that hypnosis is a form of attachment, which is the outcome of attunement, empathy and connection as a result of a collaboration based on mutual trust between therapist and patient. In a word, familiar to all hypnologists, hypnosis is characterised by that special 'rapport', that being with the patient in their uniqueness and complexity as a human being, embedded in their socio-cultural environment and whose well-being is based on a harmonious balance between mind, body and soul. In

other words, Guantieri's holistic vision saw the hypnologist as a scholar of human sciences, capable of stimulating in patients a process of self-healing and freeing them from a dependency on the hypnotist perceived as *'magician'*.

Guantieri was committed to removing any hint of superstition or trace of magic from hypnosis in order to restore its full sense of dignity as a human science. Hypnology is a discipline influenced by the studies of medicine and neurology, anthropology, sociology and on the interpersonal relationships that define and support man through psychoanalysis, psychosynthesis, transactional analysis and Gestalt. All these must be integrated into a humanistic approach that also embraces a spiritual component, with a systemic vision in which every single factor influences and is influenced by the others.

What is hypnosis if not being present in the *"hic et nunc"*, the here and now, with a patient whose attention is focused, allowing the hypnologist to collect information on relevant events which emerge from the exploratory dialogue carried out with attunement, with a conscious curiosity, the intent of which is to create connection and resonance in order to better understand the request? Resonance, based on the kind intention of helping the patient, in a loving and effective way, to re-discover a lost psycho-somatic well-being and to start to pursue new life goals once again.

Guantieri's teaching did not intend to bind his followers to a copy-and-paste methodology, nor did he want to create clones of himself, but he expected to bring out the unique potential and resources within each interlocutor, whether patient, student or colleague.

The holistic vision that Guantieri promoted correlates to the trust in the self-healing process that the patient puts in motion thanks to the trust they place in the therapist, who in turn shows trust in him/her. This recursive and virtuous circle arises from the rapport that also adapts to Guantieri's practice, which is characterised by empathy, connection and resonance with psychological and therapeutic dynamics, with the aim of making the patient independent in their healing process.

Guantieri conceives each individual as an inseparable psychosomatic entity made up of emotions, sensations, feelings, moods, constantly evolving thanks to the acquisition of self-awareness that emerges, especially in modified states of consciousness. In a hypnotic state, it is possible to stimulate a regression at the service of the ego, achieved through sensory, motor and ideational deprivation and with the activation of adequate motivations that focus attention on the areas which, in that particular trance, stimulate the therapeutic process.

Guantieri, with both patients and students, chooses words whose evocative power heals by awakening empowerment and feelings of participation; words that soothe restless souls, that inspire by motivating the recognition of one's own resources, that renew the compassion to welcome without judging, carefully-spoken words that speak directly to the heart and soul of the people to whom they are addressed. And in its inductions it revives not only the five senses but also the visceral sense of intuition, the natural sense of instinct, the celestial sense of harmony, that of vitality, resilience, benevolence and generosity. Well-considered words that evoke the spiritual sense of values and experiences of universal wisdom learned, respecting the laws of nature.

Guantieri with his multidisciplinary approach has opened the hypnotic field to the integration of the conscious and unconscious, to existential questions about the meaning of life, to mystical reflections with which patients and students can come into contact during the process of creative imagination, and to the realm of the possible, which opens the doors to desire and which prepares to transform itself into action.

His paradigm of a multidisciplinary hypnology open to epistemic doubt and curiosity welcomes the contributions of disciplines that can enrich a global vision of man in health or illness of the body or psyche, helping to provide innovative therapeutic suggestions. A holistic view of a person who has a body that feels joy and pain, who feels emotions and thinks thoughts, who lives in an environment where they are influenced, who can mature that awareness that promotes evolutionary changes, supported by a soul which protects virtues and profound values. With his paradigm, Guantieri wanted to preserve the scientific distinctiveness of hypnosis so that it is not limited to becoming complementary to other disciplines. And so far we can say that he has succeeded.

What is Guantieri's legacy to new generations who intend to learn hypnosis?

It is to take care of the interpersonal relationship, as without such care, any technique becomes inert and any suggestion becomes sterile if it is not presented with due respect towards the person with whom we are building a therapeutic path.

It is this Guantierian hypnology – his way of teaching, his idea of promoting continuing training courses for hypnologists already active in the field, or in training – that this essay by Pier Giorgio Malesani, Massimo Guantieri and Carlo Piazza intends to bring to the fore. The purpose of the book is to revive Guantierian hypnology in the scientific memory of those who recognize the depth of hypnosis, highlighting its clarity and concreteness, so that this cultural heritage continues to blossom and to bear new fruit.

Those who wish to undertake this exciting profession of hypnology will have to ask themselves how much attention they intend to devote to their continuing education, to the awareness of a knowledge that is based on theory, on the knowledge of the teachings of the founders of hypnology, but also on the knowledge of the human soul, because, as Terentius says: *"all that is human belongs to me"*.

And it is this belonging to humanity that makes us compassionate towards human suffering and willing to study the disciplines inherent to the human sciences, medicine, humanistic philosophy, existentialism and psychology, which for centuries have been committed to treating the body to heal the mind and to treating the mind to heal the body. Care that also passes through an awareness of the role of the hypnotherapist who acts as a filter, who uses not only their theories on psychopathology, well-being and ethics, but also enters into an empathic connection with the deep needs of the patient — by choosing, in a flexible manner, the best hypnotic technique for that patient and in that particular phase of his/her therapeutic path. The intimate and engaging relationship that is created between therapist and patient, and also between teacher and students, must be safeguarded from incursions of wounded parts of the self, not sufficiently elaborated, or arbitrary encroachments on areas of investigation not requested by the patient.

The main role of the therapist, as well as that of the teacher, is to protect the patient from anxiety and suffering no longer necessary for their personal and professional development.

Guantieri also worked on identifying some personal and professional behaviours that can help improve therapeutic practice, starting with the attitude towards hypnosis, the intentions that guide its use and the commitment to continuous learning. To this, we can add continuous learning not only surrounding hypnotic techniques, but above all about what promotes greater universal wisdom shared and based on flexibility and the ability to adapt with elasticity to each patient and their problems, and becoming increasingly ready to recognize and respect the specificity of each individual patient or student.

The "maternal" method that Guantieri was keen to offer his students was characterised by closeness, a welcoming manner and confidence, based on reassuring trust in the ability of students and patients to have the necessary resources. It is this mutual closeness that creates trust and, with it, the wisdom based on direct, personal experience, not only mediated by the reading of texts. The students of the training courses in hypnosis learn from direct experience through the observation of teacher demonstrations, but also through exercises on induction or suggestion techniques. They learn, from the ability to observe and participate while maintaining a critical sense, so as not to fall into the trap of those who make what is the result of commitment and honesty appear magical, ready to unmask those who cloak themselves in mystery, those who use smoke and mirrors to conceal the work they are not able to explain with scientific logic. Guantieri did not want to either deceive or be idealised. On the contrary, he stimulated the comparison of the creative meeting of different minds and experiences.

Patients also learn from their own experience, and after the beneficial effects of the hypnotic process in their first trance, they increasingly rely on the therapist and learn to go deeper and deeper. The hypnologist is a therapeutic agent whose goal is to stimulate the patient's evolution, not their dependence, in a safe place created in the therapeutic setting. The goal is to water the roots of the patient's tree of knowledge and at the same time invite them to taste its nourishing fruits.

Thinking about the Guantieri's teaching, this metaphor comes to mind:

"Once upon a time there was a student who admired his teacher to the point that he wanted to become like him. He followed his lessons carefully, memorised his sentences, imitated his style of communicating. One day, the teacher died and the young man at first despaired, then consoled himself by reviewing the numerous recordings of his courses. He looked at all the recordings of the teacher's lessons, with the intention of making them his own, of integrating them into his own way of being. One day, the young man dreamed of his teacher who told him: *"Do as I have done: I have never imitated anyone"*. The young man did not understand the meaning of this dream and went to another teacher for help. The new teacher explained what the young man did not understand about the phrase: *"Do as I have done: I have never imitated anyone"*. "Once understood, the new teacher said to the young man: *"When your time has come, no one will ask you if you have become like your father, like your mother, like your teacher. They will ask you if you have become yourself."* *"Become what you are"*, is also the encouragement used by Pindar with Nietzsche; it could also be the teaching that Gualtiero Guantieri, with his intellectual honesty, wanted to pass on to patients and students and to future generations, inviting them to deepen this stimulating discipline with solid roots and nourishing fruits."

In Memoriam
Dedicated to Gualtiero Guantieri,
by Giuseppe de Benedittis

Giuseppe De Benedittis is Professor at the State University of Milan, Vice President of the Italian Society of Hypnosis (S.I.I.), Past Vice Chairperson of the International Society of Hypnosis (I.S.H.), At-Large Board Director of the same Society.

I am very pleased that the figure of Professor Guantieri is being brought back from the oblivion into which, unfortunately, many significant figures have fallen, and restored to the rightful dimension that historical perspective has assigned to him. I met Professor Guantieri on a couple of occasions, appreciating his skills and professionalism. His 1973 book on Hypnosis has been a reference point for me...

Thus, I wish every success to your (authors of this book, Ed.), commendable publishing initiative.

I have recovered from my papers an obituary I wrote in 1995 for the *"International Journal of Clinical and Experimental Hypnosis"*, published by Taylor & Francis Inc., Philadelphia, (USA), *"in Memoriam"* of Professor Guantieri.

Here is the document: *"In Memoriam of Professor Gualtiero Guantieri. It is with deep regret that we note the passing of Professor Gualtiero Guantieri on October 20th, 1994 at the age of 67. Professor Guantieri was a Fellow of the International Society of Hypnosis and Past President of the European Society of Hypnosis. Born in 1927, he gained his medical degree from the University of Padua in 1951. After a decade practising internal medicine, he became interested in understanding hypnosis and its use, particularly in psychosomatic medicine. In 1963 he became associate professor of psychopathology. In 1970 he was appointed professor of psychiatry at the Universities of Padua and Verona, where he taught extensively on the role of hypnotherapy until 1979. In 1965, Professor Guantieri founded the Centro Italiano di Ipnosi Clinica e Medicina Psicosomatica 'H. Bernheim', (The 'H. Bernheim' Italian Centre for Clinical Hypnosis and Psychosomatic Medicine), where he taught the theory and clinical application of hypnosis to doctors, dentists and psychologists. He greatly contributed to the field of clinical hypnosis in Italy and Europe for many decades. He has been considered as one of the most outstanding clinicians and teachers in his country, since 1963, when he first introduced 'painless childbirth in hypnosis'. He was Fellow of many national and international scientific societies (e.g., the Royal Society of Medicine, London) and Member of the Board of several others. He published over 100 scientific papers on basic research and clinical application of hypnosis and conducted workshops at national and international scientific meetings. In 1993, he was the recipient of the 'Franz Anton Mesmer Award' for Leadership and Achievement in the Field of Hypnosis, by the European Society of Hypnosis. His untimely death is an enormous loss to the profession and to his many colleagues and friends".*

Notations

1. Preface[1]

Gualtiero Guantieri left important testimonies of his professional activity and his scientific knowledge in the world of global hypnology; he did so with tenacity, awareness, and an unmistakable touch of humanity. That is, he related to all those he met in his work, beyond private spheres, frequently reaching not only their rational minds, but also their hearts and affections, promoting positive emotions and feelings with gentleness and human nobility.

He therefore gave humanity, as a great protagonist, small and powerful seeds capable of germinating and producing good fruits which would continue to reproduce and leave a positive mark on the world.

His works speak of him first of all – also echoed across various scientific congresses and in some digital libraries – while many people who knew him hold him in high regard, testifying to positive memories of him.

Some of their contributions follow, as we have been able to recover them, in some cases summarising them and adapting them to our 'mission' of illustrating the figure and thought of Gualtiero Guantieri.

Guantieri was the promoter, the main architect, the founder of a school of scientific thought, study, research and training, which produced knowledge, developed methods of use, provided training in the world of hypnology, both nationally and internationally, with extraordinary effectiveness and in a very original form, very difficult to replicate and sustain, and especially to improve.

Since his death, the 'H. Bernheim' Institute of Clinical Hypnosis and Psychotherapy [2], which he built, has over time continued to experience an increasing sense of fatigue, discouragement and loss, despite many of his followers having shown a strong desire to proceed, to move forward, to resist.

It was an inevitable crisis for his followers, after his departure in 1994, occurring on all levels and which, over time, inevitably grew, making it increasingly difficult for them to continue on the path that their master had mapped out.

Objectively, it is no easy feat: Guantieri was a charismatic leader, well known in the medical and psychological world; he dialogued with everyone and proposed his thoughts in pleasant and convincing ways and was an indefatigable animator and organiser, processor of ideas and actions for the renewal of medicine and human sciences with great, enviable and irreproducible charm.

He was a strong point of reference for a multitude of professionals who were in need of scientific development, eager for professional and personal growth, and for innovative knowledge of their skills.

---

[1] Graphics and proofreading by Marisa Malesani and Carlo Piazza.
[2] The history of the 'Bernheim' Institute is covered in Chapter 2 of this text.

Guantieri frequented the world of hypnology far and wide; he often travelled abroad as a scholar, professor or when presenting the latest results of a knowledge that was being gradually acquired.

In both Italian and foreign universities and international hypnology institutes, he was particularly active, often with presidential or managerial responsibilities, and was often coordinator of and participator in the congresses that systematically took place here and there across the various continents.

Guantieri was in this sense an honorary citizen and scientist of the world.

He had feeling, a strong predilection, a keen affection, a great understanding and critical attention towards a wisdom that he loved: he asked himself questions and undertook studies and reflected, certainly on hypnosis, hypnotic states and the effects that it determines, but also on the very man who considers it, lives it, practices it.

In doing so, he gave scientific foundations to what he was considering, following a certain track, indispensable for an investigative procedure that has a philosophical and epistemological basis.

He was equipped with a compass to orient himself in the definition of conditions by means of which it was possible to achieve knowledge that was important to him, according to methods and procedures capable of dissecting knowledge as complex as that of hypnology, and that involves specific scientific methods.

The 'Bernheim' Institute is certainly the first heir to hypnology that he was able to create, but now there is exists a serious task, or more precisely, an immense task of keeping it alive, cultivating it, making it grow, bear fruit and reviving it.

This can be done by starting again from an awareness: that a Schoolmaster like Gualtiero Guantieri is no longer with us and that – as orphans of his – one must recognize the grief that has affected the fragility of those who want to follow him, the poverty of the resources available to them, the modesty necessary to proceed.

We can only start again from him, considering that this chronic crisis that has been going on for a long time has somehow clouded the very image of the Founder and his knowledge, with the inevitable risk of dissipating the same scientific paradigm that he left behind.

This book has a specific purpose: that of rediscovering Guantieri, of rediscovering the roots of his teaching, of recognizing him as a venerable pioneer, worthy of the utmost consideration, and a respectable source of pride for his followers. They can proceed modestly, retracing his practice, re-establishing national and international scientific connections, rethinking a Guantierian Hypnology that does not disdain complexity and therefore involves strenuous work, but which nevertheless deserves to be done. Guantieri not only has a relevant place in current affairs, but also deserves a revival in the future of hypnology.

2
Considerations and memories, by hypnologists who were acquainted with Gualtiero Guantieri

Directors of national and international institutes of hypnology

The Gentleman of Hypnology,
by Walter Bongartz

Walter Bongartz, Psychotherapist, Director of Klingenberger Institute for Clinical Hypnosis of Constance, Past President of the German Society of Hypnosis and Hypnotherapy, of the European Society of Hypnosis (E.S.H.) and of the International Society of Hypnosis (I.S.H.), in a nutshell writes:
To me, Gualtiero Guantieri was always the 'gentleman' of hypnosis, endowed with this special Italian nobility. I remember him as a true friend, a colleague and a luminary whose contributions were so valuable to the science of hypnosis.

The Bridge,
by Maria Paola Brugnoli

Maria Paola Brugnoli, is Surgeon, Specialist in Anaesthesia and Intensive Care, Pain Therapy and Palliative Care, Neuro-bioethics, Hypnotherapist; PhD in Neuroscience, Psychology and Psychiatry; Past Research Fellow at the American Government National Institutes of Health (N.I.H.) Medical Research Centre, Clinical Centre, Pain and Palliative Care, Bethesda, U.S.A., Coordinator of the International, Interdisciplinary, Inter-religious, Consciousness Studies, Research Centre of Neuro-bioethics GdN, at the UNESCO Chair of Bioethics and Human Rights, Pontifical Athenaeum Regina Apostolorum, Rome, Italy, Director of the Ethics Committee of the Italian Scientific Society of Clinical Hypnosis in Psychotherapy and Humanistic Medicine (S.I.P.M.U.), Member of the American Society of Clinical Hypnosis (A.S.C.H.), European Society of Hypnosis (E.S.H.) and International Society of Hypnosis (I.S.H.).
In the 1960s, my father Angelico introduced us to his friend and colleague Dr.Gualtiero Guantieri, a medical doctor, psychotherapist and hypnotherapist. At that time, I was a child attending elementary school. I remember my father often inviting his friend Gualtiero to our house, with whom he discussed an innovative therapy: clinical hypnosis. Gualtiero's wife, Anna Maria, soon became one of my mother's closest friends. Even though I was a child, I was very intrigued by hypnosis, because I saw great enthusiasm in Gualtiero and in my father. Gualtiero had just founded the 'Bernheim', and had invited my father Angelico, and other

Italian doctor-scholars of clinical hypnosis, to enrol [Brugnoli would later become a founding member of the 'Institute', born out of the transformation of the Centre, in 1968, Ed.]. For many years my family frequented the Gualtieris assiduously: my brothers and I were friends with their children Massimo and Francesca, we spent the summer holidays together in Jesolo (Venice) for many years, or we spent Sundays at their country house 'La Fasanara', in Valpolicella (Verona). Gualtiero, Angelico and other colleagues thus had the time to diligently study international publications and hypnosis books, such as those of the psychiatrist Milton Erickson, who in 1963 had founded the American Society of Clinical Hypnosis (A.S.C.H.) in the U.S.A.

Guantieri, who for many years and until his death directed the 'Bernheim' Institute, laid with great commitment the important foundations for international and interdisciplinary collaboration, for the study of hypnosis in medicine and psychotherapy. We recall the presence of Gualtiero Guantieri and the members of the 'Bernheim' Institute in 1973 in Uppsala, Sweden, where the International Society of Hypnosis (I.S.H.) was founded by the congressmen on the occasion of the World Congress of Clinical Hypnosis. Then we also find Guantieri and members of 'Bernheim' at the first international congresses of the European Society of Hypnosis (E.S.H.): in 1978 at the first E.S.H. congress in Malmö (Sweden), and in 1981 at the second E.S.H. congress in Dubrovnik, Croatia.

I remember the participation of Guantieri, my father and the doctors of the 'Bernheim' at the 9th International Congress of Hypnosis and Psychosomatic Medicine on 22nd-27th August 1982 in Glasgow, organised by the I.S.H. and sponsored by the University of Glasgow, Scotland, and the Royal Society of Medicine, London.

Guantieri organised the 3rd E.S.H. International Congress in Abano Terme in 1984, with the patronage of the Italian Ministries of Health and Education, the Health Service of the Italian Army, and the University of Padua. In 1985 he organised the National Congress of Clinical Hypnosis at the University of Verona, in which all the clinical hypnosis societies then existing in Italy participated. Guantieri, a man and doctor of great vision, was therefore the important catalyst, not only in Italy, but also internationally, of clinical hypnotherapy and modern hypnological psychotherapy. In fact, as early as the 1960s in the 'Bernheim', there was already an active interdisciplinary collaboration with many Italian doctors specialising in various sectors, [thus creating], in the 'Bernheim' and in Italy, a multidisciplinary and innovative study group of hypnosis. I well remember many of the doctors and friends of the 'old guard', [among them] the first Italian founding members of the 'Bernheim', who collaborated with Guantieri [from the beginning], and their hypnological studies:

- **Walter De Stavola**, born in Rome in 1921, Neurologist and Hypnotherapist, who lived in Vicenza, author of scientific publications and books on clinical hypnosis, and protagonist of singular sporting feats on the African peaks and in Northern Europe: he declared that he had succeeded in great sports'

performances through self-hypnosis;
- **Mario Montanari**, Neurologist, at the time head of the Neurology department of the Civil Hospital of Verona, who organised the first courses in clinical hypnosis for doctors with the 'Bernheim' Institute at the same hospital. At that time there were still very few psychologists, in fact in Italy a degree course in psychology was only established in 1971.
- **Bruno Caldironi**, Psychiatrist, Psychotherapist and Hypnotherapist from Ravenna, who had gained vast hypnotic experience in the treatment of schizophrenic patients, through introspective and spiritual hypnosis techniques. Caldironi was the author of many scientific articles and books on clinical hypnosis in psychiatry;
- **Werther Ferioli**, Pediatrician, Psychotherapist and Hypnotherapist from Ferrara; a psychosynthesis scholar, who together with Dr. Bruno Caldironi in 1971 had interviewed the psychiatrist Roberto Assagioli, founder of psychosynthesis, to understand the connection between states of introspective hypnosis and spirituality, and in particular in the study of psychiatry. He was the author of many scientific articles and books on clinical hypnosis;
- **Gastone Benatti**, Medical Specialist in Internal Medicine, Psychotherapist and Hypnotherapist, from Modena, a great scholar of hypnosis in Psychosomatic medicine. He was the author of many scientific articles and books on hypnosis in internal medicine;
- **Piero Parietti**, Milan Doctor, Specialist in Anaesthesia and Resuscitation and in Psychiatry, Hypnotherapist, who was: President of the PIIEC Study Centre (Centre for Research and Integrated EMDR Psychotherapy) and President of the 'S.I.M.P.' (Italian Society of Psychosomatic Medicine) ... [who died in 2020], author of many scientific articles and books on clinical hypnosis in the various fields of psychosomatic medicine and psychiatry;
- My father **Angelico Brugnoli** (1929-2015), Family Doctor in Verona, specialist in Psychotherapy, Medical hydroclimatology and Hypnotherapist, scholar of Modified States of Consciousness and Hypnosis in Psychosomatic Medicine and Pain Therapy, who in 1972 and 1973 published in his first scientific works on hypnosis in pain therapy in scientific journals, later indexed on PubMed, and he was the author of many scientific articles and books on clinical hypnosis and on modified states of consciousness: from hypnosis to meditative states.

In the late 1970s and in the 1980s, during my degree in medicine, I was admitted as an auditor to the clinical hypnosis courses organised by Guantieri and Montanari at the medical institutes of Verona. When I graduated in medicine in 1985, I participated in the National Congress of Hypnosis, organised by Guantieri at the University of Verona and finally I was also able to attend the 'Bernheim' two-year theoretical-practical clinical hypnosis course. Guantieri and all the doctors [...] mentioned above, who have been friends for many years now, were my lecturers in clinical hypnosis.
I recall Guantieri's particular technical-practical imprint on clinical hypnosis well:

Guantieri's hypnosis was absolutely innovative, due to many of its characteristics. I just want to mention one particular aspect which struck the hypnotised subject: despite being a non-directive hypnosis, Guantieri's particular characteristic was very important in managing hypnotic communication; specifically he modulated his voice in a very unique and incisive way: his hypnotic induction was like listening to a great actor in a play! Guantieri's hypnotic suggestions thus became self-fulfilling prophecies for the patient. During my specialisation in anaesthesia and resuscitation in the late 1980s, Guantieri was also my professor of hypnosis in anaesthesia at the University of Verona.

Guantieri therefore coordinated numerous courses, lectures and congresses on clinical hypnosis, trying to integrate not only the study of hypnosis in the various fields of medicine and psychology, but also the studies of the various national and international hypnosis societies. He was therefore a great personality and represents a milestone in the field of modern clinical and psychotherapeutic hypnosis, both in Italy and abroad.

Unfortunately we lost him far too soon; in 1994, I knew he had a very advanced tumor. I worked as an anaesthetist and resuscitator at the Verona hospital, and Gualtiero was hospitalised as a terminally ill patient. I went to his bedside not only for a pain therapy consultation, but mostly as a friend to say hello: the doctors treating him (along with his friends) didn't really understand how despite having such an advanced disease, he never complained about the pain of metastasis. I thus had the 'gift' of being able to spend more time with him, and accompany both with silence and with chats, a dear friend who had taught me a lot, and who unfortunately was leaving us.

It was a great sorrow to lose him, but he died not only leaving us a great legacy of teachings, but also a great strength and the peace of one who had known much about the field of introspective consciousness, through clinical hypnosis.

We are very grateful to you, dear Gualtiero, for having had the strength, perseverance, energy and enthusiasm to create an important bridge between the hypnosis of the past and that of the future.

For Gualtiero Guantieri,
by Camillo Loriedo

Camillo Loriedo is a Psychiatrist, Psychotherapist, Professor of Psychiatry and High Qualification Expert of the University of Rome 'La Sapienza', Scientific and Didactic Director of the Italian Institute of Relational Psychiatry (I.I.P.R.) of Rome and of the Italian School of Psychiatry (SIPSIC), President of the Italian Society of Hypnosis (S.I.I.), Chief Editor of the Journal of Relational Psychology and of the Hypnosis Journal, Past-President of the International Society of Hypnosis (I.S.H.) in which he retains important leadership roles.

Although I do not feel I can define my contact with Gualtiero Guantieri as prolonged over time, and I would not even feel I could define it as intense, I believe that the impact that his person and his being in the field of hypnosis exerted have been particularly significant and profound for me and for my choices in the field of hypnosis.

The first time was in Rome, in the first half of the 1970s, when I had recently succeeded in graduating in medicine and I was still looking for a precise location within the boundless galaxy of guidelines offered by the psychiatry of those years. At that time, the study of Psychosomatics was starting to pique my interest and seem particularly attractive to me.

Ferruccio Antonelli, who was the undisputed protagonist of the field in Rome, with his sensitivity and his commitment, managed to bestow it with great charm. Thus, at a Conference (the 5th S.I.M.P. Congress, held at the Catholic University of Rome, 1975) on Psychosomatics, in which hypnotic therapy still had a leading role, I became acquainted at the same time with hypnosis, in one of my very first contacts with this discipline, and with Guantieri's elegant impetus. My first impression as one of great sympathy, mainly due to the immediacy, clarity and degree of conviction with respect to the ideas he presented, which revealed an infectious passion for hypnosis.

Although on that occasion I was simply one of the many participants who attended and although we had not even spoken to each other directly, it is precisely to that infectious passion that I attribute the value of the first real stimulus to develop a strong interest in hypnotherapy.

Following that impulse, I began to take it up and study the subject at Sapienza, the University where I was specialising in psychiatry and where Danilo Gerardi taught with great generosity and humility. And it was again because that drive that was now part of me that I faced the very tiring but extraordinary challenge of translating the book 'Uncommon Therapies' with which Jay Haley presented Milton Erickson's hypnotic therapy to the world.

From then on, it was Erickson's words and the richness of their semantic complexity, very difficult to render in a language other than the original one, that led me definitively towards hypnosis, to read, study and participate in seminars, congresses and courses and everything related to the topic.

Unfortunately, due to a scheduling overlap with the competition that enabled me to gain a place at the university as a researcher, I was unable to participate in the historic Malmö Congress, which was held in 1978 — significant because it practically coincided with the birth of the current European Society of Hypnosis (E.S.H.), then called the European Society of Hypnosis and Psychosomatic Medicine. The birth of this new association had already been announced during a previous congress, that of the International Society of Hypnosis (I.S.H.) in Philadelphia in 1976, with the aim of increasing the interest in hypnosis including among colleagues from Europe, who had not previously been involved.

Even though I wasn't there at that moment, I was filled with pride by the decisive participation of Guantieri, whose internationalist spirit, that I had come to know in the meantime, always animated him and who — thanks also to the collaboration of other convinced pro-Europeans such as Peo Olof Wikström and Marjan Pajntar — finally succeeded in founding the E.S.H., a very important society in Europe.

The effectiveness of his cultural and political action made me think for the first time what I had previously considered impossible: the passion and determination of an Italian were able to influence knowledge, destinies and the spread of hypnosis on a global level.

At that time, the international scene was mainly dominated by English-speaking hypnotists, especially Americans and Australians, but today we can say that from that moment on (I feel I can say: from Guantieri onwards), European hypnosis began its growing affirmation until it reached an excellent, not to say prevalent, level of participation that would today prove very difficult to question.

Today it seems only right to give Gualtiero Guantieri the credit of being the innovator, the one who managed both to be the first Italian scholar to believe in the possibility of bringing Italy and Europe to the fore as a whole, and the first to be able to make this possibility feasible.

A few years later, in 1984, I was finally able to fully realize this. That year, for me, marks the definitive transition from a marginal and influential Italian and European participation to a fully-fledged presence in the world of hypnosis: a transition made possible by Guantieri's intelligent international strategy.

I had already taken part in the first International Ericksonian Congress in Phoenix, Arizona, in 1980, the organisation of which was certainly impeccable, with a very rich and very interesting program, where, however, there was not a single European speaker and no more than four Italians in an audience of almost two thousand participants.

Only three years later, in Abano Terme, at the 3rd E.S.H. Congress, for the first time the tune changed, radically. Guantieri's comprehensive opening address, as President of the Conference, heralded a vast array of content and participants from almost 30 countries, from four different continents and, as far as we were concerned, there was an excellent Italian turnout: in addition to the 'Bernheim' Institute chaired by Guantieri, the Italian Medical Association for the Study of Hypnosis (A.M.I.S.I.) also made a contribution and approximately 20 speakers from our country were present.

That time, I too was among the speakers with a contribution entitled "The Use of Metaphor in Indirect Hypnotherapy" which I presented very timidly and which did not arouse enthusiasm in the audience, who were for the most part taken with the great names of international hypnosis present on the occasion. In a completely unexpected way, as soon as the my speech was over, Guantieri came to meet me and congratulated me with a big smile and an energetic handshake that I still remember to this day.

Unfortunately, I don't recall the words he said to me, but they certainly had to do with the therapeutic relationship (a theme dear to both of us) and, at the same time, warming the enthusiasm of a young neophyte and instilling the energy necessary to carry forward his message of openness and integration.

I carried that determination with me in my mind and heart, and that smile capable of convincing anyone, and from then on, even within my limited possibilities, I always tried to do everything I could to continue supporting the ideas and the persuasive force that had been transmitted to me in a few short meetings, during which the deep passion of this uncommon man managed to rub off on me.

And it is for this reason that, as I was unable to do so at the time, I would like to take this opportunity today to thank Gualtiero Guantieri for everything he managed to transmit to me, in a very small number of very important moments.

An Unforgettable Man,
by Marjan Pajnter

Professor Dr. **Marjan Pajntar**, ["The Pajntar" as Gualtiero Guantieri called him, Ed.], is a Doctor of Gynaecology and Obstetrics, Psychologist, Senior Health Counselor, Co-founder and Past President of the European Society of Hypnosis and President of the Slovenian Association for Medical Hypnosis.

Gualtiero Guantieri: a professor, medical doctor, scientist, hypnologist, a true friend, but above all a great and good man. We met at an international congress and quickly found out that, at a time when orthodox medicine in our environments had not accepted the values of therapeutic work in a hypnotic state, we had a lot in common. We both saw the potential of hypnosis as an incredibly useful tool for pain management and treatment of psychosomatic disorders. We frequently discussed how to promote the use of hypnotherapy among professionals and lay people. In Slovenia at that time we were mainly engaged in research work on the use of hypnosis in patients with locomotor problems, so we agreed to exchange our knowledge and promote hypnosis in both countries. Guantieri and his colleagues lectured on hypnotherapy for pain management and psychosomatic disorders in Slovenia, and we presented our findings of the treatment of various locomotor problems to colleagues in Italy. This collaboration was highly successful, as we all benefited from it and made the first steps towards a formal recognition of hypnosis in both countries.

We also shared an interest in reducing childbirth labor pain with hypnosis, as at the time I was desperately trying to help my daily patients at the maternity hospital in Kranj, working as an obstetrician. So in the early 60s, we both started experimenting with hypnosis and shared our experiences and examples of good practice with each other, which helped us develop a comprehensive and effective program for working with birthing mothers.

Guantieri proved to be a shrewd man who relentlessly explored hypnotic phenomena and the possibilities of psychotherapeutic work in the hypnotic state.

The importance of his work was also identified by The International Society of Hypnosis, which ranked him among the leading international experts in clinical hypnosis. His critical approach to traditional medicine was of great importance for the development of an integrated approach to treatment. I must also acknowledge Guantieri's great contribution to the establishment of the Clinical Hypnosis Study Centre in Verona and later the 'Bernheim' Institute, which were very important milestones in the development of scientific research on hypnosis in Italy.

What I also greatly appreciated about Guantieri was the fact that he never hid his knowledge and was always willing to share it with all those colleagues who were interested in the many lectures he organised. Without any secrets or reservations, he was merely trying to make a change.

Guantieri was simply a man that one can never forget. And I will keep him in my fondest memories.

Fantastic,
by Jeffrey Zeig

Jeffrey Zeig is Founder and Director of the Milton Erickson Foundation of Phoenix, Arizona, (M.E.F.), Professor of Arizona State University and professor of the Italian Society of Hypnosis (S.I.I.).

I am honoured by your information on 'Guantierian Hypnology': Hello, Giorgio and Massimo! I find the work you are doing fantastic. It's great that you are continuing such important work.

Executives and Members of the 'Bernheim' Institute

We now come to the people who have known and interacted directly with Gualtiero Guantieri, or who have been able to appreciate him through his writings; we have looked for many that we knew to be a rich source of memories about him, who are full of gratitude towards him especially for the professional training received, and who are bearers of relevant considerations on this human and scientific figure. Some of these people, among others, we will mention again in the following paragraphs. As active participants of conferences and congresses in which Guantieri was celebrated, for many of them our search was painfully in vain because the wheel of life has inexorably continued turning and they have since died, but many others have willingly responded, some even with enthusiasm, often with abundant, deeply felt notes (a number of which have been edited by us as we said, to better focus them in line with our goal, centred on Gualtiero Guantieri). Below we report the salient passages of each.

The Master, the Friend, the Older Brother,
by Rocco Cacciacarne

Rocco Cacciacarne is a Surgeon, Psychotherapist, Specialist in General Medicine and Diseases of the Digestive System, PhD in Community Medicine, Director of S.I.A.N. (Food Hygiene and Nutrition Service) and the Health Education Service at the ULSS company in Venice, Past Coordinator of the Verona branch of the 'G. Guantieri' S.I.M.P., Author of various Scientific Publications.

As a young reserve medical officer for the armed forces, on 29 June 1969, after having attended the A.U.C. in Florence, I was assigned to the Military Hospital of Verona. During that summer, I was able to read some reviews on Professor Gualtiero Guantieri from the press. He was talked about here and there for his interest in the application of hypnosis in the medical field. I was impressed and decided to call him; even from that first conversation he appeared to me a concrete and essential professional; he was not the type to waste words; concise and exhaustive in speech; in a way, it inspired awe and deference; he left you free in your decisions and respected any point of view you presented to him; during my brief interview, he immediately went to the heart of the various questions I posed; short and complete answers. During that first contact, I perceived him to be very knowledgeable and scientifically reliable; in my heart I felt that I was not yet ready to follow him.

In the Autumn of 1973, following the achievement of my first specialisation, that famous phone call came to mind; so, I did not hesitate and I participated, first, in a conference in the Marani Room of the Civil Hospital of Verona and, then, in a Clinical Hypnosis Seminar; both events were organised under the auspices of the 'H. Bernheim'. When I met Professor Guantieri in person, I was struck by his slender physique, as well as his deep, almost magnetic gaze; he immediately remembered the phone call that had taken place four years earlier and I was amazed, to say the least.

The encounter with that particular scientific world represented the classic epochal turning point in my professional life; without any hesitation I attended the two-year course in Medical Hypnosis and the other events connected to it.

We continued to frequent each other and, in 1975, Guantieri asked me to accompany him to the 5th National Congress of Psychosomatic Medicine in Rome, at the Catholic University, which took place from 15th-20th September as part of the "Third World Congress of the International College of Psychosomatic Medicine"; my mentor was one of the most illustrious Italian speakers; from Verona, he took me with him as a young pupil of his – at just over 30 years old – and introduced me to Professor Ferruccio Antonelli, President of the S.I.M.P., who welcomed me with great enthusiasm precisely because I was introduced by him; Guantieri was speaker and chairman of more than one workshop; he was fluent in the English language. To my immense amazement, Guantieri subsequently asked me to maintain contact with the upper echelons of the Italian Society of Psychosomatic Medicine, about which he had high expectations, precisely with regard to the research conducted by him and his team on the use of hypnosis in psychosomatic diseases. It was for this scientific interest that in 1977 he was elected National Vice President of the Society and re-elected in '81.

In those years he tried to set up, involving me in the project, a Venetian branch of the S.I.M.P., with frequent training and cultural meetings at the headquarters of the 'H. Bernheim' Institute in Verona.

At that time hypnosis and the 'Bernheim' associates were under special observation by the Italian Medical Association; however, Guantieri was esteemed everywhere for his scientific rigor and seriousness; his teachings and his writings were considered impeccable. He has always been held in the highest regard by patients, colleagues and students for his seriousness and for his undoubted ability to relate to people, without any distinction.

He had a deep respect for the medical knowledge of his colleagues and he liked to compare himself a great deal, always maintaining a loyal and symmetrical attitude, equal to the esteem we had for him, especially when he discussed hypnosis in Anaesthesiology, Dentistry, Gynaecology and Psychotherapy. He was unmatched in authority on those topics and, when you conversed with him, you became aware of his incredible goodness and his spirit, which I would dare to define as prophetic. These aspects can be distinctly perceived, even now, from his writings. I jealously preserve, as proof of this, the dedication he wrote, also signed by fellow work colleagues, attached to the reproduction of a tile from the portal of the St. Zeno Basilica which was given to me when I left the Health District to go and take up a very prestigious position in Venice, in 1989. During our professional experience, side by side, his monolithic solemnity began slowly melting away, until one day he offered me his unconditional friendship, even inviting me to share some rare moments of his precious free time, of which I retain indelible memories. We spent a few beautiful afternoons in the company of other friends and in freedom of thought in his country house in Valgatara where, in order to gain access, the condition he set for his guests was: "... we can go, as long as we don't talk about medicine or anything connected to it".

He introduced me to his father Macedonio, who died at the age of 100; that reserved and always elegant elderly man attended all of his son's conferences, in a corner of the room, without ever intervening: a precious icon in that cultural context.

Guantieri was also my analyst and supervisor for psychotherapeutic activity; we knew almost everything about each other; he loved me very much, to the point of becoming affectionate brothers[...]. His premature death on December 20th 1994 left me, culturally, orphaned.

Guantieri, Master par excellence, focused on hypnosis for its ability in by-passing the control of the cortex on all the main domains of the mind. He intercepted the body language of others with his vibrational vocal charm and his personal magnetic gaze, thus managing to change the person's state of consciousness. In light of the discoveries of neuroscience, subsequent to his death, I am convinced that if he had lived, he would certainly have carried out a reasoned review of his particular way of understanding hypnosis. In his day, people were debating whether permissive hypnosis or directive hypnosis was more effective. Guantierian hypnosis had and still has the prerogative of being neither directive nor permissive.

A few further considerations on the relationship with his colleagues: he always listened to everyone and attended national and international congresses as a good listener; when he spoke he did so with wisdom, citing his own copious personal case histories. Today, we could define him as an evolved therapist, who practiced analysis mainly with silences and the addition of something else - between words and gestures - imbued with meta-messages; never with peremptory orders in violation of everyone's sacrosanct right to freedom of thought and action; he often resorted to the use of metaphors; with his voice and gaze he induced hypnosis and waited for its effects; sometimes I found myself sending him patients (who proved difficult for me) and observing how they changed over time; his method also worked because it was structured as I have described it above; I have never met others similar to him in terms of ethical and upright stature as a doctor, teacher... man. Through his somatic language he inspired righteousness and values, because he was essential and serious. He never got angry; calm by nature, it was natural for him to teach relaxation to reach peace of mind; he was a person who always understood others. Not much inclined to forgiveness, instead he sought solutions to errors with the compliance of the patient and/or students.

Endowed with a prophetic spirit, he read your destiny in the depths of his soul but did not reveal it; he let you make your way in utmost freedom; in a nutshell: he was not a manipulator; rather a forerunner of the enormous potential discovered later, belonging to the fields of empathy and epigenetics.

Obsessed with the idea that unreliable subjects could seize that tool to make fraudulent use of it; he did not tolerate freak shows, as he used to sternly assert, he was a zealous and faithful guardian of hypnosis.

When, in 1998, together with other friends, I reconstituted the Verona branch of the S.I.M.P. and gave it his name, with the approval of the National President Piero Parietti, as a fiduciary exception to the bylaws; on the day of the collective celebration of the 50 years of graduation, promoted by the Order of Surgeons and Dentists in the province, on 16th November 2018 at the Palazzo della Gran Guardia in Verona, I honoured Gualtieri in a report entitled: *'Gratitude for my Masters'*, concluding the passage about him with these words : *"Over the years, from Master to student, our relationship, due to a series of professional circumstances and beyond, turned into mutual fraternal friendship"*.

On the Figure of Gualtiero Guantieri,
by Giuliano Guerra

Giuliano Guerra, is a Psychiatrist, Hypnologist, Former Director of the Psychological Consultancy of the Military Hospital of Verona, and Past President of the 'Bernheim'.

I place myself in a meditative attitude of relaxed vigil to allow considerations, images and memories to emerge, at the centre of which is the figure of Gualtiero Guantieri, both from a professional point of view and regarding his personality as a man. In this altered state of consciousness, I welcome an infinite number of 'inputs' connected to his teachings, fragments of life lived through many years spent in a profound relationship of friendship, collaboration and hypnological experiences learned as his student enrolled in the training courses of the prestigious School of Hypnology he directed. I am immediately overwhelmed by many memories that take me back to episodes, experiences, photographs, scientific and informative articles, hypnological days and national and international seminars. I try to put in order and give a place to these numerous ideas, so as to trace and reveal a biographical profile of my friend Gualtiero that has something particular and that is not too common or similar to the descriptions that have certainly already been outlined in other writings of colleagues and people who got to know him and spend time with him.
I think I was 30 years old when my first meeting with "the Master" took place. I was immediately impressed by his deep, charismatic, penetrating and non-judgmental gaze. Straight away, I was fascinated by his genuine desire to create a relationship as free as possible from masks or defence mechanisms, and one which would enhance the dimension of the soul. The power of his unique and inimitable way of looking directly deep into the eyes of his interlocutor, at a very close distance, penetrated my inner self and set in motion thoughts, emotions and feelings, which generated a cascade of psycho-reactions and somatic and biochemical reactions throughout the body. The response that arose in my neuronal networks was immediate, short-circuited and textbook Pavlovian. In a few seconds the decision was made: I would enrol in the 'Bernheim' courses that took place in Costagrande in Verona and I recognized Professor Guantieri as a guide and training teacher from whom I would learn the disciplines related to the technique of medical hypnosis.
My last meeting with Gualtiero, when I was nearly 50, took place in his hospital room in Verona (Borgo Trento) with him enticed as he tried to oppose, with dignity and courage, the disease that was consuming him. At that moment there was no longer a teacher-student relationship, but a meeting of souls, a profound human relationship within which, with clarity and firmness, he transmitted his thoughts to me about the future of the prestigious institute he presided over.
There was wisdom, maturity and much humility in him. It was nice to see in that

moving atmosphere, even amidst human suffering, his altruism, devoid of power games, his frustration, egoic structures and regrets. He was a serene man, satisfied by his professional successes and by the knowledge acquired in the field of hypnosis and psychosomatic medicine. He wondered aloud what might be the best solution for everyone: members, students, colleagues, members of the Board of Directors. That was Gualtiero.

From my point of view, I'm eager to describe him as a humble, elegant, cultured, intelligent, altruistic man, capable of generating love with respect and prudence, capable of creating true bonds of friendship. From our first meeting he transmitted to me, so charismatically, his being there as a person who wishes to generate loving experiences for humanity and to train his students, as an authoritative researcher and in a profound manner, in the knowledge he had acquired on the subject of hypnosis in particular. Notably, in that last meeting, just a few days after which his soul left his body, he transmitted to me feelings of freshness, purity, honesty and beauty. During the many years in which I had the privilege of sharing his company, I remember the research we conducted together and his personal confidence relating to patients and initiatives of the 'Bernheim' Institute. Our professional relationship began at the Military Hospital of Verona, since I held the role of chief medical director, in charge of psychological and psychiatric facilities. I am always keen to recount that Gualtiero was the first civilian researcher to study the effects of hypnosis on people suffering from various forms of physical pain in the military. He conducted experiments with volunteers, both military and civilian subjects, at the hospital's analytical laboratory, and these studies he conducted in collaboration with universities, were pioneering at that time, in that they measured the blood levels of endorphins before and after the induction of hypnosis.

He also gave conferences and seminars at the Officers' Club in Castelvecchio in Verona, in which he promulgated the importance of self-hypnosis, autogenic training, various relaxation techniques to achieve well-being and better efficiency on the part of the military personnel on permanent active duty. He coordinated training courses to learn medical hypnosis, aimed at medical officers working in the psychological and psychiatric fields in various military environments.

Gualtiero was always punctual, elegant, concrete, exhaustive and he carried out his teaching with clarity. Always modest, humble, professional, efficient, generous, far-sighted [...] His lessons were engaging; his experiments serious, rigorous, well thought-out. I like to remember him passionately dictating letters in English to his secretary Mrs. Grazia, addressed to important international figures in the scientific and hypnological world, with whom he was in contact.

I remember his enthusiasm, when in the councils of the board of the school he chaired, he tried to get his future projects and thoughts across to his friends Ferioli, Brugnoli, Caldironi, Parietti, De Stavola, Benatti, Castagna [...] with human warmth, with vivacity, but always with respect, civility and a conciliatory attitude. It is pleasing to think of him when, at number 65 in Via Valverde in

Verona, he welcomed his patients with humanity, empathy, dignity and readiness [...] and also when he allowed himself a short coffee break at the cafe next door, or for "popping round" to his nearby home to greet his children Francesca and Massimo and his dear wife Anna Maria. They were his world, and in his heart undoubtedly in first place, alongside his beloved hypnosis. Hypnosis was so central to his life that it took him everywhere [...] I remember an anecdote from when we spent New Year's Eve together at 'Fasanara', his beautiful country house: the bells were chiming midnight, we were waiting to raise a traditional toast and he was busy inducing hypnosis in a family friend!

The flow of memories is now unstoppable, images and scenes experienced continue to be associated with him [...] but the dominant theme is always the same: Gualtiero Guantieri's boundless love for the study, research and application of medical hypnosis.

Thank you for everything dear Gualtiero, I acknowledge you as a Master, I thank you for the training you gave me, and I will remember you as a good, loyal man who was able to generate dynamics of love in his life.

The 'Bernheim' Group,
by Guglielmo Gulotta

Guglielmo Gulotta, is a Lawyer and Psychologist and was Professor Emeritus of Psychology at the University of Turin, until 2009.

I was invited to present memories and reflections about Gualtiero Guantieri who gave so much to the knowledge and study of hypnosis as a therapeutic technique and tool for the knowledge of psychological and psychopathological phenomena.
I am one of the few survivors who shared the moment when the birth of the interest in hypnosis came about, in Italy. I talked about it, albeit briefly, in an article written with Camillo Loriedo entitled 'Hypnosis in Italy' in the volume 'Hypnosis in Europe' edited by Peter Hawkins and Michael Heap[3].
The first to deal with it extensively was Franco Granone, a psychiatrist at the Vercelli hospital, who began publishing hypnosis essays in 1962, together with Giampiero Pavesi, a gynaecologist from Milan. Even earlier, in 1960 in Pavia, thanks to the initiative of Professor Giampiero Mosconi, Doctor, Psychologist and Psychotherapist, the A.M.I.S.I. Italian Medical Association for the Study of Hypnosis was founded, operating largely in Milan.
In 1965 Guantieri founded the 'H. Bernheim'. The Bernheim group published a large number of scientific articles and earned a good reputation in Europe and around the world.

---

[3] Loriedo C., Gulotta G., *Hypnosis in Italy*, in Hawkins P., Heap M., (edited by), *Hypnosis in Europe*, Whurr Publishers Ltd., London, 1998, pp. 128-140.

The orientation of the three groups was based on research and training, as well as on concrete clinical applications, and although among them were some differences of opinion regarding certain aspects, they contributed to the advancement of what we can consider the hypnological culture of our country[4].

My acquaintance with Guantieri, from which I developed great respect and admiration for the man, was essentially based on my participation in numerous congresses, including some in Verona — a place that consolidated the interests of scholars, thanks in part to the 'Bernheim' Institute.

The impression that I gleaned, and that remains now that I have looked at those "old documents", is that while I drank in international literature — so much so that I was acknowledged to have been the first to make known the therapeutic and hypnotic methods of Milton Erickson — Guantieri was the most inclined, and perhaps the only one, to cultivate personal and scientific contacts with non-Italian and prestigious authors, as shown in the volume "Hypnosis in Psychotherapy and Psychosomatic Medicine" which collects the scientific articles presented at the 3rd European Congress on Hypnosis in Psychotherapy and Psychosomatic Medicine in Abano Terme (Padua), held on 22nd-27th May 1984, during which I had published "Techniques of hypnotic influence upon the subject: argumentative and mystifying aspects". Guantieri's hypnology has a future: I believe the 'Bernheim' Institute is a Centre that has much to say and write about the development of the theory and practice of hypnosis in Italy.[5]

Paternal Guantieri,
by Giuseppe Hinegk

Giuseppe Hinegk, is a Psychiatrist, Medical Doctor and Hypnologist in Verona.

A short time ago, a patient who, at the time, had turned to Guantieri for anxiety problems, made me listen to the beginning of the recording of the induction that had been proposed. The memory of his figure came back to me: slender, with a low, baritone voice - certainly helped along by an ever present lit cigarette - the welcoming and helpful attitude that I was constantly greeted with, during a time when, as a recent graduate, I had the opportunity to collaborate with him on some secretarial work, finding myself alongside a precious formative presence and, as I perceived it, a paternal one. I remember his willingness to share some

---

[4] Gulotta G., *Techniques of hypnotic influence upon the subject: argumentative and mystifying aspects*, in AA. VV. (edited by Guantieri G.), *Hypnosis in Psychotherapy and Psychosomatic Medicine*, Proceedings from the Conference of the 3rd European Congress on Hypnosis in Psychotherapy and Psychosomatic Medicine, Abano Terme, (Padua), 22-27 May 1984, Editions Il Segno, Negrar, (Verona), 1985, pp. 67-79.

[5] One of the last editions in which the historical entry of hypnosis in Italy is reported was edited by Edoardo Casiglia: *Trattato di ipnosi e altre modificazioni di coscienza*, published by Cleup, in Padua in 2015; Guantieri G., in particular proposed — with respect to differing positions — a dialogue-based, permissive, informative and reassuring clinical hypnosis, before the prescriptive kind, and "maternal" rather than "paternal," as an alternative to authoritarian medical attitudes.

professional experiences and to supervise me in certain situations that I had proposed to him. I was impressed by how he spoke of the head physician of the medical department he had attended, recounting with amazement that he tended to patients by passing his hands over their bodies, almost without touching them. On the occasion of John Paul II's visit to Verona, he admired the Pope's communication skills. I also had the chance to share   pleasant moments with him, when the occasion arose and he would stop to chat to me and Mrs. Grazia, secretary of the 'Bernheim Centre', during a break, or when, at the time of the Abano Congress (1984), at the end of the day, he joked with Werther Ferioli and Andrea Gambacciani [executive members of the 'Bernheim' Institute, Ed.], with me looking on. It was certainly fascinating, as well as exciting, to play the role of "test subject" for a time, on occasions when the true potential of hypnosis was still to be demonstrated in various fields, and especially in training, when I enjoyed receiving a certain attention from Gualtiero in particular.

The "Psalms" of Guantierian Hypnology,
by Giulio Martinelli

Giulio Martinelli, is a Doctor, Dentist and the former director of the 'H. Bernheim' Italian Institute of Clinical Hypnosis and Psychotherapy in Verona.

Since the early 1970s, I have held in my hands the first edition of 'Hypnosis' by Gualtiero Guantieri and admired it as a "bible" [...] Unfortunately I did not [...] meet him personally [...] I only [...] heard about him with esteem and affection from the members of the 'Bernheim' Institute at the time.

I am a Hypnologist: Thanks to Guantieri,
by Michele Modenese

Michele Modenese is a Psychologist, Psychotherapist and Past-President of the 'H. Bernheim' Institute of Hypnosis.

It gives me great pleasure to share, among the many moments that I spent with him, a brief personal memory of Gualtiero. It was the late 1980s and after my graduation, we were returning from Bologna, where we had been for a S.I.M.P. congress. For me it was a very important occasion, as I had won the S.I.M.P. award for the best poster and I received the congratulations of the most important characters in the world of hypnosis and psychosomatics at the time. I remember Gualtiero feeling proud of this young pupil of his. He proposed to return to Verona together by train. I had a second class ticket; he had a first class one. He did not hesitate for a moment to change his ticket and travel with me, with the simplicity and humanity that always distinguished him. It was on that occasion that he invited me to address him with the informal "tu", or "you" in Italian, which told me that I was growing up and that he thought highly of me. He welcomed me as a young pupil, helping me to grow hypnologically, involving me alongside him in several conferences. He will always remain my teacher.

Medicine on a Human Scale,
by Piergiorgio Muzi

Piergiorgio Muzi is a Philosopher, Psychiatrist and Hypnologist.

Gualtiero was the only friend whose friendship did not cease, as it did with a few others, because of drastically increasing spiritual differences. We have been distanced by tragic events, first in Verona and then in the whole country. Our collaboration was dictated not only by a shared interest in medicine on a human scale but was also fuelled by the emotional closeness of our families and the exchange of mutual information and comparisons about emerging clinical problems within the same professional catchment area.

I think that the point of greatest convergence is that concerning the setting of hypnosis within the sphere of psychosomatic medicine, the formation of Balint groups, and a balanced de-medicalisation when the increasing use of psychotropic drugs, as well as analgesics, was feeding iatrogenic neuroses and drug addictions. But on this point, I must say that the progress of medicine in recent decades has not only failed to take advantage of that potential paradigm shift, which we hoped for, but has plummeted back into the same bottlenecks, which we currently see exacerbated in complete subservience to the pharmacological industry with all related implications, on a planetary level.

Another fundamental point which unites Guantieri and I, from a scientific point of view, is having taken mental reality seriously as suggested by the epistemological position of Popper and Eccles in 'The Self and its Brain',[6] currently in fact repudiated by the notion of science circulating online (see Wikipedia, etc.), as a by-product of materialism functional to economic empires.

---

[6] Popper K.R., Eccles J.C., *The Self and its Brain*, Springer-Verlag Berlin and Heidelberg GmbH & Co. K, 1977.

The Waves,

by Alessandro Norsa

Alessandro Norsa, Psychologist and Psychotherapist, is a lecturer in hypnosis at IUSVE University (Venice), an ESH member and founding member and President of SIPMU (Italian Scientific Society of Clinical Hypnosis in Psychotherapy and Humanistic Medicine). Researcher in the field of anthropology, he is also teaching fellow in Modern History (University of Verona) and Coordinator of the subgroup of Neuroaesthetics and Neuro-bioethics research group in UNESCO Regina Apostolorum University (Rome).

As waves bring shells or objects from distant worlds to the beach, so time brings people to come to know each other. In absence, memories are built, at times due to the constancy of the continuity of the frequentation, in other conditions fragments, occasions or single contacts remain. I remember meeting Guantieri, alas only once, at one of his conferences. It was 1987, I was 17. My father and his friend Romolo Lodetti [7] accompanied me. Obviously I had not yet started attending the faculty of psychology […] I had started to volunteer in social work, and then there were only dreams, ideas and projects of a future profession. Of that meeting I remember his many, learned quotes, a calm tone, a strong handshake. Then nothing more, until the tide of life brought me, through one of his patients, an old cassette tape with his voice: it was a hypnotic suggestion that Guantieri had left him for his home exercises. It was nice to hear: a professional, a man, a colleague at work. Although in a somewhat particular way, he was like a Master to me for an hour: "Imagine a plane that draws words in the sky," thus began the suggestion... Then nothing more. And today as I'm reading the book I inherited from Angelico Brugnoli by Gualtiero Guantieri: "Ipnosi, come oggetto di studio e mezzo di impiego in medicina" ('Hypnosis, as an object of study and a means of use in medicine') published by Rizzoli, to gather ideas and teachings for a book I am writing, the tidal wave of the internet brings me a message in a bottle: "This is Pier Giorgio Malesani […] and Massimo Guantieri […] We would be very honoured if you would consider the possibility of offering us a very short piece in writing with your memories of Guantieri". Some, recalling the Jungian theory of synchronicity, believe that these episodes have a profound significance. I am among them.

---

[7] 'Mio padre medico studioso mistico: *La scienza a servizio della pace'*, is the biography of Romolo Lodetti, published by his daughter Maria Paola Lodetti, a doctor and scholar from Verona, who was born in 1921 and died in 2007.Throughout his life he researched and meditated on the dialogue between science, faith and spirit, and left it to his descendant to bear witness to his experience. The result of a long work of preparation and evaluation of the copious written testimonies left by Lodetti (diaries, scientific texts, letters), the volume harmoniously alternates episodes from real life and references to spirituality, studies and encounters with people of faith who helped him in his research journey.

The Myth,
by Giancarlo Odini

Giancarlo Odini, is a Psychologist, Psychotherapist and Board Member of the 'Bernheim' Institute.

I met Gualtiero Guantieri in 1990, in the midst of many unfamiliar colleagues. I felt welcomed and well liked: he talked to me and listened to me with pleasure. I felt at home.

My interest in hypnosis had been born some time before, after reading the fictional life of F.A. Mesmer.

At the end of my university studies in psychology, personal analysis and supervision of clinical cases, I believed I had mastered this subject.

The meeting with Gualtiero reshaped my preconceptions, enlightening me towards new paths.

Gualtiero knew how to convey enthusiasm; he illustrated this strange world of hypnosis, aware that there were important people before him, with profound and innovative ideas.

What struck me most was his affirmation that our psyche could be reached and understood through the body. That is, he was able to paint a vital uniqueness that is rarely glimpsed in so many scholars.

His teaching made it possible to share and live in a world that took into account the body and soul.

But what was most captivating was his ability to make us open to surrender and therefore for mutual trust in relaxation and in the hypnotic state to learn from our unconscious, to be the light through sudden intuitions.

A few days ago, I was walking alone and a pleasant thought occurred to me: Gualtiero is a myth for us. He is like the cosmic tree that crosses the world with its trunk, touches the sky with its branches and sinks its roots in the unconscious world.

There are three roots that support the cosmic tree and can be recognized in Gualtiero: Freud, Jung and Bernheim.

Each made an exceptional contribution and the result was the 'Bernheim' Institute.

On the leafy branches of the cosmic tree amongst which once upon a time the gods sat in the evening, now we imagine that our friends and associates sit to discuss, to seek new ways of completing the hypnotic world.

On the branches of the cosmic tree we feel we are united in diversity, we live as a family that knows how to collaborate by recognizing the complexity of our unconscious world.

The Light of Hippocrates and Guantieri,
by Carlo Piazza

Carlo Piazza is a Psychiatrist, Medical Doctor, Pain Therapist, Criminologist, Psychotherapist, Honorary President, Teacher and Supervisor of the 'H. Bernheim' School of Psychosynthetic Psychotherapy and Ericksonian Hypnosis of Vicenza – Trento (founded in San Martino Buon Albergo - VR), and President of the 'Bernheim' Institute.

I had "many medical fathers", my birth one Alessandro, a radiologist, and two grandfathers: the maternal one, Pietro Castellani wrote, in 1962, 'La luce di Ippocrate', ("The light of Hippocrates").[8] I owe everything to them first of all, but the most intuitive and enlightened of my extra-familial fathers — the reason for my becoming a psychotherapist and hypnotherapist — was Gualtiero Guantieri: I met him in 1982, just after graduating in Medicine. Looking at the many options I had, before enrolling in a specialisation in Psychiatry, I encountered his gaze, which hypnotised me professionally even before I met him in person. It was enough for me to listen to him at an introductory course in Hypnosis, he looked at me only once and something ignited in me. I attended the seminars he opened and organised for two years, and the courses held by him for another four, before becoming a hypnologist and psychotherapist, in parallel with achieving the title of psychiatrist, in 1988; I continued with the supervision and initial collaboration with him and other teachers of the 'Bernheim' Institute, from the late De Benedetti, Parietti and Brugnoli, to Gambacciani, Zenoni, Odini, Malesani, Bottoli, Alquati Pasoli, Cacciacarne, Modenese and Guerra, and the majority of us, when on his deathbed due to a serious illness, expressed our affection, loyalty and testimony to him, taking over the reins of the Institute.

He left us in 1994, and in 1997, after three years of humble grief and loss, together with Giuliano Guerra we inaugurated "Acta Hypnologica", a quarterly magazine about Hypnosis which continued until 2010; in 2002 the 'H. Bernheim' School was born, recognized by the Ministry of Education, University and Research also thanks to the enormous national and international credentials of Guantieri. Since then, it has offered the four-year specialisation in Psychosynthetic Psychotherapy and Ericksonian Hypnosis Diploma Course, and in 2012 the School was accepted as a member of E.S.H., the European Society of Hypnosis.

Long before then, since 1965, Gualtiero Guantieri and his 'Bernheim' Institute were characterised by their own original psychotherapeutic approach for the teaching of hypnosis; they were among the first Italian pioneers, with Franco Granone and Giampiero Mosconi, to propose the study of hypnosis in Italy.

---

[8] Castellani P., *La luce di Ippocrate*, Cisalpino, Milan-Varese, 1962.

The Guantierian Hypnological path emphasises the uniqueness of every therapeutic relationship and is an integral part in the training of future therapists, so that they can acquire a unitary vision of the patient and of the various psychological and psychotherapeutic contributions, both as individuals and in groups, paying particular attention to the psychodynamic and interactive relationships and interpersonal communication: a conception of the human being therefore inspired by a unitary, global and integrated vision of psychotherapeutic practice.

I am now honoured to hold a title which is very dear to me, that of Honorary President of this school, and I am also co-founder and supervisor. In the Institute, which continues its activity together with the School, in the memory and in the continuous cultural, ethical and human enhancement of Guarneri, I am now - in 2024 - its Director, and there is the significant and testimonial presence of Gualtiero's son, Massimo Guantieri, among the other councillors: Malesani, Mometti, Odini, De Mattia, Filippozzi, Novarese, Rosson, Tagliati (last five all graduates in the last 20 years of the Bernheim Psychotherapy School).

Previously, alongside Giovanni Gocci, the first Director of the School, introduced to me twelve years earlier by Gualtiero when I asked him for the recommendation of an analyst, and whose entire history as Vice I witnessed, then took his place for four years; with him I prided myself on an intuitive aura, and hovered beside him humbly but very aware of being my usefulness to him, as a modulator; with him, first as my analyst and then supervisor, I entered the Jungian kingdom and rediscovered 'Memories, dreams, reflections by C.G. Jung', published by Il Saggiatore in 1965, the same date as my father's signature on the title page of the book he left me on his death in 1985, twenty years later; on closer inspection it was also the same year as the foundation of the Institute. Gradually I discovered that I could open my professional empathy to the soul, live cosmic experiences in a timeless synchronic dimension, something great and indefinable, a full immersion in a modified state of consciousness, out of time and space, a new and sublime dimension of hypnosis taught to us by Guantieri.

Thanks to "my fathers" Alessandro, Pietro, Clearco and Gualtiero, thanks to the past, in the present and in the future, made up of infinite presents, out of time, this from Gualtiero Guantieri onwards has been and continues to be my hypnotic timelessness.

3
Memories of Gualtiero Guantieri at various conventions and congresses.

XX Congress of the Italian Society of Psychosomatic Medicine (SIMP), dedicated to Gualtiero Guantieri
Anxiety in the clinic and in today's society,
Verona, 21-23 October 2005

The 20th Congress of the Italian Society of Psychosomatic Medicine (S.I.M.P.), specifically dedicated to Gualtiero Guantieri and held in Verona in 2005, was an important scientific occasion to commemorate him.

The Abstract Book of the congress includes a presentation of the meeting by the then President of the S.I.M.P., Pietro Parietti (who was one of the founders, alongside Guantieri, of the 'H. Bernheim' Institute of Clinical Hypnosis and Psychotherapy in Verona, and Psychiatrist, Director of the School of Specialisation in Psychotherapy with Psychosomatic Orientation of the Riza Institute in Milan), in which it reveals that the choice of Verona as the venue for the 20th Congress dedicated to Gualtiero Guantieri [...] through a celebration of the 'Bernheim' Institute, his creation which survived him and keeps his memory alive, while continuing his teaching "was a tribute to the scientist and his Institute".

He also writes, in summary of one of the reports to be presented at the congress, that "the continuous, close [and courageous - he adds -] collaboration experienced with Guantieri since the foundation of the 'H. Bernheim' Clinical Hypnosis Study Centre was fundamental for both his personal and professional training".[9]

During the session on the last day of the congress, talks relating to personal and professional recollections of Guantieri were planned by colleagues who knew him and worked and studied with him, as well as other scientific contributions, the inspiration for which arose from several years of attending the 'Bernheim'.

One of the protagonists (co-founder of the 'Bernheim', Angelico Brugnoli, said: "Gualtiero Guantieri [was] my life teacher and research friend, [with him] I shared the early days of the study and the application of hypnotic training. Sometimes there were also difficult moments, especially due to the fact that in those days, and we are talking about the 1960s, hypnosis was almost entirely experienced as a phenomenon to be practiced in the living room and certainly not approachable to clinical applications of even considerable importance. Those were the years in which even psychosomatic medicine, in Italy, was taking its first steps, not without great difficulties [...] Guantieri, with his tenacity, perseverance and also a certain amount of resourcefulness, was able to provide an historical turning point [...] in the learning and implementation of the various phases of hypnotic training, particularly in the field of somatoform disorders, depression due to

---

[9] Abstract Book of the 20th S.I.M.P. Congress. Dedicated to Gualtiero Guantieri, *Anxiety in the clinic and in today's society*, Italian Society of Psychosomatic Medicine (S.I.M.P.), Verona, 20th-23rd October 2005.

environmental factors and the various aspects of anxiety associated with the state of hyper-stress. [...N]ationally and internationally [...] motivated in research[...]. His intuitions and expectations are still proving to be of great relevance today. [It was his] mental stature [which led him] to [...] illuminations and discoveries in the field of hypnosis".

Pier Giorgio Malesani proposed an idea of Guantieri as a "Modern benevolent shaman" and described him as an "epistemological scientist [...] with a psychosomatic and multidisciplinary orientation [...] as an innovative pioneer [...] who looks to the future and as a teacher".

Gastone Benatti, another of the founders of the 'Bernheim', in his speech 'The First 40 Years of Guantieri's Bernheim' , began by wishing "a long and fruitful scientific life at the 'H. Bernheim' Italian Institute of Clinical Hypnosis and Psychotherapy Studies, founded by Gualtiero Guantieri in way back in 1965. In fact", he added, "Guantieri still identifies himself in the most concrete way, with the last 40 years of clinical hypnosis as a research activity in the field of psychosomatics, where as testament to him, many scientific creations, intense teaching, congresses and honours, including foreign ones, remain. Inspired by Hyppolite Bernheim as founder of the Nancy school for her contributions to medical-psychological progress, also proposing hypnosis [...] as a specific relational reality between operator and subject which is impossible to ignore [...] the 'Bernheim Institute' " – says Benatti – "has found progressive consensus in the academic and medical environment, both nationally and internationally, for the many practical applications of hypnosis in medicine and not only as a communication tool in the doctor-patient relationship but also as a useful means of anamnestic-diagnostic investigation, in addition to the real modification of certain functional organic realities", specifies the author, "Guantieri has motivated all of us collaborators and students, to the modern idea of no longer centring the treatment on the disease and not even on the sick, but on the person [...] A greatly respected teacher and master", continued Benatti, "[he paid great attention to the training of hypnologists and] certainly favored the most appropriate ways in Italy so that doctors and psychologists could better adapt hypnosis [to] psychotherapy and [to] research. If a man disappears", concludes Benatti, "the evidence of his work certainly does not disappear, nor do the merits that have honoured his personal relationship with others and above all in favor of others. All of us at the 'Bernheim' institute, colleagues, collaborators, disciples and former patients [...] we must preserve [...with intensity, these] memories [...] and [such] beautiful professional and human images of Guantieri".

Conference of the 'Bernheim' Institute:
Guantierian Hypnology and its developments over time,
San Martino B.A. (Verona), November 15, 2008

Another opportunity to commemorate Gualtiero Guantieri that we remember was the conference "Guantierian Hypnology and its developments over time", held in San Martino B.A. (Verona) on 15th November, 2008.[10] During the conference there was a brief introductory review that recalled the 40 years since the birth of the 'Hyppolite Bernheim'.

Angelico Brugnoli once again opened proceedings with tales of a touching relationship full of memories and focused on the characteristics of courage, intuitiveness, genius and loyalty of his friend and fellow medic.

In that report, Brugnoli hinted at the scientific confrontation that took place between Guantieri and Franco Granone, a renowned hypnologist from Turin, and of their different ways of using hypnosis — the latter of the authoritarian type, the first of the "maternal" type.

He cites Guantieri, a "man of great willpower" who affirmed that the "patient should not be tamed... nothing should be imposed on them... [rather, they should] be guided towards a slow awareness of their psychic condition. For us novices", continues Brugnoli, "it was very important to rely on him precisely because of the way of conducting the induction. Few words, many pauses, and, an innovative feature for us: to end the word in one breath, as if it were lost in the air forever". And he adds: "His 1973 definition of trance [...] as [...] a state-relationship passing through the body, anticipates and accompanies [...] towards the future the most advanced discoveries in psycho-neuro-immuno--endocrinology [...]. Guantieri had a brilliant intuition", continues the speaker, "with intuition in fact, you reach the heart of the subject [...] [and create] that interpersonal relationship [...] [of] fundamental importance [...]. Gualtiero [was creative and] always brought [...] new ideas [... and provided] useful advice [... He] certainly did not disdain to learn or discuss [...]; his way of life was Spartan: study and work, alternating with the preparation of courses, events, congresses and conferences [...] Guantieri left a great void in the 'Bernheim' [...] as a doctor, as a great human being, as a friend".

After Brugnoli, the aforementioned Rocco Cacciacarne remembered Guantieri as a stalwart researcher and defender of hypnosis with respect to its improper uses and dwelled on how the teacher also conceived it in the form of learning, using the suggestive metaphor of the teacher of the arts who stimulates talented students through with practice. "In founding the 'Bernheim' Institute", continues Cacciacarne, "Guantieri intended on the one hand to study the potential of the

---

[10] AA.VV., Proceedings of the Conference *L'Ipnologia Guantieriana e i suoi sviluppi nel tempo,* San Martino B.A (Verona), November 15, 2008 in *Acta Hypnologica* magazine, Edited by the'H. Bernheim' Italian Institute of Clinical Hypnosis and Psychotherapy - Research and Training School, S. Martino B.A., (Verona), Year XII n. 3, 2008 and Year XIII, n. 1, 2009.

hypnotic state to better apply it in the therapeutic and rehabilitative processes to be used with patients and, on the other, to snatch it from the ill-intentioned, accustomed to making it an instrument of manipulation to the detriment of other people's freedom, without even sparing the characters of the spectacle [... He was a] leader like Hyppolite Bernheim and Milton Erickson [...] in favour of equal dedication, methodological, scientific seriousness and honesty, profuse in research and clinical application [...] He was a great master who made it possible to face with greater ease any relational difficulties that may arise in the setting [...] He considered hypnosis a very strong and effective tool in the hands of the therapist; today he would consider it equal to a life-saving drug".

Vittorio Grecchi, who was also president of the 'Bernheim', in his speech instead emphasised the developments of Guantieri's intuition, a "revolutionary scientist" hypnologist whom he also compares, in a different yet equal form, to Milton Erickson. "In commenting on the Master", says Grecchi, "I consider it my precise duty to mention another author who, with him, built modern hypnosis [...] dictating the teachings that today allow for truly effective psychotherapy and measurable results: Pierre Janet. For this author, between psyche and soma, there is continuity at every level, starting from elementary sensitivity and movement: however the psychic functions differ more and more from the organic substrate as their complexity increases. [Well,] in Italy the 'revolution' towards the dominant conceptions of hypnology was carried out by Guantieri [...and] his intuitions [...] are still fundamental to the current conception of hypnosis for its applications in psychotherapy ... [Relevant, then, was the ability to] understand that the unconscious is often expressed through images, and [to understand] how the brain structures perceptions even when they come from within the psyche rather than from the outside world".

Following on from that, Pier Giorgio Malesani recalled Guantieri as the "Master Shaman" of the 'Bernheim' Institute, the "place-laboratory of investigation and technological application [of hypnosis] where didactic value [... was] fundamental [...] to Guantieri's great School of Hypnology, on which he [...] imprinted [...] charisma [...] in dialogue, in lively, colloquial, confidential confrontation [... thus realising] lived experiences that gradually became true wisdom. [... A school, a forge, a central place for training and structuring the original paradigm of Guantierian Hypnology]".

Michele Modenese, another previous president of the 'Bernheim' , then recalled the didactic-formative history of the Institute and the reflections and scientific journey carried out there, in particular on the themes of pain therapy and progressive hypnosis developed under the impulse of Guantieri.

In these proceedings of the San Martino B.A. conference, the aforementioned Carlo Piazza recalled some quotes, not received in writing, but equally intense and not to be forgotten – as he states – for example, the "passionate" one by co-founder Pietro Parietti, "the moving letters written by friends and founders Gastone Benatti and Bruno Caldironi", the affectionate and moving tribute to the "strong impression of historical, scientific and cultural continuity" that there was between the 'H. Bernheim' Institute and the 'H. Bernheim' School of Psychosynthetic Psychotherapy and Ericksonian Hypnosis (S.P.P.I.E.), due to Giovanni Gocci, psychologist, psychotherapist, director of the same school, and again, Giuliano Guerra, doctor, psychotherapist, and hypnologist, who testified to his spiritual hypnological gaze inspired by the masters Guantieri and Assagioli.

Carlo Piazza himself then presented, at the conclusion of the conference, the report: "Hypnosis in progress, from Guantieri to Neuroimaging", and said "I owe a lot to Guantieri" and concluded thus: "the psychodynamic, psychosynthetic, Guantierian and Ericksonian Hypnology orientations [...] merged into the same school [thus binding] past and present: the fathers of scientific hypnosis and of the most brilliant neurophysiological intuitions".

The 10th National Congress of the Italian Society of Hypnosis.
The languages of hypnosis: A bridge between mind and body, between past and future and between imagination and reality
Verona, 21-23 October 2016.

It was in this national congress of the Italian Society of Hypnosis that a report by Pier Giorgio Malesani entitled "Gualtiero Guantieri: the Master Hypnologist" was presented. In it – taking up and elaborating themes already touched upon in the aforementioned conference in San Martino B.A. (Verona), 2008 – he stressed that the residential courses of the 'Bernheim' Institute had gradually become more and more over the years, for the participants, a context of psychophysical immersion in which individual and group dynamics, experiences and knowledge developed simultaneously and synergistically, supported and coordinated by a cohort of teachers led by a master who guaranteed the originality of a school that was at the same time a place-laboratory for research and theoretical, operational, personal training.

Guantieri 'the Master' was in fact a researcher and scientist, a hypnologist with a dynamic and humanistic orientation, a charismatic educator-trainer, particularly sensitive and attentive to the personalities of his followers, while distinguishing himself as a good, reassuring and effective clinician-healer.

The study of hypnosis, in this way, was contextual to the training of the hypnologist while Guantierian hypnological epistemology, which intended to give structure to its own science, associated itself with a pedagogical epistemology that succeeded in increasingly refining the concept of a man-hypnologist project, suitable for delicate and efficient clinical and training tasks.

The report then, focusing on the details of the didactic training, the responsibilities of the teacher, the qualities of the student, the skills that the latter must acquire and the relevance of the interpersonal relationship that is established between one and the other, on the themes of transference and countertransference, concluded that what united one and all was the common involvement in research training and the dissemination of knowledge that was acquired on a national and global level.

With some emphasis, Malesani highlighted how the 'Bernheim' Institute had been a great school of Hypnology, a school of encounter and dialogue, and of global confrontation, where creativity and intuition were also gradually integrated to build a 'corpus' that he was training within the framework of a vision of hypnosis projected towards the future.

4
Gualtiero Guantieri reconsidered in current hypnology, by Andrea Angelozzi: Forty years later *"Hypnosis: a foundation and a perspective"*.

Psychiatrist Andrea Angelozzi was, in one of the most prosperous phases of the 'Bernheim' Institute, one of the protagonists who, along with Guantieri, gave the scientific foundation to an original hypnology that was gradually coming to life as Guantierian.

In his in-depth reflections and meditations, which have taken shape in a paper still in the process of publication, entitled: 'A memory of Gualtiero Guantieri and his rich and fruitful teaching',[11] Angelozzi states: " To think back to the role that Gualtiero Guantieri played in my training is a mix of both memories and perspectives [...] linked to an encounter that proved essential in a period in which I was intensely looking for therapeutic models and a personal and professional identity. In fact," he continues, " the encounter with hypnosis and the collaboration that was established with Guantieri, after I was a student of his, were decisive for me ".

That was a very dense period in the world of research in hypnosis: the debate was alive between the "state" and those of the "non-state" (or relationship) and often between clinicians and experimentalists; "We witnessed the emergence of Ericksonian models, with their charm but also with their problematic systematisation; Neuro Linguistic Programming had appeared, with its seductive and (sometimes over-) simplified models. Many reflections had emerged from this which found their way into a body of work that we wrote together, Guantieri and I, illustrating both in Italy and abroad, thanks to its Italian and English editions, the path that the 'Bernheim' Institute was following.

Angelozzi points out that "Guantieri has always remained – faithful to hypnosis as an explicit practice, always bringing it back to the Centre of his clinical activity and his scientific insights. And even if my path," he adds, "is different, moving away from hypnosis as a 'formal' practice, the link with what hypnosis suggests along the path to change and the many horizons it has opened up has remained".

Angelozzi continues to write: "Forty years after my first meeting with Guantieri,

---

[11] Guantieri G., Angelozzi A., *(A foundation and a perspective. The 'H. Bernheim' and the conceptual evolution of hypnosis)*, Edited by the 'H. Bernheim' Institute of Clinical Hypnosis and Psychotherapy — Research and Training School, Verona, 1985.

I realize how much hypnosis has influenced my path, only seemingly different. I therefore thought that the best way to honor and thank Guantieri was to retrace the many aspects that were at the Centre of his teachings and our reflections, and describe the various new horizons, unpredictable at the time, to which they led me. This document seeks to be a postscript to that common work of 1985, an ideal continuation of it almost half a century later; unfortunately, lacking that confrontation with Guantieri, always so full of ideas. But I'm sure that, with the human and mental generosity, desire to deepen and the curiosity that always distinguished him, he would have been happy to discuss these issues, as we have often done in the past".

Having said that, Andrea Angelozzi develops his theses, articulating them on the themes of the importance of hypnosis, the nature of hypnosis, the various models that consider it and the possibility of their integration, susceptibility to hypnosis (stable and modifiable) of the affective involvement of the hypnologist and the effects of hypnosis on them, of the relationship and its specific aspects, delving into the themes of the influence of gaze, eye fixation techniques, contact, attention and association, with extensive research documentation carried out all over the world.

After an extensive excursus relating to hypnological research, he considers the clinical approach to the induction of hypnosis, focusing on the specific topic of the "deconstruction" of the state of consciousness.

Again, he considers the new contributions of social psychology, commitment theory, cognitive dissonance, intrinsic and extrinsic motivation, central and peripheral persuasion and the sparing of cognitive resources.

Another subsequent chapter is dedicated to hypnosis in psychotherapy, distinguishing different models, "therapy as acceptance, transformation and use, the therapeutic dynamics: mis-identity, metaphors and narratives".

Angelozzi concludes with an enlightening chapter on learning hypnosis.

Of Angelozzi's in-depth studies, two fundamental issues are focused on here in particular:
1) that of the interpersonal relationship between hypnologist and client;
2) that of the hypnologist training school.

Going into the specifics of the arguments developed by the author, relating to the first highly debated topic of hypnosis understood as a "state" or as a "non-state" (or interpersonal relationship), Angelozzi recalls the efficacy that Guantieri reached (together with others, such as, for example, Milton Kline (1923-2004), with whom he had scientifically interacted for a long time) through an innovative integration paradigm, clearly delineated since the 1960s, of hypnosis as a dynamic interaction (with reciprocal and continuous influence) between state and rapport.[12]

---

[12] Guantieri G., *Ipnosi medica. Introduzione allo studio e alla pratica dell'ipnosi in medicina*, in *Opera medica magazine*, edited by A. Wassermann SpA, Milan, LVI Year, April-September, n. 130, 1968;

"Guantieri's position", writes Angelozzi, "seeks to integrate hypnosis, recognized as a specific state of consciousness, with relational aspects, which become an essential element in its realisation and the form it can take"; whereby "the state and the hypnotic relationship are inseparably linked: the relationship in fact helps to initiate and maintain the state; the state, in turn, influences the relationship, similarly to what happens in many other vital situations".[13]

– The Author reminds us that this approach, reaffirmed in the 1985 paper by Guantieri and Angelozzi, fo und experimental support and evolution in Éva Bányai,[14] who demonstrated how the development of the hypnotic condition is influenced by the personal characteristics of both the hypnologist and the subject, from their relationship, and also from the physiological, experiential, behavioural and subjective changes that accompany the induction process in both.

This approach therefore does not privilege individual causal aspects between the different components and considers hypnosis as an integration that arises from the interdependence of its elements.

This paradigm, Angelozzi observes, is very close to the approach of Guantieri, it is the very development of it, and is closely linked to his - predominantly clinical - vision, , where he defines hypnosis as a "process that involves the whole organism, conceived as a psychosomatic unit in intimate contact, action and reaction with its surrounding environment".[15]

For Guantieri, a clinical approach indicates that induction is a function of the interpersonal relationship existing between the subject and the hypnotist and that any inductive technique that allows for adequate and prompt cooperation is effective, as is further underlined in the deeper states of hypnosis, known as somnambular, where the operator becomes the only intermediary for the external environment, as well as in hypnotherapies where relationship and possibility of induction advance in parallel.

Moreover, recently[16], a model of hypnosis entirely focused on relational aspects has been proposed, retracing the mother-child interaction and considering hypnosis as a mechanism for unfavourable childhood situations, supporting this hypothesis with neuroanatomical and neurochemical aspects.

Subsequent studies on restructuring have also largely confirmed these early emphases. Restructuring is the process that transforms beliefs into knowledge,

---

[13] Guantieri G., *L'ipnosi, come oggetto di studio e mezzo di impiego in medicina,* Rizzoli, Milan, 1973, p. 50.
[14] Bányai É. I., Mészáros I. e Csókay L., *Interaction between Hypnotist and Subject: A social Psychophysiological Approach, (Preliminary report),* in Waxman D. Misra P.C., Gibson M., Basker M.A., *Modern Trends in Hypnosis,* New York, London: Plenum Press, 1985.
[15] Bányai É.I., *Theories of Hypnosis. Current Models and Perspectives,* New York, London: The Guilford Press, pagg.564-598, 1991; Bányai É.I.,*On the Adaptive Value of Hypnosis: A Social Psychobiological Model,* Invited address presented at the 12th International Congress of Hypnosis, Jerusalem, Israel, 25-31 July 1992; Bányai É.I., *The Interactive Nature of Hypnosis: Research Evidence for a Social Psychobiological Model,* in *Contemporary Hypnosis,* 1998
[16] Varga K., *Possible Mechanisms of Hypnosis from an Interactional Perspective,* in Brain Sciences, 2021; Sugarman L.I., Schafer P.M., Alter D.S., Reid D.B., *Learning Clinical Hypnosis Wide Awake: Can We Teach Hypnosis Hypnotically?* In *The American journal of clinical hypnosis,* 2018.

thus modifying personal beliefs susceptible to doubt into elements taken for granted, with a "naturalisation" that makes them obvious and implicit, and as such, removed from doubt.[17]

"Among its many aspects", continues Angelozzi, "the reference to a common sense 'ontology' is interesting, by which people take for granted the existence of a material world with its rules, and the very existence of each person and others; a common sense 'physics' that allows us to handle medium-sized objects in everyday life; the 'rationality' of common sense, which, as reasoning, is characterised by the ability to adapt to the individual case by violating universal rules of classical logic; and a 'psychology of common sense' where we find the aspects relating to mental functioning and identity in everyone. A particular case is the reconfirmation of dissociative lines already preformed as 'your unconscious' as opposed to 'your conscience': where the certainty in our identity is altered, demarcating the limits of awareness or the difference between conscious and unconscious ('it is not necessary for you to listen to me with your conscious mind'). But still the dissociation may concern spatial representations, in which one sees oneself".[18]

Angelozzi then comes to the second, relevant issue highlighted here: learning hypnosis.

And on this point, he recalls how Guantieri was not only a great theorist of hypnosis and a great clinician of its application, but he always dedicated himself to teaching and integrating it into his overall hypnological paradigm: there can be no research and study, he argued, if not within a school and training community where the continuous confrontation between teachers and learners is a creative and scientific propellant.

Guantieri and Angelozzi published a list of the Bernheim Institute's completed studies up to the end of 1988.[19]

In this sense, it should not go unnoticed, Angelozzi points out,–that Guantieri managed to create the first university-level teaching of hypnosis at the School of Specialisation in Anaesthesiology and Intensive Care of the University of Verona. And then the great work at his 'Bernheim' Institute in which generations of doctors and psychologists have been trained in the use of hypnosis, where -better- true hypnologists have been molded.

The teaching method that Guantieri has created over the years is interesting, favouring residential courses in which people could not only receive theoretical

---

[17] Muzi P., Angelozzi A., *Building the trance. Linguistic Means and Illustrative Models*, in *Acta Hypnologica*, 'H. Bernheim' Italian Institute for the Study of Clinical Hypnosis and Psychotherapy -- Research and Training School, San Martino B.A (Verona), Year I, n. 2, May 1997;
[18] Kirsch I., Lynn S.J., *Dissociation theories of hypnosis*, in *Psychological Bulletin*, 1998; Green J.P., Lynn S.J., *Hypnotic responsiveness: Expectancy, attitudes, fantasy proneness, absorption, and gender*, in *International Journal of Clinical and Experimental Hypnosis*, 2011.
[19] Guantieri G., Angelozzi A., *Hypnosis: a Base a Way Forward*, edited by The 'H. Bernheim' Institute for Research in Clinical Hypnosis and Psychotherapy – School for Research and Training, Verona, 1988.

elements and practice using them, but they could also directly experience hypnosis on other course-mates, and above all on themselves.

Gualtiero Guantieri paid particular attention to all these aspects, recalls Angelozzi. Similarly, dangers have also been reported for the hypnologist who has a very powerful tool at their disposal, which risks dispensing them from the need to listen to and solve problems, and deludes the patient that it is possible to evade their responsibilities in therapy, by placing all the burden on the therapist. It is important then to recognize, process and manage the pleasurable and seductive experience of omnipotence associated with the hypnologist-hypnotist.

For all this, formative training is needed, and not just the informative kind, in which the personal experience of hypnosis plays an important role. And this is how Guantieri organised his courses and teaching, excluding the idea that a 'pure' learning of techniques leads to an efficient use of hypnosis.

The aspect of direct knowledge of hypnosis as subjects played an essential role in Guantieri's teaching methods, representing a new element. There was an awareness of the value of knowledge and trust in hypnosis that is acquired with one's direct experience as a subject.

Pardell[20] noted that a good number of his colleagues expressed some degree of reluctance to be hypnotised and very few had actually been so. Moreover, few references appear in literature in this regard, making Guantieri a pioneer in this as well, considering direct personal experience an essential tool for learning, experimenting on oneself the various phenomena and emotional aspects that are connected to hypnosis and relaying this to the group, with its capacity for support and understanding.

In other respects, this didactic-training proposal which integrates in training the role of interpersonal aspects and experiences in hypnosis as central elements, for those who induce it and for those who experience it first-hand, is fully in tune with the vision of hypnosis as a state and relationship that Guantieri had always pursued: consequently paying attention to the patient, the duty to understand their needs, adapting the technique on a case-by-case basis, in order to grasp the patient's subjective needs and desire for change, and combine training in hypnosis with adequate psychotherapy.

In all these areas, concludes Angelozzi, Guantieri emerges as forerunner with great stature as a researcher and clinician on the Italian and international scene.

---

[20] Pardell S.S., *Psychology of the hypnotist*, in *The Psychiatric quarterly*, 1950. Lankton S.R, *Training in Therapy-Induction Without Scripts*, in *The American journal of clinical hypnosis*, 2017.

5
Gualtiero Guantieri and his hypnology in virtual encyclopaedias.

There is important information about Guantieri and his hypnology on Wikipedia,[21] Among other things, it states: "According to Gualtiero Guantieri (1927-1994), hypnosis, like any other discipline, has two phases that gradually pass into one another: from an empirical, prescientific phase, based exclusively on observation of phenomena, we pass to a scientific phase, characterised above all by the description and classification of the phenomena detected, as well as by the research of how and why they can occur.

The pre-scientific phase of hypnosis begins in prehistory, of which there is no written evidence, but the study of the archaeological finds discovered, and of the customs of the current primitive peoples, testify to the possibility that hypnosis phenomena and related manifestations were already present then, induced in various ways and for divinatory or therapeutic purposes".

In delving into the historical theme of hypnology, we are reminded of a Guantieri that mentions in his work events that "accompany the Bacchic mysteries of the Magna Mater and Terra Madre mentioned in the Attis of Gaius Valerio Catullo [... and] the ceremony of initiation into the arcane of Silenus, painted in the Pompeian Villa of Mysteries, which involved the protracted fixation of a mask depicting Silenus himself reflected in an illuminated cup, involving hypnotic phenomena".

The text explores the theme, taking up Guantieri's thought, and cites Franz Anton Mesmer (1734-1815), also in reference to the condemnation he had to suffer from the Academy of Sciences and the Faculty of Medicine of Paris at the time (1784) and goes on to recall the subsequent revision of Mesmer's theories proposed by the English physician James Braid (1785-1860), and later still the developments in hypnology instigated by Ambroise-Auguste Liébeault (1823-1904) and by Hippolyte Bernheim (1837-1919) , who founded the Nancy School — which opposed the ideas and methods of Jean-Martin Charcot (1825-1893), who worked at the Salpêtrière hospital in Paris. The discussion continues on a Guanterian track, recalling John Elliotson, Sigmund Freud (1856-1939) and others, up to Milton Erickson (1901-1980).

The text then states: "Thanks to Milton Erickson, in the U.S.A., and to other important international figures, such as Franco Granone and Gualtiero Guantieri in Italy, hypnosis underwent a progressive development in the second half of the 20th century, finally acquiring the status of a scientific, medical and psychological discipline". And there are further interesting considerations, referring in particular to the developments of hypnology in recent years: the birth of national and international hypnology societies, the current scientific debates in progress, the development of brain 'imaging' techniques, which make it possible to visualise the

---

[21] https://it.wikipedia.org/wiki/ipnosi

changes in brain activity during a state of hypnosis, the themes of ideoplasias (plastic monoideisms), hypnositherapy, hypnosipedia, i.e. the use of hypnosis in learning, most relevant aspect of the hypnotic relationship – so dear to Guantieri – as a fundamental factor involved in the generation of the clinical-hypnotic condition characterised by deep and sincere collaboration between the hypnologist-hypnotist and the patient, in order to achieve the personal goals of the latter, and the topic of self-hypnosis as an important skill that the person can acquire through learning conducted under the guidance of experienced hypnologists. The current considerations of hypnosis as a "plastic manifestation of the properly oriented creative imagination" are also reported.

The culturally rich text, worthy of careful and critical consideration, contains extensive bibliographic references, including the masterpiece by Gualtiero Guantieri: 'Ipnosi, come oggetto di studio e mezzo di impiego in medicina' ("Hypnosis as an object of study and means of use in medicine"), published by Rizzoli in Milan, in 1973.

CHAPTER 1

Gualtiero Guantieri: biographical notes[22]

1. Origins

Gualtiero Guantieri was born in Verona on September 9th, 1927, to Macedonio Guantieri and Maria Gasperazzo. He was the eldest of two children; his younger brother, Carlo, was born in 1928.

His family had ancient noble origins: aristocrats and the upper echelons of the bourgeoisie, medieval knights, lawyers, state accountants (although there were never any doctors before Gualtiero, an unusual discovery, of which he was proud) bestowed dignity and prestige upon it.

There are records of Guantieri's ancestors dating back to the 14th century. The lineage of these predecessors had Austrian ancestry and Venetian relatives including that of Giovanni Dolfin (1303-1361), doge of the Republic of Venice.

Filippo Guantieri's father, Nicolò, was mayor of Florence in the first half of the 14th century. Filippo was economic advisor to Cangrande II della Scala (1332-1359).[23]

Among these illustrious relatives of the past, there was also an Austrian citizen, of Italian origin, Luigi Negrelli (1799-1858). The famous engineer, among countless other works, designed the Suez Canal.

Guantieri was quietly proud of his genealogy. The father of two children, Massimo (born in 1965) and Francesca (born in 1968), he hoped his family could have a line of continuity, He was awaited grandchildren who were born, sadly for him, only after his death. They are Leonardo Gualtiero, born in 2003, Eleonora Anna, born in 2005, children of Massimo and then Anna, born in 2007, the daughter of Francesca.

Even Carlo, Gualtiero's brother, could have made his own contribution to this family tree, but in the end, he only had one daughter.

Gualtiero's father, Macedonio, was a bank employee. He died in 1993, a year before the death of his son, at the age of almost 100. He was a meek man; he was rarely angry. It is said that only twice in his entire life was he able to express his opposition to something: the first time was during World War II, when his home was bombed. It happened that, having made all his family members take refuge in the basement of the house, he calmly spent the night in his own bedroom. That night, however, a bomb gutted the building, destroying the stairs, preventing him

---

[22] The contributors to the collection of these notes are his children, Francesca and Massimo Guantieri, and Drs. Rocco Cacciacarne, Serena Rosson and Federica Tagliati.

[23] The tomb of Cangrande II della Scala, from 1432, frescoed by Antonio Badile (1518-1560) is located in the church of Santa Maria della Scala in Verona.

from going down the next morning, except by makeshift means. He then became very upset, but only due to this restriction in his freedom of movement.
In the second case he had quarrelled with his wife, disagreeing about the hiring of a maid whom he defined – obviously manifesting his point of view – as an "unpleasant presence".
In his late. years, he closely followed the exploits of his successor and was well known in the world of Italian hypnology. He had the appearance of a neat, clean old man. He liked to assiduously his son's lectures, without ever intervening, however, he became a sort of icon in that setting.
Gualtiero's mother was a traditional housewife; she dedicated her life exclusively to the family.
His relationship with her was conflictual.
Gualtiero recounted how his mother was very strict with him, always demanding exceptionally polite behavior and excellent academic results.
If he were to receive, for example, a mark of nine out of ten, rather than ten, she would lock him in the bathroom to study (she inflicted these punishments despite her husband's disappointment, and would not forgive her for such behavior, even if he recognized that his wife's tyranny did indeed have positive side effects, in terms of his son's commitment to study and research).
A very close childhood friend of Gualtiero used to describe such events from the opposite perspective. As far as he recalled, during Gualtiero's "imprisonment", the friend would intervene — as both witness to and protagonist of the event — placing a tall ladder under the window to allow him to climb down, so that together they could venture out into the countryside.
According to this friend, Gualtiero's mother was actually very nice and sweet: in the story recounted, she would seemingly have understood everything and, smiling to herself, would have pretended not to see the boys' crafty escape, letting it go.
However, this episode would seem to reveal a relational style of little confidence between the mother and her son, inevitably leading to certain consequences on the psychic development of little Gualtiero.
In any case, she was a mother who cared a great deal about her son's upbringing and education; she steered him towards high-level education, first through the 'Liceo Classico' high school and later the medical faculty at the University of Padua, so that he would become a good doctor, who was able to   establish himself more and more.
Maternal pressure undoubtedly had good effects on her son, who became assistant head doctor at the age of 31, with an excellent reputation (colleagues nicknamed him "Doctor Murri", alluding to the famous scientist Augusto Murri (1841-1932), one of the greatest clinicians of his time).
Guantieri's mother encouraged her son so that, once he became a doctor, he would acquire the title of Head Doctor, telling him that he would become important, famous and rich. It also happened that Guantieri participated in a

competition to become hospital head doctor, winning it, despite his reluctant participation.
Moreover, he hated the idea of holding that professional title, due to the pompous nature that he believed it had. So it was that, immediately after receiving this professional proclamation, he resigned. His aspirations were certainly neither public appearances nor financial enrichment.
When he returned home, evidently irritated with his mother for having pushed him beyond measure, as he saw it, to deal with things he did not like, finding himself alone in the living room, he covered the floor with large banknotes, gluing them to the floor and thus severely damaging them. He sat down and waited for his mother. When she came back, he said to her: "You see, Mum, now you should be happy, I have become a Head Doctor, I will earn a lot of money. Well, I just want you to know that, upon receiving this promotion, I have resigned from the hospital".

2. Childhood, adolescence and youth

Gualtiero was a physically frail child, perhaps suffering from a mild form of rickets. Little inclined to physical activity, he was instead very curious, perceptive and intellectually active.
Nature attracted him, he sought to know and understand it.
At the age of ten he collected various small animals, such as butterflies or other insects, lizards and frogs. He studied them, dissected them and preserved them, fixing them on wooden boards and writing observations and considerations about them.
Since he was a little boy, he liked to spend time with his peers. Not only schoolmates but also, indiscriminately, the children of peasants or noble people and wealthy families, especially at weekends the during the summer holidays, when he went with his family to their countryside residence.
A good pupil, of notable intelligence, he was very creative, imaginative and inventive.
He also liked to engage in very whimsical behavior.
It is said that, from a very young age, he gathered friends of the same age to carry out experiments on them with verbal and non-verbal communication. For example, he asked his accomplices to assume certain postures, to perform certain movements, to express sentences in a certain way.
He did these things with a playful attitude, but always with an underlying intent aimed at getting to know people's characters, the traits and nuances of their personalities, the reactions and collective behaviours that derived from them[24]

---

[24] In the manner of the protagonists of the 1975 film *Amici Miei,* by Mario Monicelli.

He and his friends, who imitated him, participated in these good-natured pranks using strange verbal language, apparently meaningless, also involving unknown passers-by.

Once, while he was waiting for a train in a railway station, Guantieri put a match between his lips, then, turning to a gentleman near him, he asked if he had a light. The poor man, a little bewildered, replied: "What? Do you want to smoke a match?", implying that requests of this kind were completely insane.

Gualtiero replied that the lighting of the match was not what he had requested, but simply whether the person had something to light it with, thus wanting to see how easily misunderstandings can be created due to stereotyped, unreflective, non-critical common thoughts.

Once he stood alongside a person who was looking at a pipe display case. Turning to him, he exclaimed: "Beautiful pipe! But, you know, I prefer a white limousine". His interlocutor (there by chance) replied: "But what do cars have in common with pipes?". The reply was: "You know, I don't like white meat!", at which point, the stranger was totally astonished. Gualtieri then summed up the conversation by exclaiming: "Too many weirdos around!" .

Conversations like this could continue with Guantieri fuelling it with syllogisms, further misleading questions and meaningless words, tending to bring about unpredictable outcomes, a bit like a cultural anthropologist engaged in field research.

There was an episode in which he wrote a letter to a friend, neglecting to stamp it. He simply drew the stamp on the envelope, writing next to it a note addressed to the postman stating that the stamp was inside, so as to avoid licking it, so that he, or the recipient, could preserve it — given the fact that nobody could find this out. The friend appreciated the joke so much that he kept the letter which his wife later returned to the Guantieri family.

Years later, the protagonist was able to comment on those episodes, claiming that our world is also a place of madmen in which it is common for people to be amazed or dumbfounded!

3. The student

Guantieri, thanks to his own skills and also to a favourable upbringing, not least the attention and solicitations of his mother, always achieved excellent grades in school.

He was extremely curious and lively, he studied a lot, but he also dabbled in experiments in chemistry, physics and psychology (in this case, as mentioned, involving cousins and friends).

He liked Latin and Greek very much. During high school he won three scholarships thanks to which he was able to spend long periods of summer study in Cambridge, so that, at the age of 18, he already knew the English language perfectly (later recognizing that these skills had been very useful to him, both in terms of personal growth and as facilitating tools for the many international relations that involved him throughout his life, especially with the international world of hypnology).

Ingeniously, despite his young age, in order to avoid leaving for military service, which would have taken place during the Second World War, he completed an additional year of high school during the summer holidays, thus graduating early. This stratagem, combined with his congenital frailty, enabled him not to leave for war In November 1951, at the age of 24, he obtained a degree in Medicine and Surgery from the University of Padua.

4. The Man

Personality

Guantieri was a man of integrity, both as a doctor, teacher and trainer and, in general, throughout his entire life.
He inspired confidence.
He was upright, not only in moral terms, but also metaphorically, and physically, with his straight posture, with his thinness and his casual clothing, being as he was an enemy of neck ties.
He was generous and helpful, never failing to fulfil a promise he made.[25]
Seemingly very emotionally controlled, he never appeared to get angry, and he showed great calmness (despite his inner torments), so it was easy for him to teach the process of learning relaxation.
He was also sympathetic to people who could make mistakes, which he disliked, but tended to correct by supporting those who needed help.
He was an intelligent and cultured man, of surprising humility; very synthetic and concrete, he did not waste words. Extremely concise and incisive, he had an intense and penetrating gaze, and seemed to read the soul of his interlocutors; to many he was awe-inspiring; he did not flatter or plead with anyone.
His statements were exhaustive: they were short, concise, essential sentences.
He was renowned for his great charisma. Although hypnosis and the group of doctors who practiced it, with whom he founded the 'Bernheim Centre' in 1965

---

[25] We recount various anecdotes in this chapter about Guantieri's generosity, his attention to others, and how he sought to protect the weak and persecuted who were dear to his soul Here we recall an episode told by his daughter Francesca of an American boy who came to visit them on vacation, referred by a fellow hypnologist of her father. The family became a base for this young man's Italian excursions, visiting them almost every week and for a long time, welcomed as if he were, not only a welcome guest, but an important person, to be assisted and protected with respect.

(later transformed into the 'Bernheim' Institute), were regarded with caution or even with mistrust in the 1980s, he was respected by all, well-liked by many, and by others he was even praised.

A great visionary, he was nevertheless methodical, precise, and punctual (preferably showing up early for prearranged meetings). He suggested, for example, going to the train station early, to have the chance to catch the previous train that would in any case likely have been late (a life choice, which meant he passed unscathed through Bologna station, on his way to Rome, just half an hour before the deadly terrorist attack that took place on 2 August 1980).

He had a prophetic spirit, he knew how to read into the depths of people's souls, as if he could know the fate of each, without ever revealing it, thus avoiding any manipulation and allowing his patients and students to freely take their therapeutic or training course.

If he had any intolerance, it was for unreliable people, such as those who use hypnosis dishonestly, for example.

He did not lack fragility; he smoked a lot, for instance, but he did not tolerate those who preached to him about it, or calls to quit. He defended himself simply by saying that: "We all have to die of something".

Relational style

Guantieri was a fairly extroverted man, very interested in the human condition, and extremely sensitive to the suffering of others.

In his relations, he acted with leadership and was attentive to the communications of his interlocutors, showing incredible goodness.

Of his friends, and his youth, much has already been said.

Later in life, he mainly associated himself with people he had met in a professional context, therefore many people working in hospitals (it was during a recurring conference, called International Medical Days, where he met his future wife Anna Maria, there in the role of organisational manager) and then with partners and attendees of the 'Bernheim'. He also had many foreign friends, going abroad several times (even as a boy, as we have seen) and then frequenting the world of hypnology.

His seriousness and ability to relate to the people who needed him clearly distinguished his personality. Greatly appreciated in the health districts where he worked in those years, and in the clinical laboratories he attended, he always presented himself in line with his areas of absolute competence: psychotherapy first of all, thus emanating serious and unquestionable professionalism.

At national and international congresses, many of which he organised himself, he always participated in the work sessions, and always as an active listener. When he then spoke, he did so as a master, talking about the cases he worked on and with immediate reference to what he had previously heard from other speakers.

He was capable of analysing more with silence than with words.

He was also a seducer, he liked women (his wife, however, considered him harmless from this point of view, perhaps because he really was, or otherwise because she believed that her place beside him would never be questioned).

He was a charming man and he himself believed as such. Whenever he intended to be so, he was aware that his intense gaze was something that very few people could handle.

Social and political orientation

Those who knew him in this respect considered him a liberal socialist.

In any case, he believed that all people deserved the same opportunities and the same treatment by public institutions, while believing that merit should be recognized and valued.

He did not actively deal with public affairs, he limited himself to following them, informing himself about them, reading the newspapers and only occasionally watching the news on television. He had been asked several times to be mayor of the town where he had his summer residence, but he always refused.

In fact, he, a free and pure spirit as he was, perceived politics as a compromising transaction, absolutely opposed to his way of being.

During the Cold War, at a time of tensions between Eastern and Western Europe, Guantieri was able to help some skilled doctors from Eastern countries escape from their countries, moving to the West.

While still a child, during the Second World War, he took it upon himself to provide food to Jewish people persecuted by fascism, who were occasionally kept hidden in a cave as "displaced persons", near his countryside home.

He was not only critical of but also indignant towards Italy during the 1980s, which he considered a "Banana Republic": a state adrift, in the hands of some incompetents, lacking vision but very adept at imposing taxes and duties (he said – with disdainful satire – that all that was left was for the State to impose a tax on the air we breathe), so much so that he encouraged his children to try to move abroad to fulfil themselves.

He hated the tv, which he called an "infernal machine" even if, at times, he watched it and agreed to participate in it for interviews that he conceded with the sole intent of spreading knowledge about clinical hypnosis, as opposed to "freak-show hypnosis" as he would define it when related to magicians, illusionists and stage hypnotists.

Ethics, spirituality, religion

Family, righteousness, freedom, modesty, moderation, generosity, altruism, reality, consistent behavior and keeping to one's word and commitments were moral pillars of his existence.
For him, honesty, fairness and ethics were essential values.
His virtuous imperative was to be able to be satisfied. He used to say: "The less you want, the happier you will be."
He held culture, study, and research in high regard (aware that "the more you know, the more you are convinced that you don't know"), and while he believed that knowledge had such contradictions, in any case one should not give it up.
He invited some of his students to consider that: "the farther we walk (on the path of awareness), the more we will remain alone".
He believed that embarking on a path of meditation on human issues and the study of what is unknown, certainly involves a profound and never exhaustive knowledge, but this endeavour increasingly distances the subject from everyday life and people.
He was a relatively religious man, attending places of worship; he defined himself as deeply Christian but not very Catholic. That is, he felt closer to Christ than to the Church.
He believed little in the narrative miracles which he mainly considered extraordinary human events such as those which he and his fellow hypnologists would often see in their medical practice.
Curiously, he considered Jesus to be an expert hypnotist.

Hobbies

He loved contact with nature, animals and agriculture, was a good gardener, delighted in the cultivation of flowers - particularly dahlias, begonias and nightshades.
He contemplated the growth of trees, he liked to plant them (every Christmas he purchased a Christmas tree that, right after the holidays, he re-planted in his garden), cultivate them and make them grow.
He loved life; he allowed himself to enjoy beautiful days of freedom with friends in his country house. However, if they were doctors accompanying him, he would say to them: "let's go there, but let's not talk about medicine".

He liked to sunbathe, by the sea, in the mountains, in the countryside, but also on the balcony of his house when he watered his plants, sometimes naked (deliberately heedless of onlookers). He liked to be constantly tanned.[26]

---

[26] When his wife reprimanded him, asking for a little modesty, he replied that the balcony was his and that whoever might be watching could happily do so, otherwise they could simply turn away. By free, or perhaps silly, association, the anecdote of Archimedes might come to mind, coming out naked from the public baths

He drew very well, both in color and in black and white, but without ever having fostered this great ability. In the years 1963-1965, when he was assistant head doctor of the hospital, he won a drawing and cartoon competition three times in a row, at the Hospital Institutes in Verona. His depictions often featured, as a recurring theme, a parody of the national health system, sometimes to the annoyance of certain colleagues and superiors. In an award-winning caricature, he depicted an arrogant and imperious head physician, whose aids, doctors, and postgraduates, kneeling down around him, were shining his shoes.

He did not engage in any kind of sport except long bicycle rides. Only as a father did he make occasional and unsuccessful attempts to learn to swim with his children. Alongside his son Massimo, he collected stamps, partly for pleasure and partly to share an interest with him. Over the summer weekends he often took his son fishing by the lake or the sea.

He was fond of classical music, and had a particular appreciation for Tchaikovsky.

He began, under the guidance of a teacher, to take piano and pianola lessons, when he was already in his late fifties.

He enjoyed his weekends mainly in his countryside house, where he used to go with the entire family, or the children, where he spent his time gardening or researching, studying and writing, always on the theme of psychosomatic medicine and hypnosis.

He was not averse to following, with much moderation, some theatre or television shows, preferring mainly national comedians of the time or the first satirical and irreverent television broadcasts of the late 1980s.

He disliked holidays conceived as crowded beaches or nightlife. He owned a beachfront apartment near Venice. He used to say that: "if you go for a seaside vacation, better to stay a few days less but enjoy a sea view, and not the view of a wall". He believed that no wall should be in front of him, if it would prevent him from looking far ahead, just as he liked to do in his life.

---

of Syracuse and running through the streets and shouting "Eureka! Eureka!". Who knows if knowledge has to do not only with truth, but also with nudity!

5. The family

The husband

As husband and wife, they had an intense, vigorous, deep, even a little transgressive relationship, ever since they got engaged.
Once, they were on the shores of a lake in the mountains, when he suggested they go skinny dipping together at night (a hazardous thing, at that time in a deeply catholic Italy in the 1960s).
In 1964, Guantieri married Anna Maria Oddone, born in 1928, and already a mother to daughter Lindarosa, born in 1950. His bride was the daughter of Secondo Oddone, from Piedmont, a member of a family of hoteliers and manager of the state railways and of Rosa Elisa Lonardi, a commercial entrepreneur in the food sector.
A very intelligent woman, humble and wise, with a practical and sunny disposition, she was a mother in the true sense of the word. Protective and affectionate with anyone who was part of the family, including all those belonging to the 'Bernheim' Institute.
She loved life and always put herself forward positively, making the best of of things, although she was destined to a premature death in store for her, in 1992, after undergoing multiple surgeries for breast cancer.
Always by her husband's side, she knew how to support him, effectively collaborating in the promotion and creation of the 'Bernheim', the success of which was certainly down to Guantieri and his medical friends, but in which Anna's role and her concreteness played a significant and decisive role.
It was mutual: he took great care not only of her but also of her family.
She had two brothers, both accountants; the younger was diligent, mature, funny and responsible, while the elder one was rather a loafer, fortunately somehow convinced by his brother-in-law to finally assume his responsibilities, in his 40s.
Husband and wife integrated perfectly: the former was an idealist, a scientist; the latter was the one who, always at her husband's side, would concretely and materially organise his life. She was the one who, for the 'Bernheim' Institute, promoted contacts with institutions, sponsors and banks to obtain patronage, as well as concessions of meeting places, the dissemination of material and economic contributions. She would proofread her husband's writings and balance the family and Institute budget each night, after sending the children to bed.
Guantieri could spend up to five years organising a congress. He obsessively planned every detail in advance, striving for an excellent level of research presentations and publications, for every colleague at the 'Bernheim' Institute.
He was very demanding of himself, frequently preparing, along with his colleagues, masterful reports that, being so profound, often couldn't be completely understood by other participants.

Such an approach, however, would imply a waste of energy that was at least partially contained by his wife's concreteness . She knew how, with careful guidance, to point decisively and clearly to common goals.
Their relationship was relevant in a human way, beyond any inevitable limitations that each may have had.
Her husband wrote an affectionate tribute to her, in the preface of the 1968 book "L'ipnosi".[27] Dedicated to his "parents, his wife, children, every pioneer and every man who suffers", he wrote: "I express heartfelt gratitude to my wife Anna Maria, who in many ways has constantly and lovingly accompanied me along the impervious path that was indispensable for me to follow, so that this modest work could see the light".
Some relatives and friends believe that, without his wife, Guantieri would not have been able to achieve the professional results he did.
He would frequently argue with her, almost as if to replicate what he had experienced with his mother in the past. Such regular confrontations were incomprehensible, given that they were based on trivial reasons.
In truth, without Anna who was like vital oxygen to him, he was lost. In fact – it may seem like a strange coincidence – after she died, within days he fell ill with lung cancer.

The father

Guantieri was an affectionate father, in his own way. Francesca, his daughter, says that he was a father who was very absorbed in his thoughts, a little distracted, yet rather indulgent, who granted trust and allowed his children to grow up responsibly and independently. Heartily committed to the upbringing of his children, he was at the same time loving and apprehensive, demanding and permissive.
In any case, he knew how to underline inalienable principles and ethical values; those he held dear. He patiently and respectfully accepted complaints from his children and was able to support and direct them toward the right decision, without invading their private life.
Disputes between them were not rare, but the outcome was usually that of a father who almost always aimed to please (for example, he bought his son a motorbike when he was only eleven years old), only trying to encourage reflections such as: "Do you really want to buy something? Buy it! But do it tomorrow, for now think about it carefully and consider whether you really need it".
His son Massimo says that his father scrutinised the friends he brought home and in a few minutes he read their psychological profile. He didn't impose his point of

---

[27] Guantieri G., "L'ipnosi, come oggetto di studio e mezzo di impiego in medicina", 1973, Edito da Rizzoli Milano, Italy

view, but only suggested reflections. Even if he didn't believe it at first, in the long run, he couldn't help but recognize that Dad was right.

Guantieri was the kind of father who criticised but did not interfere in the choices of his children. He secretly appreciated them, bragged about them, especially to his wife and friends, although generally never in front of his children.

With his adopted daughter, Linda, who was much loved, he always had difficulty expressing his affection so much so that she, unfortunately, was never aware of it.

In any case, he was concerned about their future, their excesses, their rebellions, their aspiration for freedom which he himself considered an essential existential principle.

He had adopted a sort of Montessori method with his children, having a clear understanding that if he forbade something, it would have the opposite effect.

He was always there when his children needed him, whether for a school assignment or a quarrel with other children in the neighbourhood. He indulged their every desire; when it was concrete, he supported it right to the end, and when he realised it was fleeting he made them believe he was supporting, it until it spontaneously fizzled out.

Always open, free of prejudice, innovative and a little crazy, he was affable with his children's friends. He stopped by to chat with them on whatever topic was requested of him, in an open and equal manner and they were both flattered and amazed by so much attention from "such an important, busy and esteemed professor". At Gualtiero's funeral, as well as that of Anna which preceded his, all their children's friends were present, more for their passing than to be close to the friends affected by the loss.

He spent almost every weekend, except those when he had conferences or training courses, with his children, until their teenage years. He took his family with him to every convention that wasn't held in his hometown. He wanted his children to open up to the world, he called himself a "man of the world". And this is how his son Massimo came to spend a good part of his life working abroad, especially in Asia.

6. The doctor, the hypnologist, the psychotherapist

Very faithful to the Hippocratic oath, he stated that he deeply respected any suffering person, as a true doctor should do. For this reason, he preferred qualified and measured psychotherapies and a great deal of research, to the simple and convenient, non-responsible administration of drugs.

He used to say, with a hint of mockery, that "the patient, from the Latin patiens, is the one that suffers and often has to endure not only the pain but also indulge the attempt that we doctors make in trying to heal them. For this reason, we must respect patients and not be arrogant towards them."

He argued that a doctor should not chase money or consider the patient as a client and used to say: "I also like tailored clothes and beautiful cars, therefore if I see the patient as a client, I only feed my external needs and I lose sight of my true reason for being a doctor. If, instead, I remember that I am dealing with a patient, I simply take charge of them, I want to understand them, be close to them and help them to heal. This should be the purpose of a doctor."

His concept of being a doctor meant understanding the deepest origins of the illnesses of his patients, studying them, therefore analyzing them but also humanly involving himself by entering into a state of profound empathy with them. Sometimes, however, this state of deep sharing led Gualtiero to great internal suffering, not always being able to distinguish the psychotherapeutic moment from the empathic emotion.

The hospital, the criticism of traditional medicine, hypnological interests

The very young recent graduate Guantieri had already long expressed important hypnological interests.

His attraction to hypnosis deepened during his hospital internship to prepare for the state exams.[28]

Once he became a hospital doctor, he built up his training, distinguishing himself as a psychosomatist and hypnologist.

Among other things, as early as 1963 he had been dealing with psychoprophylaxis at childbirth, and was the first in Italy to prepare women in labour for a painless birth, through hypnosis.[29]

---

[28] Among his relatives, some tell how this man's inclination for hypnosis was, even before becoming an object of study in his eyes, a sort of drive, an attraction, a desire, which he possessed since he was a boy when he hypnotised animals or experimented with similar things with companions and friends, with whom he created conditions of an authentic trance. The suggestion game, which we considered in those singular behaviours of Guantieri, a university student at train stations or in front of shop windows, was nonetheless the induction of modified (and perhaps somewhat disturbed) states of consciousness of a hypnotic nature.

[29] Regarding the use of hypnosis in gynaecology, psychosomatic medicine and surgery, a record was achieved thanks to one exceptional surgery, whereby, for the first time in Europe, with extensive media, journalistic and television coverage, on the 31st January 1980 in Rovereto, a woman in a hypnotic state was operated on

The discussion he had with the sick convinced him deeply that a large number of their problems were very often of a psychological rather than somatic nature. According to Guantieri, traditional methods of treatment could be revised.
Ten years of medical experience in hospitals (he remained no longer than that), caused increasing discomfort in him. He perceived and criticised in a progressively more severe way a certain inadequacy of the medicine that was practiced at the time, with respect to the emotional experiences of the patients.
At the same time, he therefore experimented with alternative methods of treatment, noting how other types of medical action produced sensational results on a clinical level and with precise scientific value.
He administered placebo substances, i.e. without specific active ingredients, to many patients, achieving resounding healing results in 85% of cases and thus avoiding pharmacological treatments that were not always necessary.
This was perhaps the moment of his psychosomatist enlightenment.

Private practice and the foundation of the 'Bernheim' Institute

Uninterested in a bureaucratic career, on the same day he was informed of his success in becoming Head Doctor, he resigned.
Upon his resignation from the hospital, he vigorously embarked on the path of hypnology, despite being attracted to phytotherapy. He motivated his choice on the grounds that, in the latter case, there would be a commercial element to it, while with hypnosis money would have played a marginal role.
Thus, his contact with a multitude of national and international institutions and protagonists of hypnology and psychosomatic medicine intensified.
It was in those years, around 1966, when Ferruccio Antonelli (1927-2000) founded the Italian Society of Psychosomatic Medicine (S.I.M.P.) and his friend Guantieri joined him as vice president.
Later, in 1968, Guantieri followed in his footsteps and started up the Verona branch of S.I.M.P. (a branch that has since become an important point of reference for psychosomatology in Italy, to this day).
Previously, in 1965, together with other talented the talented and visionary doctors Walter De Stavolta, Mario Montanari, Bruno Caldironi, Werther Ferioli, Gastone Benatti, Piero Parietti e Angelico Brugnoli, Guantieri founded the 'Bernheim' Italian Centre for Clinical Hypnosis, which was later transformed into the Institute.

---

in a private clinic in that city. The lady was prepared for the event by means of appropriate training that had lasted a couple of months and was closely followed during the surgery by a medical team, by Guantieri, who supervised. Positive results were, as he declared, *"to avoid the complications of impaired breathing that disturbs the abdominal skein, reduced bleeding and consequently a lower risk of bleeding, faster wound healing, postoperative lack of vomiting, a prompt restoration of abdominal function, better rest, a reduction in or abolition of pain"*. He added: *"Surgery has taken a notable step forward, all the resistance that the medical profession has always placed against what is unorthodox has been overcome"*.

The scientific work, the research, the ideas, the theories of Guantieri and of the whole Institute were disseminated and published with great prominence throughout the scientific world, through cultural meetings, conferences, congresses, training courses, scientific articles, books and manuals, making continuous comparisons within the international community and between the various societies for the study of hypnosis. Among others, the prestigious International Society of Hypnosis (ISH)[30] of which he was co-founder in Uppsala, Sweden, in 1973, with, among others, Ernest Hilgard, Martin Orne, Peter-Olof Wikstrom and Erika Fromm, and of which the Bernheim Institute was the first Italian constituent society. In 1978 he was an active participant in the establishment of the European Society of Hypnosis, alongside Wikström (Peo), Basil Finer, Vladimir Gheorghiu and Marjan Pajntar, with whom he actively collaborated until his death.

Guantieri underlined, in every context and forum, the importance of the doctor-patient relationship as an essential therapeutic moment.

Round tables and conferences on the meaning of the "Balint" and "The Psychological Training of the Doctor" groups were set up at the Civil Hospital of Borgo Trento in Verona from the 1970s onwards.[31]

Those were the years in which the scientist and scholar Guantieri gave body and paradigm to his own hypnology, defined its foundations, worked on its definition and gave impetus to its cultural diffusion and to the training of his students.

It was the result of a journey that began from very far away.

After becoming a doctor, he immediately began to follow and study international experts on the subject, from his first contact in the early 1960s with Milton Kline, subsequently publishing in the "Journal of Clinical and Experimental Hypnosis" ,and then with John C. Watkins, PhD, secretary of the ISH (International Society for Clinical and Experimental Hypnosis).

He gradually understood more and more how that particular modified state of hypnotic consciousness, if induced by the voice of a trained and serious professional, could constitute an important means of clinical use for multiple pathologies and also a medical and psychological professional training tool.

---

[30] The I.S.H. is now made up of 33 national companies. The organizational headquarters are in Berwyn, Pennsylvania, United States.

[31] Among the issues that were evaluated in all hypnological Centres worldwide, at the 'Bernheim' it was considered and debated whether to open clinical hypnosis societies to other professional categories, other than doctors. Some proposed welcoming psychologists, others argued that it was not appropriate, yet others would have liked to open up to teachers, nurses, physiotherapists, masseurs, chiropractors or other social health categories. There were those who argued that only a doctor could have a complete somatic and psychic vision of the symptoms, that is, a psychosomatic orientation of the disease. It was retorted that the question remained open whether it is the doctor who must acquire more psychological knowledge or the psychologist who must give himself the minimum medical skills and there were those who also claimed that the hypnologist was mostly approached by desperate patients after having tried all possible and imaginable ways to heal. In the end, the time came when, at Guantieri's Institute, and largely thanks to him, this openness to others began to take place.

He spoke (and wrote) with fervently about the things he knew in depth. He spoke about his studies, his research, his discoveries, the need for further medical progress, arousing much interest among those who knew him.

And so it was that, a small group of people, united by this common founding ideal of hypnology, gathered together and then grew into a sort of cohort, of people bearing a common characteristic: that of being a little "crazy".

That group founded the 'Bernheim' Centre - Institute. They were united by innovative ideal affinities, they were holistic and predominantly psychodynamic in orientation, all essentially convinced of the need for considering the patient and their overall humanity, with whom to interact with great dedication and empathy, according to a totally different approach that broke away from the concept of cure, at the time.

A position that in in some ways was sectarian and therefore unpopular within institutional medical colleges, but courageously supported.[32]

He devoted himself to psychotherapy in moderation. He did not want the profession of his being a therapist to take over the space dedicated to research and study.

He had many interests, preeminently hypnology and therefore its study, the school of clinical hypnosis and the training of hypnologist students, research, his relationship with many colleagues from all over the world, the national and international organisation of scientific meetings and congresses, but also his family and free time for hobbies such as music or country life.

For this reason, after leaving the hospital and opening his private practice, he devoted himself to the care of his patients only a few days a week and never beyond Thursday.

His basic orientation was dynamic and he was convinced that if it was the psychoanalytic type of therapeutic action, it could be greatly accelerated by hypnosis, emerging from the mire of endless psychotherapies, thus approaching hypnoanalysis.[33]

For precisely these reasons, he followed a particular care strategy aimed at limiting intervention times as much as possible. So, if necessary, he taught his patients self-hypnosis, so that they could manage their problems independently, as soon as possible.

However, being well-renowned, he was sought out by a multitude of potential patients.

---

[32] Guantieri also considered hypnosis as a means of overcoming rational and logical rigidities and opening the mind to intuition, creativity, imagination and the artistic dimension of the person.

[33] Hypnology, in progressively establishing itself more and more as a science, has continuously engaged in and oriented itself over time to the development of new methods of using the modified state of hypnotic consciousness in the field of brief therapies. For further information, see the text *'Hypnosis and hypnotic therapies. Mysteries revealed and myths debunked'*, written by the four famous therapists Giorgio Nardone, Camillo Loriedo, Jeffrey Zeig and Paul Watzlavick, Salemi Editore S.p.a., Milan, 2012.

To limit these solicitations, he ordered his secretary — and his wife who received many home phone calls — to respond to requests for psychotherapy saying that he would be available no sooner than 12-18 months.

He was a psychotherapist who, once he took charge of a patient, devoted himself to them with great clinical and empathic skill and with magnanimity, while absolutely avoiding considering the subject as a profitable, collectible item.[34]

He was, in his own way, in his dealings with people, a generous Robin Hood.

His professional fees varied according to the economic conditions of his patients. He applied charges related to the wealth of those who were landowners or children of wealthy families, while assisting those who were destitute for free — proposing occasional secretarial duties at the 'Bernheim' Institute to those who had the capacity.

7. The professor

Guantieri held various, prolonged teaching positions at many foreign and Italian universities as well as at the 'Bernheim', of course.

He was a greatly appreciated, widely followed and much admired teacher and trainer.

---

[34] The following anecdote is an example of his way of conceiving clinical activity: In the early 1990s, a Venetian countess, business partner of a very rich prince of Persian origin, went one day to the United States to contact a famous hypnologist and begin a psychological journey with him. The latter pointed out to the lady that it was not appropriate to start a clinical relationship with him, given the enormous distance that separated the residences of the two, and especially considering that a few hundred metres from her home in Verona, there was an excellent hypnotherapist — his dear colleague and internationally renowned researcher — who could help her adequately. The clinician, a colleague and friend of Guantieri, informed the latter of the issue. Guantieri thanked his colleague, but when the very wealthy noblewoman began to call him insistently, he felt a little uncomfortable. He then informed his wife and secretary, who usually received requests for help by phone, that if this person called, the waiting time for her would be even longer than usual. The called multiple times, relentlessly for several weeks. The noble lady, used to being revered by obliging people, she could not bear the idea of having to wait for so long. However, realising Guantieri's prevarications , she made a very attractive and flattering contractual offer to his wife, proposing weekly meetings for which she would go to Verona, during the period in which she lived in Veneto, while from May to September, the period in which she moved to the Costa Smeralda, it would be Guantieri who would travel to her in Sardinia, every seven days, transported by a private helicopter provided by the countess. The financial compensation for this service would have been 10.5 million lire! A huge sum in those days, especially for four hours of therapy. At that point, Guantieri felt that this lady, accustomed as she was to buying everything and everyone, might not have true psychotherapeutic needs, but simply wanted to have him at all costs. He therefore asked his wife and secretary to respond the the next phone calls with a simple denial, due to a full schedule. After a few weeks of further insistence, the house phone began ringing one Saturday morning and, as chance would have it, Guantieri himself answered. The lady began showering him with words of praise, uttering flattering words, and made her insistent request. The answer she received was the following: *"Dear madam, I do not believe that you need psychotherapy, but rather a court jester. In any case, you can find people of the kind simply by leafing through columns or professional registers. You will undoubtedly find someone available. Thank you for your compliments and good luck"*. When he hung up the phone he said: *"Let us remember that freedom is the most important value in life"*. There were obviously various comments from family family members, especially from his wife Anna who managed the accounts and tried to explain to Gualtiero how that offer would allow him to devote himself almost completely to the research and study he so loved, while guaranteeing total financial serenity for the family. There was, however, no follow-up to the matter, other than the strong imprinting of this absolute value in the minds of those present.

A unique lecturer, always absorbed in his thoughts, he loved teaching and devoted himself to his students with great attention and generosity.

He made himself available to his students not only while sat at his desk in the classroom, but also by offering personalised meetings for pedagogical listening and, if necessary, personal help.

For example, he did not hesitate to propose to the student addressing him possible psychological introspection, sometimes with the aid of hypnotic inductions, in a manner that courageously integrated pedagogy and clinical practice.

His exams were further training opportunities, and his final assessments were notoriously very encouraging and gracious.

He spoke about hypnosis by truly living it, proposing and inducing it, so that the result was at once a theoretical and experiential form of teaching.[35]

Already a professor before dedicating himself to hypnosis, he was a professor of General and Developmental Psychopathology and Psychiatry at the University of Padua, in the early 1960s. A position which he no longer renewed after actively dedicating himself to the study of hypnosis — at the time considered almost an esoteric practice.

Professor and trainer, Guantieri became president of the Committee for the Implementation of Permanent Training of the European Society in Psychotherapy and Psychosomatic Medicine in 1981.

Thanks to his tireless efforts, he introduced the teaching of Psychosomatic Medicine and Clinical Hypnosis to the University of Verona, first at the Postgraduate School of Psychiatry and then at the Postgraduate School of Anaesthesiology and Intensive Care. In 1984 the official courses for Psychosomatic Medicine and Clinical Hypnosis were established, as part of the School of Specialisation in Pathophysiology and Pain Therapy. From then on, he continued to teach General and Developmental Psychopathology and Psychiatry at the same universities.

Much earlier, in the United States, he attended the Institute for Research in Hypnosis and Psychotherapy in the state of New York where he taught from 1967. Later, from 1973, he held teaching positions at the Faculty of Psychology of the International Graduate University of Florida in Gainesville. He then collaborated with the Royal Society of Medicine and the American Association

---

[35] A former student, today an acclaimed doctor, recounts how, at the end of the first lesson of a seminar on 'Clinical Hypnosis and Pain Therapy' which Guantieri held as part of a specialisation in anaesthetics course at the Faculty of Medicine at the University of Verona in the 1980s, he complained to the professor who was already saying goodbye to the class as he was about to leave, urging him to stay so that he could start the lecture and begin to define what hypnosis was. Guantieri's response to the entire class was "Would you kindly observe the clock on the wall?". When the student, astonished, realised that almost an hour had passed since the start of the lecture, Guantieri simply explained that   hypnosis was the very thing that the student and his classmates had just experienced during that hour, which had now ended. He believed that, by inducing direct experience of it and not simply providing theoretical explanations, it would catalyse interest and the attention of all attendees. given that they had all seen, in a relevant hypnotic state, a particularly sensational subjective temporal distortion. The Professor won their immediate trust and credibility. The time spent in that classroom was perceived by all to have been very brief, as if it had been a matter of minutes, and the former student still remember that episode to day as one of the most impactful on his life.

for the Advancement of Science and, from 1979, at the Florida Institute of Technology in Melbourne, Florida where he had the chance to interact with Charles Corman (1920-2000), who was the founding dean of the School of Psychology at the same institute.

8. The scientist

International relations

From the time that the 'Bernheim' Centre for the Study of Clinical Hypnosis and Psychotherapy was founded, Guantieri had the sensibility (which he deemed necessary) to spread the hypnological knowledge that he and his collaborators were acquiring, both in terms of research and from a pedagogical point of view, when teaching hypnosis. This outlook, this orientation and this intent looked to national and international horizons from the very start, so much so that the 'Bernheim' was almost immediately awarded with recognition by and affiliation to the Institute for Research of Hypnosis and Psychotherapy of New York (an emanation of the University of the State of New York), later becoming its Italian headquarters.

At the same time, strong connections with the International Society of Clinical and Experimental Hypnosis were formed.

The stages of this transnational exposure were marked by the participation in many international congresses on hypnosis and psychosomatic medicine, including, among others, those held in Mainz, Germany, in 1970 and in Uppsala, Sweden in 1973, on the theme "The Other Medicine". On that occasion, as previously mentioned, Guantieri and others founded the International Society of Hypnosis (I.S.H.) of which Ernest Hilgard (1904-2001) was the first President.

In 1974, the 'Bernheim' became the Italian National Constituent Society of the International Society of Clinical and Experimental Hypnosis.

The following year, participation in the 'International Psychosomatic Week' in Rome and, in 1978, in the Malmö congress in Sweden, the foundations were laid for the establishment of a European association of hypnosis in psychotherapy and psychosomatic medicine which took shape a few years later under the name "European Society of Hypnosis" (E.S.H.). Gualtiero Guantieri was one of the founding members.

Further initiatives were created, around the same time.

In 1978, the 'Bernheim' Centre gave its patronage to the "Pan-American Congress of Hypnosis and Psychosomatic Medicine" in Rio de Janeiro, Brazil.

In 1983, in collaboration with the Slovenian Society of Clinical and Experimental Hypnosis, the 'Bernheim' organised the first Italian-Slovenian Conference on Hypnosis in Psychotherapy and Rehabilitation.

In 1984 the 'Bernheim' Institute organised, in collaboration with the aforementioned European Society of Hypnosis, the Military Healthcare body and the Italian Medical Association for the Study of Hypnosis (A.M.I.S.I.), the 3rd European Congress of Hypnosis, in Abano Terme (Padua). The Chairman was the President of the Institute, Guantieri, and it was sponsored by the International Society of Hypnosis, the Italian Health and Public Education Ministries and the University of Padua. 27 countries from four continents participated; 78 contributions were presented, of which 19 by Italian authors, 12 of whom were members of the 'Bernheim'.

From 1984 onwards, increasing numbers of conferences, conventions, congresses were organised across the world, with the constant active participation of the Institute, pertaining to various themes of a hypnology that was becoming more widely recognized, not only as a subject of study, but increasingly as a means of clinical and pedagogical-training. Parallel to this, the organisation was increasingly consolidated, research on hypnology topics was assiduously supported and hypnologists were systematically trained with courses, initially on a two-year then on a four-year basis. Such training programs were officially recognized in 2002, thanks to the executives who succeeded Guantieri, who died in 1994, at the 'H.Bernheim' School of Psychosynthetic Psychotherapy and Ericksonian Hypnosis (S.P.P.I.E.). The school gained the recognition of the Ministries of Education, University and Research, with a decree on 30th May, 2002, officially enabling the 'Bernheim' to train psychotherapists.

It all began in the 1960s: Guantieri's the horizons of knowledge were global from the start, thanks to the many international hypnosis institutes where he met and could interact with renowned hypnologists from all over the world, such as his Japanese friend Gosaku Naruse from Kyushu University in Fukuoka, his Australian university colleagues Graham Burrow, Lia Kapelis and Keith Page, his South Africans colleagues from the University of Pretoria, David Fourte and Stanley Lifschitz, or from Israel, Moris Kleihauz and Barbara Beran from the Community Mental Health Centres in Jaffa and Tel Aviv.

In the United States, he worked with many hypnological scholars and researchers, in particular with Milton Vessel Kline[36] and his dear friend Erika Fromm, from the University of Chicago, with whom he collaborated and published in the International Journal of Clinical and Experimental Hypnosis. He questioned the concept of Freudian analysis with her, seeing hypnosis as a more brief, effective and affordable than psychoanalysis.

---

[36] Milton Vessel Kline was a prestigious hypnologist at the Institute for Research in Hypnosis and Psychotherapy in New York; he became famous in particular for his book 'The Roots of Modern Hypnosis,' which he wrote at the 1st International Congress on Hypnosis in New York in 1961 and which was published by Bloomington's publisher, Xlibris Corp, in Indiana. The Vice President of the New York organization at the time was H.W. Marcus, a world-renowned hypnologist who has shown how hypnosis could offer valuable help in the field of dentistry. It was he who wrote the preface of the first hypnology textbook by Guzzieri in 1968: 'Medical Hypnosis: An introduction to the study and practice of hypnosis in medicine', published by the journal Opera medica, edited by Wasserman S.p.A., Milan, 1968.

Other American colleagues (and great friends) were Martin Orne from the University of Pennsylvania and Ernest Hilgard from Stanford University in California (particularly famous for his research on hypnosis. In Italy he is known mainly for the diffusion of his institutional textbook: 'Psychology – An Introductory Course', Giunti, Florence, 1971).

In 1988, both Guantieri and Hilgard wrote two different introductory notes to the third textbook release of David Waxman's (1917-1994) 'Hartland's Medical and Dental Hypnosis', Baillière Tindall, London[37]. In this book Waxman takes up important works by John Hartland, dentist and hypnologist, author of a popular manual for medical and psychiatric hypnotherapy, also known in Italy, where he published the compendium 'Hypnosis in medicine and dentistry', with Monduzzi in Bologna, in 1977.[38] For the sake of completeness, it should be noted that in the previous edition of Waxman's work there is an introduction by Milton Erickson, in which he cites a professional guide capable of inspiring, through hypnosis, a medical art, then verifiable in its effectiveness, by means of a return to the text, in order to further learn what the medical reader needs; this, to improve the relationship with his patient, to better understand their personal values and promoting greater conditions of well-being and development in them.

Hilgard, in his prologue, emphasised the hypnotherapeutic aspect of Waxman's hypnosis as an ample means of use in short psychotherapies, across all theoretical areas of psychology, becoming, in the case of psychoanalysis, a hypnoanalysis capable of accelerating traditional psychotherapy, often undermined by its own limitation of being infinite.

Guantieri, nonetheless, noted in the text he was analyzing a whole series of convergences, that he felt between the author he was presenting and his own hypnological cornerstones.

Therefore, he underlined the idea of:

1) A scientific hypnology enriched with an openness to the comprehension of one's own limits, to research, to creativity that can make it grow, to art that vivifies it, to technique, which cannot be an exclusive space, otherwise reducing hypnology to a technicality, but which must also be recognized and respected;

2) A hypnology that is in itself therapeutic, if known and used with ethical seriousness by adequately trained professionals (in this sense Waxman, with his considerations, is suggested as a guide for fellow readers);

3) The humanism of that text, concretely expressed in its holistic consideration of the human being;

4) A multidisciplinary vision of hypnotic phenomena;

---

[37] Waxman D., Hartland's Medical and Dental Hypnosis, Baillière Tindall, London, 1988.
[38] Hartland J., Ipnosi in medicina e odontoiatria, Monduzzi, Bologna, 1977.

5) A psychosomatic consideration of the given patient's troubles;

6) A psychodynamic and interpretative orientation, in the case of psychotherapeutic hypnology;

7) The necessary sensibility of the psychotherapist towards the person suffering, characterised by feelings of acceptance, welcoming, understanding and empathy, so that between the two a deep, intimate, particular relationship can take place, that is to say that special, hypnotic rapport which brings unity, both in the help being offered and in the exchange of affection and humanity.

In addition to the aforementioned foreign authors, on the basis of our inevitably incomplete memories, we recall various doctors, neurologists, psychiatrists, psychologists, researchers, professors, and especially hypnologists.

In America, Guantieri met and engaged with many other characters in the world of international hypnology. We remember: Jeffrey Zeig, of The Milton Erickson Foundations in Phoenix, Arizona; the Californians David Dargileleth, Alan Jensen, a doctor in Malibu, Ray London and Antonio Madrid, from the University of San Francisco in California; Laers-Eric Unesthal, a doctor in Iowa Dale Harding. And again: Paul Biederman, professor at the University of Maryland in Baltimore, Maryland; Denis Pelon of the city of East Lansing in Michigan; the New Yorkers Marianne Anderson, David Frauman, James Holland, Dario La Rocca and Paul Sacerdote; again, John Casey, Siman Chiasson, Meir Gross, David Frauman, Stevan Jay Lynn, Michael McKee, Michael Nash, Suzanne Penzien, Judit Rhue, Jack Steele, Moshe Torem of Ohio, Frank Schmidt from Somerset, New Jersey, Kay Thompson from Pennsylvania, the Texans Harold Crasilnek, president of the American Society of Clinical Hypnosis and professor at the University of Dallas, and Scott Grover, physician at The Glover Clinic in Houston.

In the United States, Guantieri also came to know and have dealings with Milton Erickson (1901-1980).

His American experiences also included encounters with Canadians Alan Banak from Toronto, Germain Lavoie from the Louis Lafontaine Hospital and the Université de Montréal, who was President of the International Society of Hypnosis in the 1980s, Jaan-Roch Laurence, from the University of Waterloo, Neill Malcolm, from the Leduc Hospital of Alberta, Campbell Perry from the Université de Montréal, Douglas Ringrose, from Edmonton, Alberta, and Thomas Verny.

In Europe, Guantieri had scientific relationships with the Austrians Gerhard Barolin from the Neurological Department and Psychiatric Department of the Hospital in Rankweil and Henrich Walnoffer from the University of Innsbruck, with the Czech Stanislav Kratochvic from the Psychiatric Hospital in Kroměříž

(Czech Republic), with his great friend Walter Bongartz from the University of Constance and with other German scientists and researchers such as Vladimir Gheorghiu, from the University of Giessen, Frank Schmidt, from the University of Maryland, from Heidelberg and Zbgniew Pleszwski, from the University of Hamburg and with many great names in the world of hypnology in England, where Guantieri was Fellow of the Royal Society of Medicine in London and member of the Board of Directors of numerous national and international scientific associations. In addition to the aforementioned David Waxman from the Central Middlesex Hospital in London, he met and collaborated with Peter Blythe from the Institute for Neuro-Physiological Psychology in Chester, DW Ebrahim, from Coventry, Brian Fellows from the University of Portsmouth, Geoffrey Graham from Newcastle upon Tyne, Frans Lohman from Colchster, John Mackett from the Isle of Wight, Prem Misra from Gartloch Hospital and the University of Glasgow, Howard Samuels from Leeds. Later, Guantieri professionally interacted with Dutch colleagues R. Van Dyck and C.A.L. Hoogduin, with Jerzy Aleksandrowicz, Jerzy Siuta and Janina Zmeltyma from Poland, at the Psychotherapy Research Unit Department of Psychiatry and of the Academy of Medicine and Centre for Treatment of Neurosis, in Krakow, Stefan Baron, doctor in Parodnia, Maria Pachalska, from the hospital in Krakow, Kazimierz Szatanik, doctor of Parodnia, Zbgniew Pleszwski, from the Institute of Psychology at the University of Poznań, with his friend Marjan Paintar from the Obstetrics and Gynecology Hospital in Kranj and professor of the Medical Faculty at the University of Ljubljana, with the Swede Bengt-Göran Fasth, from the University of Gothenburg, with colleague and great friend Basil Finer, from the Universities of Uppsala and Samariterhwmmet, Lars-Eric Unestähl, from the University of Orebrö, C. Martinsoon and Per-Olof Wikström, a dentist from Stockholm (with whom Guantieri shared a deep brotherly bond) and with Hungarian doctors and university professors such as Anna Balázs, Éva Bányai, Gyula Biro, Istvan Boncz, Laslo Csokay, B ela Daubner, L. Fazekas, Judit Frater, Zita Kaszab, Iren Kovács, K. Gaal, Istvan Meszaros, P. Migaly, Maria Molnar, Alain Poltz, K. Taganyi, Jànos Tiba, A. Zseni and Csilla Zsombor.

This immense global human and scientific interaction culminated in 1993, at the height of his prominence. During the 6th International Congress of the ISH in Vienna, Austria, Gualtiero Guantieri was awarded, by the European Society of Hypnosis during the presidency of Eva Banyai, the highest international recognition in the field of clinical hypnosis at that time: the *"Franz Anton Mesmer Gold Award for Leadership and Achievements in the field of Hypnosis"*

Publications

With around 100 publications to his name — of which the bibliographical references are, to a large extent, reported in the bibliography – Guantieri made and disseminated concrete and remarkable hypnological work of epistemological and scientific reflection, research and experimentation, meetings, conferences, conventions and international congresses, and also simply informative and cultural meetings, didactic activities and the training of hypnologists, which represents a milestone in the history of the study of hypnosis and its diffusion as a means of clinical and pedagogical use.

The first scientific articles he published, in fact, dealt with recurring themes of traditional medicine, such as, for example, the treatment of hypertension, or the treatment of diabetes. However, his arguments were already marked by courageous and innovative ideas (such as the use of cutting-edge medication) and always of medical reform.

There were then about ten years of a sort of scientific silence, in the sense that Guantieri did not publish any work. In retrospect, it was most likely a time of meditation for him, necessary in order to official start his psychosomatist and hypnological theories, directed towards the medical and psychological world of therapies and the care of suffering adults or healthy subjects of a developmental age. Subsequent to that phase, in 1963, Guantieri published his psychosomatist and psychodynamic investigations and considerations about the origin and influence of emotions in physical suffering, with respect to the importance that the familial context has in the onset of pathogenic issues, especially in childhood and then in relation to hypnosis.

Hypnosis, recognized and deemed worthy of being the subject of study and a means of clinical and pedagogical use, is first investigated, considering the development of previous studies, both historically and anthropologically, and gradually observing it in its phenomenology, as a state and as interpersonal relationship; with particular attention and importance attributed to this latter dimension.

Hypnosis then, observed in its most in-depth levels, is examined in its expressions and in its effects, then more throughly investigated in its nature and interpreted from a multidisciplinary, neurophysiological, socio-psychological, dynamic, psychological and psychoanalytic point of view. and again about the means and modalities of its induction.

Guantieri then considers its use as a means of studying the personality, of experimental or clinical investigation, as a therapeutic tool that can be used in somatic and psychosomatic disorders, from a psychotherapeutic perspective and in practical applications in certain branches of medicine, such as obstetrics, dentistry and surgery.

He then, as a master hypnologist – also dealing with the didactics of teaching the discipline, that is the best way of teaching – dedicates extreme scrupulous, pedagogical, attention, with great sensitivity based on a holistic vision of the person, to the formation of the hypnologist and writes about the human qualities that this person must possess, warning them of the risks they face in using a tool that is both powerful and delicate, that they must first of all get to know personally, gaining direct experience of it.

All this while never forgetting the need and the will to define – or at least to contribute in this sense – what the epistemological foundations of a science that was increasingly establishing itself were: hypnology. He succeeded in offering a pioneering, scientifically relevant and absolutely original personal contribution to it. Of all Guantieri's writings, his masterpiece was undoubtedly the book that he conceived precisely for the training of hypnologists: 'Hypnosis, as an object of study and a means of use in medicine', from 1973, and the central reference of this work.

9. Old age and death

After his 60s, and in conjunction with his wife's incurable illness, Guantieri's state of mind took a downward turn: from levels of brilliance, good humor and sympathy, he became more reserved, introverted and sad, especially in the family.
According to his son Massimo, he over-processed the dynamics of his patients. It almost seemed that, by taking on others' torments, he absorbed them directly himself, psychically loading himself with a painful burden that was increasingly heavy and more difficult to bear.
More generally, he experienced frustration with regards to a world that he considered closed to authentic knowledge, especially in relation to such challenging and delicate issues as hypnosis.
Beyond the hypnological specific, the current human consortium seemed to him refractory or at least slow in applying itself to the study and understanding of and commitment to better human evolution.
He stated that none of us are willing, or at least we are slow, to commit ourselves to a better world, so changing it would be unlikely.
  He also considered how partisan, corporate, trade, medical and pharmaceutical lobbying interests were imposing obstacles to modernity, technological development, growth, and, above all, the prosperity of all mankind.
Intellect inevitably produces rationalizations such as those that elaborate subjective descriptions of man and mankind, however the consequences of these are, essentially, moods. And the consequences – often mysterious – take a toll on one's relationships, especially familial ones.

The death of his wife in 1992 was a truly shocking event for Guantieri. He went through particularly painful grief, as if he had lost part of himself, as if he had suffered an unbearable mutilation.

His father also died the following year, while his mother died earlier in 1971. Those events brought him pain and discouragement. He fell ill, although he still gained important satisfaction from life, such as the recognition and delivery of the most esteemed hypnological prize, the 'Franz Anton Mesmer Award for Leadership and Achievements in the field of Hypnosis', awarded to him in 1993 by the European Society of Hypnosis, and the recognition, also in 1993, of hypnosis as a clinical tool, officially included in the Italian Handbook of Diagnostics and Medical Therapy.

But his days on this earth were numbered yet, approaching the end of his human adventure, he was still able to practically testify to his own understanding of hypnosis. His son Massimo says that his father "went into a hepatic coma about 40 days before he passed away. In that state, however, he had unexpected and lucid awakenings, as if nothing had happened. Most remarkably, he was practically pain-free. The primary doctor who treated him at the hospital told me that the only plausible reason must be that my father induced a state of self-hypnosis capable of attenuating, to the point of almost eliminating, all his physical suffering."

Gualtiero Guantieri died, smiling on December 20th 1994, .

The news agency ADN Kronos reported his death as follows: "Guantieri, a doctor and psychotherapist, listed by the International Society of Hipnosis (I.S.H. – based in Bewyn, Pennsylvania), was one of the leading international experts in Clinical Hypnosis. He passed away at the age of 67 in Verona. Born in 1927, he graduated in medicine in 1951, and after a decade spent as an internist, Guantieri began his role as a researcher in psychosomatic medicine and clinical hypnosis, in 1963. He was professor of General and Developmental Psychopathology and of Psychiatry at the Universities of Padua and Verona from 1960-1969. In 1965, he founded the 'H. Bernheim' Italian Centre for Clinical Hypnosis and Psychosomatic Medicine". [39]

Gualtiero Guantieri, profound thinker, selectively eclectic scientist, capable of an acute and broad outlook, a great teacher [40], left the legacy of his hypnology to the

---

[39] http://www1.adnkronos.com/Archivio/AdnAgenzia/1994/12/21/Cronaca/IPNOSI-CLINICA-DECEDUTO-A-VERONA-GUALTIERO-GUANTIERI_132600.php

[40] We have had the opportunity to define Guantieri as a *"Benevolent Shaman"* (Malesani P.G., *Guantieri: Uno sciamano benefico?* In *Proceedings of the 20th Congress, Anxiety in the clinic and in today's society*, of the Italian Society of Psychosomatic Medicine, Verona, 2005, pp. 327-343). How can we understand the shamanic idea associated, metaphorically, with his name? Shamanism belongs to a higher, transcendent and universal reality [See Giuliano Boccali, Perhaps the shaman has something to tell us, Sunday supplement of Il Sole 24 Ore of 21 March 2021. For further information, also consider: Stefano Beggiora, (Edited by), *The shamanic cosmos. Indigenous Ontologies between Asia and the Americas, S.T.R.A.D.E. Series, Spirituality and Religious Traditions: Approaches, Disciplines, Ethnography*, Franco Angeli, Milan, 1919]. Are there obstacles, then, for a scientist to simultaneously be a shaman? If he is able to exercise a spiritualization of his surrounding world, if this man believes in a reciprocal and all-encompassing connection between nature and man, he already has good shamanic prerequisites.

world, an original, unmistakable, precious scientific paradigm.
The continuous evolution of knowledge will, most likely, only determine further confirmations and insights.

The shamanic ontology indicates in its essence the overcoming of the division between the knowing object and the known object, because it considers them intrinsically and inextricably linked, so that the first can only make an immersion inside the other to meet them closely, living it in themselves (the example of the knowledge of hypnosis, which occurs through the trance, fits perfectly!). Here then – at certain levels of depth – the shaman becomes a man capable of radical self-upheavals that deeply involve his body and mind and make him an exegete, a monk (even a layman), custodian of the authentic knowledge of his community, guardian of mythologies and of beliefs, signifiers and meanings and metaphors, a charismatic, authoritative and esoteric guide dedicated to initiates who are in search of themselves. In this capacity, the shaman falls into a self-induced state of modification of his ordinary consciousness, in a daring and sometimes risky condition, in order to penetrate a subtle, immaterial world where, by allowing his ordinary self to die, he transforms himself into something wider, identifying himself with a cosmic whole which makes him witty and insightful and therefore even more present in the state of initiation. And he becomes capable of knowing all sorts of negativity and malaise, and of proposing – similarly to what belongs to his own personal experience – the dismembering and recomposing of the personalities of his clients. A bit like what happens in the myth of Dionysus: the metamorphosis that occurs through the destruction of the unity of the multiple and then returns to the unity itself and which allows one to dominate the secrets of the energies that move the universe. Furthermore, the shaman, once transfigured, is able to act as an oracle because the strength and knowledge that he acquires with his abilities allow him to interpret for the cohort around him, the past, the present and the future, and to exercise skills as a life teacher, healer and therapist.

CHAPTER 2

The 'H. Bernheim' Institute of Clinical Hypnosis and Psychotherapy[41]

The history, evolution, identity, scientific and educational characterisation of the 'Bernheim' Institute of Hypnology began in the 1960s. In Italy "there were times of an official science that did not allow much space for the techniques of hypnotic psychotherapy, considered to be on the verge of moral sanctions", wrote Gastone Benatti.

In that climate – it was the year 1965 – the 'H. Bernheim' was established. It was initially a cultural and scientific circle made up of Gualtiero Guantieri, Bruno Caldironi, Giuseppe Castagna, Dino Dall'Oglio, Anna Maria Oddone and Nazario Sauro.

This first association grew rapidly, until it assumed formal legal status in 1968, signed by the first founders in 1965, who were joined by Gastone Bennati, Angelico Brugnoli, Walter De Stavola, Werther Ferioli, Jacopo Irone, Pietro Parietti and Domenico Tinti.

Gualtiero Guantieri was named as President, a role he held until his death. He was succeeded, from 1994 onwards, by Pier Andrea Gambacciani, Giuliano Guerra, Michele Modenese, Carlo Piazza, Vittorio Grecchi, Serena Rosson and, since 2017, Sebastiano Filippozzi.

As long as Guantieri was alive, the 'Bernheim' Institute saw continuous growth, in terms of the number of students and graduates of hypnology, as well as study and research activities carried out, systematic participation in national and international conferences and congresses on hypnology, and publications related to the institutionally designated discipline.

---

[41] An important contribution to the historical reconstruction of the 'Bernheim' Institute and its scientific accomplishments was made by Carlo Piazza.

From its foundation onwards, in addition to the people already mentioned, men and women from all over the world joined the 'Bernheim' organization, whether directly or indirectly: scientists, university rectors and professors, hospital superiors, directors of scientific institutes, doctors, psychiatrists, neurologists, dentists, psychotherapists, psychologists, but also military officers of the medical regiments of the Italian army, writers, journalists, curators of cultural events and of course secretarial staff.[42]

There was no lack of institutional sponsorship from the Ministries of Health and Public Education, the Veneto Region, the Municipality of Verona, the ULSS 20 (now ULSS 9, Scaligera), the CONI of Verona, the Universities of Padua and Verona, the International Society of Hypnosis and the Italian Society of Psychosomatic Medicine; there were also sponsors, mainly publishers, airlines, pharmaceutical companies and banks.

The 'Bernheim' Institute was and is a community melting pot of scientific and human passion, of many exciting moments, of fruitful and synergistic

---

[42] The following is a list (only of those whose personal or documentary memory is found, to which are added, without repeating them, all the names cited in § 8/a: *International relations,* in Chapter 1, relating to the biographical notes of Guantieri), although inevitably partial and indistinct: Paolo Agnello, Fausto Agresta, Emanuela Alquati Pasoli, Giuseppe Amari, Vittorino Andreoli, Andrea Angelozzi, Lucio Antonello, M. Arena, Chalmers Armstrong, Eugenio Arrigucci, Vincenzo Azzini, S. Baldi, Antonio Balestrieri, Paolo Ballaben, M. Baraccano, Stefano Baratta, Pietro Barba, C. Barbieri, Margherita Barone, Alberto Bartoloni, G. Belussi, Carlo Bernini, G. Bertolazzi, E. Bianchin, F. Bilone, Antonio Bogoni, Emanuela Boldrin, P. Bonfante, Cesare Boni, Silvia Bonizzi, Alberta Bottoli, Donato Bragantini, Maria Paola Brugnoli, Angelo Brusco, Giuseppe Bulgarini, Lorenzo Burti, Renato Butturini, Rocco Cacciacarne, Bruno Caldironi, Paolo Caliari, Giorgio Campanella, Rino Capitanata, Clara Carletti, Giancarlo Carli, Mirko Carollo, Consuelo Candida Casula, Donatella Cavana, Giovanni Cesa Bianchi, Marcello Cesa Bianchi, F. Champignoux, Luciana Cherubini, Giuseppe Chiaroni, E. Chiavegatti, Franco Chierego, Lino Chinaglia, F. Cipressi, Luciana Colognato, F. Consigliere, Cristina Coppa, M.G. Crisci, Giuseppe Crosa, Guido Cucciniello, Raffaella Dalla Valle, L. Dal Santo, Giovanni De Bartolomeis, Massimo De Battisti, Luciano De Benedetti, Giuseppe De Benedittis, Costante Degan, Roberto De Giovanni, E. Del Castello, Paolo De Lutti, Giorgio De Sandre, Romano Di Donato, Giuseppe Disertori, P. Donadi, Giorgio Donati, V. Erculiani, A. Ermentini, Valentino Facchini, E. Faretta, Silvano Fayenz, Fabio Ferrari, G. Finco, Pier Luigi Forghieri, Giulia Fraccaroli, C. Frogo, Lilla Galassi, E. Galdiolo, Enrico Galeotto, E. Galili, Osvaldo Galvano, G. Garofalo, Daniele Gasparini, A. Genovese, Elisabetta Gesmundo, A. Giannelli, G. Giomaccioni, Giancarlo Gobbi, Francesca Gocci, Franco Granone, Francesca Guantieri, Massimo Guantieri, Francesco Guidolin, Guglielmo Gullotta, Jan Peter Hallmark, Daniel Handel, Giuseppe Hinegk, J.G. Höyersten, Stefano Ischia, Marco Janeselli, Jonia Lacerda Felicio, Sergio Lafisca, A. Lanari, Antonio Maria Lapenta, Gabriele La Porta, Denisa Legac, A. Ligabue, G. Savino Lisanti, Sebastiano Livoti, F. Locatelli, R. Lodetti, M. Lora, Camillo Loriedo, Umberto Lucchese, Maurizio Lupardini, Aldo Luzzani, R. Maffezzoli, Roberto Magarotto, Pier Giorgio Malesani, Giorgio Manzini, Massimilla Manzini, Mario Marigo, Giovanni Marini, Daniela Martinelli, Giulio Martinelli, Elvio Melorio, Giambattista Melotto, Vittorio Meneghini, Angelo Mercurio, Pandit Shri Kanta Prashad Misra, Pandit Vishal Misra, Leonardo Mometti, C. Montanari, Mario Montanari, Giampiero Mosconi, Willy Murgolo, Piergiorgio Muzi, Cecilia Natarella, Alessandro Norsa, Giancarlo Odini, Anna Maria Oddone, Alberto Oliverio, Alberto Panerai, Jacopo Panozzo, Marco Parolini Shivchandra, Alberto Pasetto, Mario Passerelli, Ambrogio Pennati, A. Perini, G. Pescetto, Eugenio Piana, Michele Plescia, E. Polati, Sergio Poletti, Metè Poscio, Maurizio Pozzani, Ugo Pozzi, Loris Premuda, Attilio Randone, R. Ranieri, Elisabetta Razzaboni, Giuseppe Regaldo, Paolo Remondini, Laura Rigotti, M. Ringressi, C. Robazza, C.A. Robotti, Barbara Romani, Pierluigi (Piero) Roncaroli, Ignazio Rubino, Luciana Salerno, Mario Santini, Paolo Santonastaso, G. Sarao, Nicoletta Sartori, Bruno Sartoris, Gabriele Sboarina, Antonio Scanagatta, Corrado Scatolin, G. Schilirò, Alberto Schön, Thomas Schneider, F. Simonelli, Grazia Sinigaglia, V.A. Sironi, E. Sitta, A. Sodaro, Gianluca Solla, Massimo Somma, Franco Tagliaro, Federica Tagliati, Giovanni Tazioli, B. Hrayr Terzian, Mario Thanavaro, Paolo Tito, Ilaria Toso, M. Trabucchi, Wilma Trasarti Sponti, E. Vallero, Sergio Vannoni, Olga Venturini, Silvio Venuti, A. Verri, Flaviano Vighi, Marco Villamira, Rolando Weilbacher, Lea Zanotti, Waideh Zeighaminia, Loredana Zenoni.

confrontations, but also of detrimental tensions and clashes, though humanly comprehensible, because self-centredness and competition belong to man, as well as ambition, conceit and envy. Certainly the loss of its founding teacher made the Institute an orphan: weak, fragile, uncertain and even a little forgetful. However, its past, before those difficult moments, was bright, and if the present is tiring, it has no lack of founding pillars that make it solid, rich in a heritage that bears the name of its creator: Guantierian Hypnology.

Loris Premuda – one of the early members – was able to describe the ensemble, considered with some prejudice to be a bit deviant and transgressive, as a "cooperative of ardent and willing doctors who gathered in meetings that brought to mind [...] the Carboneria". Guantieri himself, with regard to the origins of the Centre, recalled how it was housed, in the early stages of its existence, at the Museum of Natural Sciences in Verona, demonstrating – he argued – mistrust among official medical and psychological circles in accepting the idea of clinical hypnosis. According to him, in that way, hypnosis in Verona was metaphorically positioned as the heritage of a "Homo Hypnologicus", at an initial stage of a science mistakenly considered to be still too steeped in magic and pre-scientific elements.

The subsequent "evolutionary link" – the author reports –was symbolically and concretely implemented with the Centre's arrival at the headquarters of the Order of Medical Doctors and then with its reception at the University of Verona, leading "up to the fundamental passage" that was, in relation to the training of hypnologists, to recognize "the need to enter into individual group dynamics through residential courses".

More than half a century has passed since then: the Centre, acquiring knowledge and experience, expanded its membership and, in 1968, became the 'H. Bernheim' Italian Institute of Clinical Hypnosis and Psychotherapy.[43]

It was increasingly characterised by original scientific specificity and was met with progressive national and international consensus in ever-widening academic and medical circles.

The cultural hypnological work of the Institute, through research and training commitment, has been widely diffused through its "Basic Preparatory Course", "Advanced Clinical Hypnosis Course", and specialisation courses (Masters) in Hypnosis, reserved for psychotherapists, doctors, psychologists, dentists, as well as promoting (in 2002) the establishment of the School of Psychosynthetic Psychotherapy and Ericksonian Hypnosis, also called 'Bernheim' – independent from the Institute.

---

[43] It should be noted that in Gualtiero Guantieri's time, the Institute was a member of the International Society of Hypnosis (I.S.H.), of the European Society of Hypnosis (E.S.H.) and collaborated scientifically with the Institute for Research in Hypnosis, Chartered by the Board of Regens of the State University of New York.

A review summarising the Institute's activities in the period 1965-1992 was published by the Newsletter magazine, (Published by the Institute itself), in Year VI, n. 1-2, September 1993, as seen below:

Year 1965

November: Foundation of the 'H. Bernheim' Clinical Hypnosis Study Centre in Verona, recognition by the Institute for Research on Hypnosis and Psychotherapy in New York, U.S.A., (Director: Dr. Kline M.V.).

Year 1966

February: Organization of the 1st Theoretical Practical Course of Hypnosis for doctors, at the Museum of Natural Sciences in Verona (Director: Professor Sandro Ruffo). The course was introduced by Professor Loris Premuda and conducted by G.Guantieri, in collaboration with Caldironi B., Castagna G. and Montanari M.

June: First conference organised by the Centre on Problems in Medical Hypnosis, Lazise del Garda (Verona).

September-December: Organization of the 2nd Theoretical Practical Course of Hypnosis for doctors, at the Museum of Natural Sciences in Verona.

October: Organization of the 2nd Conference on Problems in Medical Hypnosis, Lazise del Garda (Verona).

Year 1967

March-May: Organization of the 3rd Theoretical Practical Course of Hypnosis for doctors, at the Verona Medical Association (President: Professor Mecca M.).

June: Organization of the 3rd Conference on Problems in Medical Hypnosis, Lazise del Garda (Verona).

September: Participation in the International Psychosomatic Week, organised by the Italian Society of Psychosomatic Medicine (S.I.M.P.), under the auspices of the Catholic University of Rome.

September: Participation in the Symposium of the Italian Society of Obstetric Psychoprophylaxis, Rome.

September: Participation in the 1st National Congress of the Italian Society of Psychosomatic Medicine (S.I.M.P.), Rome.

September: Organization of the 4th Conference on from, with the participation of Kline M.V., of the Institute for Research on Hypnosis and Psychotherapy of New York and Sacerdote P., of Montefiore Hospital and Medical Centre, Albert Einstein of the College of Medicine in New York, U.S.A., Lazise del Garda (Verona).

September-November: Organization of the 4th Theoretical Practical Course of Hypnosis for doctors, at the University of Verona (Rector: Professor G.Barbieri).

Year 1968

March: Organization of the 5th Conference on Problems in Medical Hypnosis, at the Verona Medical Association.

March: Participation in the Swiss National Congress on Psychosomatic Medicine, Locarno (Switzerland).

April: Organization of the 6th Conference on Problems in Medical Hypnosis, at the Cignaroli Academy (Didactic Director: Professor Bittasi), Verona.

May: Hypnosis Lesson at the Italian Society of Psychosomatic Medicine (S.I.M.P.). Refresher Course in Psychosomatic Medicine, Rome.

May: Constitution at the Veronese Centre of the Italian Society of Psychosomatic Medicine (S.I.M.P.).

May-June: Implementation of conferences reserved for members on topics of particular scientific importance in Verona.

June: Organization of the 7th Conference on Problems in Medical Hypnosis, Lazise del Garda (Verona).

June: Participation in the 2nd Abruzzese meeting of the Italian Society of Psychosomatic Medicine (S.I.M.P.), Chieti.

June: Constitution of the Abruzzese branch of the Centre, based in Pescara (Coordinator: Dr. Di Donato R.).

September: Participation in the National Congress on Psychosynthesis, Rome.

October 1968-April 1969: Organization of the 5th Theoretical Practical Course in Hypnosis at the Order of Medical Doctors of Verona, for doctors (conferences, with practical demonstrations, for a total of 10 days).

Year 1969

January: Organization of the 8th Conference on Problems in Medical Hypnosis,, at the Cignaroli Academy (President of the Regency Council: Professor Vecchiato B.), Verona.

April: Contribution to the organization of the 2nd National Congress of the Italian Society of Psychosomatic Medicine (S.I.M.P.) in the context of which a Hypnosis Session in Psychosomatic Medicine, is held, Verona.

April: First participation of the 'Bernheim' Centre in a national television program (RAI newscast).

September: First collaboration with the Italian Medical Association for the Study of Hypnosis (A.M.I.S.I.), Vercelli.

October: Participation in the 2nd National Congress of the Italian Medical Association for the Study of Hypnosis (A.M.I.S.I.), Turin.

December 1969-June 1970: The usual Theoretical Practical Course is replaced by in-depth seminars (six days).

December: Medical Hypnology Meetings, reserved for doctors already enrolled in preparatory courses, at the Verona Medical Association.

Year 1970

March: 'Medicine of the imagination', participation in television show, TV 7.

March: The President of the Centre, G. Guantieri, is entrusted with a course of lessons in Psychosomatic Medicine at the School of Specialisation in Psychiatry at the University of Padua in Verona (Director: Professor Balestrieri A.). This position would be maintained until 1979.

April: Organization of the 9th Conference on Problems in Medical Hypnosis, with the participation of Jabush M., from the Institute for Research on Hypnosis and Psychotherapy in New York, U.S.A., at the Order of Medical Doctors, Verona.

May: Participation in the 10th International Congress on Hypnosis and Psychosomatic Medicine, Mainz, Germany.

May-June: Contribution to the 2nd Refresher Course in Psychosomatic Medicine, under the auspices of the Italian Society of Psychosomatic Medicine (S.I.M.P.) and the hospital institutes of Verona.

June: Participation in the National Congress of the Italian Society of Obstetric Psychoprophylaxis, Milan.

August: Participation in the 8th International Congress on Psychotherapy, Milan.

November 1970-January 1971: Organization of the Hypnosis and Frigidity Conference (two days), Verona.

Year 1971

May: Participation in the 3rd National Congress of the Italian Society of Psychosomatic Medicine (S.I.M.P.), Florence.

May: Organization of Refresher Course in Hypnology, under the auspices of the Institute for Research on Hypnosis and Psychotherapy of New York, at the Civil Hospital of Borgo Trento (Health Superintendent: Professor Rizzotti G.), Verona.

June: Organization of the Conference 'Meaning and Aims of the "Balint" groups' at the hospital institutes of Verona.

October 1971-March 1972: Organization of in-depth courses at the Medical Association, reserved for those who had already attended a Theoretical Practical Hypnosis course (divided into four meetings of two days each), Verona.

October: Organization of the 2nd edition of the Refresher Course in Hypnology (divided into two days: the first at the University of Verona, the second at the Verona Medical Association).

Year 1972

June: Organization of the Conference 'Psychological training of doctors today', in collaboration with the Italian Society of Psychosomatic Medicine (S.I.M.P.) and the Neurology Division of the Verona Civil Hospital (Head physician: Professor Montanari M.), Verona.

Year 1973

March: Organization of the Round Table 'Position and role of hypnosis in medicine', in collaboration with the Division of Neurology of the Civil Hospital in Arco (Head physician: Dr. Robotti C.A.), Arco (Trento).

May: Participation in the International Congress 'The other medicine', Sanremo (Imperia).

June: Participation in the 4th National Congress of the Italian Society of Psychosomatic Medicine (S.I.M.P.), Messina.

July: Participation in the 6th International Congress on Hypnosis and Psychosomatic Medicine, Uppsala, Sweden.

Year 1974

April: Appointment of members of the Centre as teachers of the Italian Society of Psychosomatic Medicine (S.I.M.P.) courses, by the S.I.M.P. and establishment of the Permanent Secretariat for S.I.M.P. at the 'Bernheim' Centre.

September: The 'Bernheim' becomes National Constituent Society of the International Society of Clinical and Experimental Hypnosis.

November: Organization of the Preparatory Course on Hypnosis, (two days), Verona.

Year 1975

February-November: Organization of Practical Hypnosis residential courses, with a psychodynamic orientation (divided into five meetings lasting two days each), Padenghe del Garda (Brescia). The Centre organises an educational model that will be followed for the following years, structured in:

a) Preparatory courses lasting two to three consecutive days;

b) In-depth technical and training seminars, of a practical nature, of a residential type, divided into six to eight meetings over a period of 16 months, lasting two days each. Those who have attended the Preparatory Course are admitted. In addition to graduates in Medicine and Surgery, graduates or specialists in Psychology are admitted. Undergraduates in these disciplines are admitted under particular conditions as auditors. The Practical Course in progress is extended until May 1976.

September: Participation in the International Psychosomatic Week as part of the 3rd International Congress of the International College of Psychosomatic Medicine, along with the organization of the Symposia 'Relaxation and Psychodynamics and Hypnosis', Rome.

September: Participation in the 6th National Congress of the Italian Medical Association for the Study of Hypnosis (A.M.I.S.I.).

September: Preparatory Hypnosis Course, Verona.

Year 1976

June: Participation in the 5th National Congress of the Italian Society of Psychosomatic Medicine (S.I.M.P.), Milan.

October: Organization of the Medical-psychological meeting 'The body and its experience in relaxation in psychotherapy', La Spezia.

October: The 1976-77 Practical Course continues.

Year 1977

January: Organization of the conference 'The nature of hypnosis in the light of communication theories', Hospital Institutes of Borgo Trento, Verona.

February: Preparatory Course in Hypnosis.

March: Organization of the Medical-Psychological meeting 'Neurodynamic bases of hypnosis, Hypotheses and perspectives', Prato.

April: Participation in the Sexuology course, organised by the Italian Society of Clinical Sexuology, Abano Terme (Padua).

October: Organization of the Psychosomatic and Psychotherapy conference, in collaboration with the Italian Society of Psychosomatic Medicine (S.I.M.P.) and the Hospital of Marostica, Marostica (Vicenza).

October: Participation in the 5th National Congress of the Italian Medical Association for the Study of Hypnosis (A.M.I.S.I.), Milan.

October: Preparatory Hypnosis course, at the Hospital Institutes of Borgo Trento, Verona, (Health Superintendent: Professor Scanagatta A.), Verona.

October: Beginning of the practical course, 1977-1978.

Year 1978

January: Constitution of the Lombardy branch of the 'Bernheim' Centre, based in Milan, (Coordinator: Dr. P. Parietti).

March: Co-sponsorship of the Pan-American Congress of Hypnology and Psychosomatic Medicine, Rio de Janeiro, Brazil.

June: Participation in the 1st European Congress of Hypnosis in Psychotherapy and Psychosomatic Medicine, Malmö, Sweden.

June: Participation in a television program (RAI2, Access Programs.)

November: Participation in the 1st Italian seminar on Hypnotic Phenomena, organised by the Italian Medical Association for the Study of Hypnosis (A.M.I.S.I.), Rome.

November: The preparatory course, implemented as usual, at the end of the year, is extended to three days, as a result of the expansion of the didactic material.

November: Practical course 1978-79. The 'Bernheim' Centre is also opened up to psychologists, in addition to doctors, provided that they have the necessary requisites. The issue of differentiating courses in relation to the various specialties and needs is raised.

Year 1979

May: Organization of the International Symposium 'Hypnosis and Sexuology', in collaboration with the Italian Society of Clinical Sexuology and the International Centre for the training of The European Doctor, Champion of Italy (Como).

May: Preparatory course in Hypnosis.

May: Practical course 1979-80.

Year 1980

May: Participation in the 2nd European Congress of Hypnosis in Psychotherapy and Psychosomatic Medicine, Dubrovnik, Croatia. On this occasion, the President of the 'Bernheim' Centre, G. Guantieri, is appointed President of the European Hypnosis Association, alongside P. . Roncaroli as Secretary.

June: The Abruzzese branch organises an Extraordinary Preparatory Course in Clinical Hypnosis, Vasto (Chieti).

July: Organization of the International Conference 'Stress Research and Clinical Applications in Psychosomatic Medicine' and of a Clinical Hypnosis Workshop, conducted by G. Guantieri, B. Finer, MV Kline ,LE Unestahl, in collaboration with the International Graduate University of Lugano, Lugano, Switzerland.

October: Organization of the round table 'Psychological needs in heart disease rehabilitation', in collaboration with the Body Psychotherapy Study Centre, Brescia.

November: Establishment of the Piedmontese branch of the 'Bernheim' Centre based in Novara (Coordinator: Dr. P. Roncaroli).

November: Establishment of the Triveneta branch of the 'Bernheim' Centre, based in Venice (Coordinator: Dr. A. Gambacciani).

November: Organization of an Autogenic Training Course, conducted by W. Ferioli, Ferrara.

Year 1981

April: Participation in the 8th National Congress of the Italian Society of Psychosomatic Medicine (S.I.M.P.), Venice.

May: Contribution to the organization of the conference 'The art of Milton H. Erickson', promoted by the Psychiatric Clinic of the University of Padua-Verona, in Verona.

June: Beginning of the collaboration with the Military Health body, Verona Military Hospital (General Director of Military Health: Lt. Gen. Med. Prof. E. Melorio), Head of Health Services and Director of Health of the RMNE, Maj. Gen. Med. Dr. P. Barba, Director of the Military Hospital of Verona: Col. Med. Dr. M. Plescia).

June: Autogenic Training Course in collaboration with the Italian Society of Psychosomatic Medicine (S.I.M.P.) and the Military Hospital of Verona, to be followed, in subsequent years, by seminars on clinical hypnosis and psychotherapy.

June: The president of the Centre, G. Guantieri, is commissioned for an annual lecture series on clinical hypnosis,, which he holds until 1984, at the School of Specialisation in Anaesthesiology and Intensive Care (Director: Prof. S. Ischia), of the University of Padua in Verona.

November: Preparatory course in Hypnosis in Verona.

November: Preparatory course in Hypnosis in Venice (organised by the 'Bernheim' Triveneta branch).

December: Preparatory course in Hypnosis in Novara (organised by the Piedmontese branch of the 'Bernheim' Institute).

December: Practical course 1981-82, Verona.

Year 1982

January: The Centre changes its name to the "H. Bernheim' Clinical Hypnosis and Psychotherapy Study Centre". The number of members of the Board of Directors increases from seven to nine.

August: Participation in the 9th International Congress of Hypnosis and Psychosomatic Medicine, Glasgow, Scotland.

October: Organization of the seminar 'Hypnosis in pain therapy', in collaboration with the School of Specialisation in Anaesthesiology and Intensive Care of the University of Padua-Verona, Verona.

November-December: Preparatory Hypnosis Courses in Venice and Verona.

November: Beginning of the practical course 1982-83.

November-December: Supervision courses are introduced.

November: Establishment of the Tuscany branch of the 'Bernheim' Centre, based in Florence (Coordinators: Prof. G. Campanella, Dr. M. Santini).

November: The symbol of the 'Bernheim' Centre is created by the sculptor Fulvio Cassan.

Year 1983

April: Organization of the Italian-Slovenian Symposium 'Hypnosis in psychotherapy and rehabilitation', in collaboration with the Slovenian Society of Clinical and Experimental Hypnosis, Porto Rose, Slovenia.

November-December: Preparatory Hypnosis courses in Venice and Verona.

November: Beginning of the practical course 1983-84.

November: A series of Guided Visualisation Seminars is introduced, led by B. Caldironi., for those who have completed the practical course.

Year 1984

May: Organization of the 3rd European Congress of Hypnosis in Psychotherapy and Psychosomatic Medicine, Abano Terme (Padua), with the European Society of Hypnosis in Psychotherapy and Psychosomatic Medicine, in collaboration with the Italian Medical Association for the Study of Hypnosis (AMISI) and Military Health body. The President of the 'Bernheim' Centre G. Guantieri is Chairman, scholars from 27 countries are enrolled in the congress, representing four continents, 78 works are presented, of which 19 are by Italian authors, 12 of whom are members of the 'Bernheim' Centre. Members of the Centre also include Chairmen of sessions (A. Gambacciani, P.L. Forghieri) and of workshops (B. Caldironi, A. Gambacciani, L. De Benedetti). 11 workshops are held on key themes. The Congress receives the patronage of the Ministry of Health, the Ministry of Education, the University of Padua, the International Society of Hypnosis and the Italian Society of Psychosomatic Medicine (S.I.M.P.).

May: The President of the 'Bernheim' Centre, G. Guanteri, is in charge of the official teaching of Psychosomatic Medicine and Clinical Hypnosis, in line with article 25 of the Presidential Decree 382/1980, in the new School of Specialisation in Pathophysiology and Pain Therapy at the University of Verona (Director: Prof. S. Ischia).

November-December: Preparatory Hypnosis courses in Verona and Venice.

November: Practical course 1984-85.

November: Guided Visualisation seminars.

November: A series of seminars on 'Personality Structures in Hypnotherapy' is introduced, conducted by B. Caldironi, reserved for those who have attended previous seminars.

Year 1985

During the year: Practical courses in Hypnosis 1984-1985, Course in Guided Visualisations (Conducted by B. Caldironi), Course in Personality Structures in Hypnotherapy (Conducted by B. Caldironi).

May: Participation in the 10th National Congress of the Italian Society of Psychosomatic Medicine (S.I.M.P.).

As part of the Congress, the organization of the Symposium 'Body Language in Hypnosis', on the occasion of the 20th year of the foundation of the 'Bernheim' Centre, Chieti-Pescara.

May: Organization of the National Conference (Verona, December 1985), 'Hypnosis in Institutions: its role and contribution', in collaboration with the Istituto Policattedra of Anaesthesiology and Intensive Care at the University of Verona, the North-Eastern Military Region Health Services Command, the Military Hospital of Verona; with the patronage of the Ministry of Health, the Ministry of Education, the University of Verona, the Veneto Region, the U.L.S.S. 20 of the Veneto Region, the European Society of Hypnosis in Psychotherapy and Psychosomatic Medicine, and the Italian Society of Psychosomatic Medicine (S.I.M.P.).

August: Participation in the 10th International Congress on Hypnosis and Psychosomatic Medicine, Toronto, Canada.

September: As a result of the evolution it had undergone, the Centre changes its name to: "'H. Bernheim' Italian Institute of Clinical Hypnosis and Psychotherapy, School of Research and Training".

October: Participation in the 13th International Congress on Psychotherapy, Opatija, Croatia.

October: Participation in the International Congress 'Hypnosis and Family Therapy', by the Italian Medical Association for the Study of Hypnosis (A.M.I.S.I.), organised in collaboration with the Catholic University of Rome and the Milton Erickson Foundation,.

December: Introductory hypnosis courses in Verona and Venice.

December: Participation in the 1st National Conference 'Hypnosis in Institutions', organised by the 'Bernheim' Institute in collaboration with the Instituto Policattedra of Anaesthesiology and Intensive Care at the University of Verona and the Military Health body, with the patronage of the Ministry of Public Education, the Ministry of Health, the University of Verona, the Veneto Region, ULSS n. 20 of Verona. The Congress is held in the Aula Magna of the University of Verona.

Year 1986

During the year: Practical Hypnosis courses 1985-1986, 'Personality Structures in Hypnotherapy' course (led by: B. Caldironi). The Ministries of Health, Public Education and the Veneto Region Health Department, U.L.S.S. n. 20 of Verona also grant patronage to the teaching activities of the 'Bernheim' Institute.

September: Participation in the first National Course of the Italian Association for Analytical Relaxation (ASS.I.R.A.), Pescara.

November: Participation in the 1st International Mind-Body Congress, Milan.

December: Preparatory hypnosis courses in Verona and Venice.

December: Practical courses 1986-87.

Year 1987

During the year: Practical courses in Hypnosis 1986-1987, the establishment of the first year of the advanced course (three residential seminars, each lasting one Friday-Saturday-Sunday, conducted by G. Guantieri, W. Ferioli, A. Gambacciani, P, Parietti, with the collaboration of ML Zenoni.

February: Participation with lecture and workshop in 'Rencontres Internationales' by the International Federation of Balint Groups, Ascona, Switzerland.

May: Organization of and participation in the Symposium 'From aggression to therapeutic communication in the hypnology field', as part of the 11th National Congress of the Italian Society of Psychosomatic Medicine (S.I.M.P.), Messina.

July: Participation in the 4th European Congress on Hypnosis in Psychotherapy and Psychosomatic Medicine, Oxford, England, with presentation of reports and organization and development of the workshop 'The Induction and Deepening of Hypnosis as a Psychotherapeutic Modality', (Conducted by: A. Angelozzi, P.L. Forghieri, G. Guantieri, P. Roncaroli).

November: Participation in the Round Table 'The lived body', as part of the 2nd International Mind-Body Conference, Milan.

December: Preparatory courses in hypnosis in Verona and Venice.

December: Practical courses 1987-88.

Year 1988

During the year: Practical courses in Hypnosis 1987-1988, Advanced Course (first year), establishment of the second year of the Advanced Course (three residential seminars each lasting one Friday-Saturday-Sunday, (Conducted by G .Guantieri, W. Ferioli, A.Gambacciani,   P. Parietti, with the collaboration of A. Angelozzi and L. De Benedetti), institution of the 1st National Course in Hypnotic Analgesics, sponsored by the Veneto Region's Department of Health, the U.L.S.S. 20 of Verona, the Instituto Policattedra of Anaesthesiology and Intensive Care of the Faculty of Medicine and Surgery of the University of Verona, the Italian Association for the Study of Pain and the Italian Society of Psychosomatic Medicine (S.I.M.P.) (two seminars lasting five days each).

January: Sponsorship of and participation in the National Congress for Research and Intervention in Sport Psychology, Verona.

April: The National Federation of the Orders of Doctors and Dentists grants patronage to the teaching activity of the 'Bernheim' Institute.

August: Participation in the 11th International Congress on Hypnosis and Psychosomatic Medicine, Leiden, Holland, in addition to papers presented with the organization of the workshop 'Relational Modes in Hypnotherapy', (Conducted by: A.Angelozzi, P.L. Forghieri, A. Gambacciani, G. Guarneri, P. Roncaroli).

Year 1989

During the year: Practical courses in Hypnosis, 1988-1989, and Course in Hypnotic Analgesics.

June: Participation in the 12th Congress of the Italian Society of Psychosomatic Medicine (S.I.M.P.), in Milan, focused on 'Psychosomatics 2000: Neuroscience and Psychotherapy to rediscover human value'. As part of the Congress, chaired by P. Parietti, a Round Table was held, 'From Relaxation to Hypnosis, organised by the 'H. Bernheim' Presidents: W. Ferioli and A. Gambacciani; participating as speakers, G. Benatti, R. Di Donato, W. Ferioli., G. Garofalo, G. Gocci, G.F. Gramaccioni, A. Lanari, U. Pozzi, and M.L. Zenoni. As part of the Round Table 'The brain and its self', P.G. Muzi and A. Angelozzi present a report.

October: Participation of G. Guantieri in the 6th National Conference of the Anthropos Study Centre, Verona.

November: 1st National Meeting 'Hypnosis in sports', promoted as part of the Introductory Course in Clinical Hypnosis at the 'Bernheim' Institute, in Verona, at the "Giorgio Marani" Medical Cultural Centre. The meeting is sponsored by the Veneto Region, the Verona Department of Sport, the C.O.N.I. Provincial, the ULSS 20 of Verona, the Italian Society of Psychology (Venetian branch), the Italian Society of Psychosomatic Medicine (S.I.M.P.), the Italian Association of Sports Psychology and the Institute of Sports Medicine in Verona. Participants: G. Benatti, P. Roncaroli, P. Castelli, F. Champignoux, G. Gramaccioni, A. Lanari and M. Modenese. Introduction to the work by G. Guantieri.

December: The publication of the 'Bernheim' Institute Newsletter begins. Editor-in-Chief: A. Angelozzi. 11 issues were published from 1988 to 1993.

December: The 1989-1990 academic year begins.

December: G. Guantieri holds conferences and lectures at the Specialisation Schools in Anaesthesiology and Intensive Care and Physiopathology and Pain Therapy of the University of Verona, respectively.

Year 1990

Practical courses in Hypnosis 1989-1990 continue throughout the year.

February: G. Guantieri and P. Parietti participate in the seminar 'Hypnosis today from a clinical point of view', promoted by the Italian Society of Psychosomatic Medicine (SIMP), Parma branch, with the patronage of the Order of Doctors and the Chair of Psychosomatics at the University of Parma.

April: G. Guantieri introduces and leads the Symposium 'Hypnosis in the psychological preparation of the athlete', as part of the 8th National Congress of the Italian Association of Sports Psychology, Senigallia (Ancona).

June: The 'Bernheim' Institute organises the conference 'Hypnosis in therapy' in Mestre (Venice) chaired by Prof. Harold B. Crasilneck, former President of the American Society of Clinical Hypnosis,.

August: Contribution to the organization of (G. Guantieri) and participation in the 5th European Congress on Hypnosis in Psychotherapy and Psychosomatic Medicine, in Costanza, Germany; reports presented by: G. Bulgarini, G. Campanella, L. De Benedetti, P.L. Forghieri, A. Gambacciani, G. Guantieri, G.F. Gramaccioni, A. Lanari, A. Pasetto, P. Roncaroli, L. Zanotti. Guantieri holds a conversation hour: 'The hypnotic approach to the psychosomatic patient'. In collaboration with Kratochvil, he organises and conducts the Symposium 'The training of therapist in the use of hypnosis'.

October: Organization of an international workshop in Verona with Basil Finer, 'The induction and deepening of hypnosis in pain therapy'.

October: The academic year 1990-1991 begins, G. Guantieri holds conferences and lectures at the Specialisation Schools in Anaesthesiology and Intensive Care and in Pathophysiology and Pain Therapy of the University of Verona, respectively.

Year 1991

During the year: Practical courses in Hypnosis 1990-1991.

G. Guantieri is appointed President of the Committee for the Implementation of Permanent Training in Clinical Hypnosis, at the European Society in Psychotherapy and Psychosomatic Medicine.

March: Participation in the 9th National Congress on Clinical and Experimental Hypnosis by the Italian Medical Association for the Study of Hypnosis (A.M.I.S.I.), 'Hypnosis Today: Evolution of the Phenomenon from Neurophysiology to Psychotherapy', Monastier (Treviso). The 'Bernheim' Institute participates, with talks by G. Guantieri, L. De Benedetti, P. Roncaroli, C. Robazza, G. Gocci, L. Zanotti., G. Benatti, A. Gambacciani. G. Guantieri moderates the Round Table 'Psychotherapy and Psychiatry in relation to Hypnosis'.

May: Participation in the Congress 'Pregnancy on the threshold of 2000: well-being and safety', Marina di Ravenna (Ravenna).

May: Participation in the 3rd National Congress of the Italian Society of Psychosomatic Medicine (S.I.M.P.), Bologna branch. As part of the 'Quality of Life' Congress, a Symposium is held, with the moderator G. Guantieri, attended by L De Benedetti, G. Campanella, P. Roncaroli, C. Robazza , G. Gocci, L. Zanotti L, G. Benatti, A. Gambacciani, P. Parietti, M.L. Zenoni. Participants in the Posters were M.L. Gramaccioni, A. Lanari, R. Lodetti, M. Modenese, M.L. Zenoni.

November: Day of Hypnological Studies 1991.

Year 1992

During the year: Practical courses in Hypnosis 1991-1992.

November: Day of Hypnological studies 1992.

Thus, many training activities have from time to time received, whether occasionally or permanently, patronage or recognition from the Ministries of Health and Public Education, the Veneto Region, the Chair of Anaesthesiology and Intensive Care of the University of Verona and the Northeast Italian Military Region Health Services Command.

Members of the Institute have published countless articles and scientific essays, some with national publishers, others appearing in their own journals (one of the first quarterly publications was "Newsletter", now replaced by "Acta Hypnologica",[44] which is currently available periodically in electronic format).

---

[44] 11 issues of the Newsletter magazine were published from 1988 to 1993: Year I, n. 1, December 1988, Year II, n. 1, June 1989, Year II, n. 2, October 1989, Year II, n. 3, December 1989, Year III, n.1, April 1990, Year III, n. 2-3, October-December 1990, Year IV, n. 1, April 1991, Year IV, n. 2-3, September 1991, Year V, n. 1, June 1992, Year V, n. 2-3, December 1992 and Year VI, n. 1-2, September 1993. 27 issues have been published in the review Acta Hypnologica, from 1997 to 2010: Year I, n. 1, January 1997, Year I, n. 2, May 1997, Year I, n. 3, September 1997, Year II, n. 1, January 1998, Year II, n. 2-3, May-September 1998, Year III, n. 1, January 1999, Year III, n. 2-3, May-September 1999, Year IV, n. 1, January 2000, Year IV, n. 2, May 2000, Year IV, n. 3, September 2000, Year V, n. 1-2, January-May 2001, Year V, n. 3, September 2001, Year VI, n. 1, January 2002, Year VI, n. 2-3, May-September 2002, Year VII, n. 1, January 2003, Year VII, n. 2-3, May-September 2003, Year VIII, n. 1-2, January-May 2004, Year VIII, n. 3, September 2004, Year IX, n. 1-2, January-May 2005, Year IX, n. 3, September 2005, Year X, n. 1, January 2006, Year X, n. 2-3, May-September 2006, Year XI, n. 1-2, January-May 2007, Year XI, n. 3, September 2007, Year XII, n. 1-2, January-May 2008, Year XII, n. 3, September 2008, Year XIII, n. 1, January 2009, Year XIII, n. 2, May 2009, Year XIII, n. 3, September 2009, Year XIV, n. 1, January 2010. Subsequently, some issues of Acta Hypnologica were published in electronic format on the website of the 'Bernheim' Institute. The complete lists of the studies published by the 'Bernheim' journals are reported in relevant sections of the BIBLIOGRAPHY. The availability of the works cited can be verified at the 'H. Bernheim' Italian Institute of Clinical Hypnosis and Psychotherapy, School of Research and Training of Verona, (www.istitutoipnosibernheim.com), or at the 'H. Bernheim' School of Psychosynthetic Psychotherapy and Ericksonian Hypnosis (S.P.P.I.E.) of Vicenza - Trento (www.bernheim.it).

The 'Bernheim' Institute, again, has organised many conferences, congresses, (of all of them, the most emblematic was the National Conference on 'The Role and Contribution of Hypnosis in Institutions' held in Verona in 1995, and the 3rd Congress on Hypnosis in Psychotherapy and Psychosomatic Medicine in 2003, held in Abano Terme, Padua), and has actively participated in many professional meetings, national and international, concerning hypnosis and psychosomatic medicine (among these, the 20th Congress of the Italian Institute of Psychosomatic Medicine Society – S.I.M.P. – in 2005, which was dedicated to Gualtiero Guantieri).

As discussed, it was Guantieri's idea to name the Institute 'Bernheim', in homage to Hippolyte Bernheim (1840-1919), French physician and neurologist, founder of a school in Nancy, active at the beginning of the twentieth century, and to whom the history of hypnology recognizes fundamental contributions in the development of hypnosis studies.

The French School contributed to the rollout of hypnology, in particular through the themes of suggestion and dynamic psychotherapy about the original theorisations with regard to that peculiar interpersonal relationship that, through hypnosis, is established between doctor and patient, capable of opening to the depth of a treatment that probes dimensions, (albeit somatic), filled with psychic and relational, preconscious and unconscious connotations of the suffering personality.

These themes, taken up, explored in depth and systematised, finally enriched with the dimensions of a philosophy of science which could no longer ignore it, ended up characterising the hypnological paradigm of Gualtiero Guantieri and the 'Bernheim' Institute.

Thus, over the years, a scientific institution unmistakably delineated and characterised by the imprint of its teacher took shape – obviously complemented by collaborators and followers who admired the leader – representing and constituting a strong, incisive and original reality of modern hypnology.

Specifically, Guantieri and his group developed an epistemology of hypnology with precise historical and scientific multidisciplinary attention, to which consistent clinical and didactic methods are connected.

Theirs was a scientific inspiration that strived to "define the possible genesis, essence and dynamics of hypnosis" to indicate important prospects for its use.

That idea was intended to outline the concept of hypnosis:

- Dealing with the possible dynamics of onset and evolution;
- Highlighting its meaning as an object and means of study, a tool for diagnosis and therapy;
- Outlining the role it can play and the contribution it can make in broad clinical and pedagogical fields.

That approach to hypnosis had to be implemented by means of a dynamic and psychosomatic orientation, because "hypnosis involves the human being in their totality, which also includes the social context", argued Guantieri.

The guiding idea was to appreciate all the possible scientific directions, while taking into account recurring contrasts, especially in order to consider the susceptibility of their mutual integration, even criticising the limits of an approach to a philosophy of research, another example, already established previously in medicine, whose principles were absolutely insufficient for the study and understanding of hypnotic phenomena.

According to the author, his hypnology (and that of his Institute) was therefore one of openness, both prudent and constructive, to the ultimate frontiers of knowledge. "It is a question of claiming for man in the face of science", in his words, "the concreteness and meaning of experiences, without cultivating the impoverishing illusion of being able to erase, by virtue of the pretext of their non-adaptability to mathematical calculations, everything that is not is organic or reducible to statistics".

And he, on the hypnotic interpersonal relationship, laid claim to a position inspired by a "legacy of a European tradition, a knowledge in which humanistic, phenomenological and existentialistic studies, as well as psychoanalytic ones, have left a very rich, deep imprint".

Thus he prepared an "overall plan for the construction of hypnology, on a scientific and cultural background in which the 'Bernheim' was the protagonist, characterising itself according to certain, essential points:

- The intertwining of hypnosis with the need for renewed tools in the doctor-patient relationship;
- The need for new languages which could lead to the rediscovery of integration between body and mind;
- The critical rethinking of old psychotherapeutic models (many of which need to emerge from the swamp of interminable time);
- The importance of keeping new trends in mind;
- The search for suitable models in training and teaching".

Here, then, is the teacher: he felt, alongside the need for research, parallel need to consistently disseminate the knowledge that was being acquired.

For Guantieri, the basic questions of hypnology are those that also arise in the field of training: for him, it is the same path, whereby he deems relevant the process aspect of effective learning that is built, through training, in the context of study and of past and present experiences of the hypnotic condition, with attention to the complexity of hypnotic togetherness.

An effective and correct application of hypnosis depends on the understanding and mastery of all this.

Guantieri's training method was attentive to the specificity of each student: close, empathic, convincing, welcoming. He argued how the hypnologist should be, with his or her own personality and conduct, a "therapeutic agent", an example of life, we would like to add. He encouraged attitudes favourable to formative experiences, motivating and guiding them, indicating how a proper use of the word remained central. He wished to facilitate collaboration, self-understanding, the strengthening of one's character, autonomy and personal growth.

The stimulus for the study and in-depth analysis of hypnology, was for Guantieri, more than a necessity, a natural consequence of this special way of understanding the 'Bernheim' School of Hypnology.

A School that was – first of all – an authentic community of real men.

CHAPTER 3

Epistemological foundations of Guantierian Hypnology

Gualtiero Guantieri was an original protagonist, a scholar, researcher, epistemologist of modern hypnology and, at the same time, a charismatic teacher of countless followers who inherited his teaching.

His contribution to the science of hypnosis was to indicate the safe path to which it must move. He traced the indispensable coordinates to follow, the essential philosophy that must characterize it. Having outlined this framework, he specified precise conditions of study, research and training of the hypnologist, using which to arrive at hypnological knowledge, according to methods and procedures, capable of dissecting very complex knowledge that requires a specific scientific paradigm. Gualtiero Guantieri provided this discipline with the seven pillars it needed:

1. The assumption that hypnosis is an entity as complex as the man who experiences it and that as such it should, a priori, be considered worthy of a study connoted necessarily by rigorous research procedures and consequent considerations that tend to grasp the complexity that characterises it, thus avoiding reductive yielding of a positivistic matrix;
2. The holistic view of the person anchored in his or her specific world;
3. The anthropological and historicist consideration of clinical and pedagogical hypnosis;
4. The multidisciplinary orientation of hypnological study and research aimed at capturing the contribution of many scientific disciplines that together better define the complexity of the phenomena involved;
5. The psychosomatist inspiration, also necessary for their understanding, because there is no psychic function that does not have somatic consequences, nor a body that, being alive, does not determine a psychic emergence;
6. The indispensability of a contextual, hypnological community of pioneering scientists, researchers and master trainers, which gives vital and cognitive thrust to an important and complex knowledge that can become common cultural heritage;
7. Attention to the evolutionary, ongoing and future projections of this knowledge.

Gualtiero Guantieri and his 'H. Bernheim' Italian Institute for Clinical Hypnosis and Psychotherapy in Verona, built on these foundations, contributed significantly to making hypnosis an increasingly sought-after object of study and an effective means of clinical and pedagogical use, from the 1960s onwards.

Guantierian Hypnology and its model, which in that sphere were therefore original and unmistakable, are characterised by a memorable, anthropological attention to hypnotic phenomena, a scientific inspiration drawn from multiple psychological and medical disciplines at the same time, and but specific operational, clinical procedures and training methods, logically derived from and correlated to the overall model.

Central to this framework is the importance of the hypnotic interpersonal relationship and the theme of a person's self, involved therein, producing a peculiar interaction that is very special, global, unitary, capable of promoting changes in states of consciousness, that is, authentic openness to emotional experiences, to strong, pleasant or painful sensations, to true feelings, to more authentic encounters and confrontations.

1. The need for a philosophical foundation of hypnology

Hypnosis is a complex entity. The science dealing with it must be able to grasp this tangle of constituent elements and harmoniously put them together. Therefore it needs, like every discipline, its specific epistemological foundations.
Every science has its foundations.
The philosophy of science aims to identify them case by case, field by field, subject by subject, in relation to natural sciences or social sciences, so that each discipline can outline and define its own identity.
This is the epistemic basis that supports each scientific discipline in a different way. Gualtiero Guantieri was an epistemologist of hypnology with undoubtedly marked pioneering and innovative connotations, of a radical challenge to the very way of approaching the phenomena of hypnosis up to that point.
We could say that he characterised an evolutionary stage of the scientific transformations that hypnosis has undergone, analogous to what has always historically happened across all branches of human knowledge.
As is well known, the path of science is marked by scientific revolutions which often upset the paradigms of reference.
The philosophy of science has been dealing with this for centuries, studying its presuppositions.
Thomas Kunt (1922-1996), gave an account of it in the 1960s in one of his famous essays.
The philosopher Karl Popper (1902-1994), perhaps exaggerating this concept, went so far as to argue that science, to be authentic, must have a structural need

for permanent revolution, and have doubt as a presupposition and starting condition[45].

Now we put these authors in an uncomfortable position, because their thinking seems to be very well suited to the scientific history of Italian hypnology as Guantieri was able to interpret it.

The medical and academic world of the time, which he knew well as a part of it, applied scientific procedures to its discipline, inspired by a positivism that – extended to hypnology – could not work.

According to Guantieri, a knowledge that we would say expired in scientism was expected to reduce the object of matter that he considered, more precisely hypnosis, as an elementary and manoeuvrable entity, such as to be able to easily analyse and replicate its manifestations, for example, as if it were of the same category as the phenomena of the expansion of physical bodies under the effect of heat, or of a chemical effervescence obtainable by adding vinegar to sodium bicarbonate.

Hypnosis, on the other hand, being a complex entity of troubling mysteriousness according to various prejudices of the time (in the middle decades of the 20th century), struggled to obtain full irrefutable academic consideration.

The scientific method necessary to achieve the objective knowledge of reality could not – for Guantieri – be limited to the mere organization of material and practical experimental data, dismissing other constituent, foundations of very composite phenomena, yet worthy of study and research.

He therefore courageously denounced the limits of that previously established methodological approach already applied tout-court, uncritically, to hypnosis, because, in their traditional structure, those principles of the human sciences were absolutely insufficient to fully grasp the breadth of the events they were intended to explore.

His thought was always inspired by the need for an open, critically constructive hypnological foundation, capable of recognizing the indisputable cornerstones on which to rest in the scientific foundations of medicine and psychology, but he also intended to look beyond, to integrate them and complement them and to push the ultimate frontiers of knowledge, without fear of crossing them.

"It is a question," he stated, "of claiming for man, in the face of science, the concreteness and meaning of his own experiences, of his own individual historical reality, of his own being in interpersonal relationships, without cultivating the impoverishing illusion of being able to erase everything with a complacent denial, by virtue of the pretext of their non-adaptability to arithmetic calculations. The truth is certainly not reducible to a statistical result, nor can thought be debased as a simple organ. On the other hand, even current epistemology is by now too

---

[45] Kunt T., *The Structure of Scientific Revolutions*, University of Chicago Press, 1970.

savvy to believe that only experimentation and the laboratory are the demarcation between science and non-science".[46]

Tracing the personal professional history of Guantieri, it is possible to trace various moments that attest to this aspect of his reflection and his methodological critique of the world of knowledge of his time.

We recall how, on the occasion of the 20th anniversary (1985) of the foundation of the 'H. Bernheim Clinical Hypnosis Study Centre, at the time already transformed into the 'H. Bernheim' Italian Institute of Clinical Hypnosis and Psychotherapy – Training Research School, Guantieri wrote of a Centre which had "intimately suffered the conflicts of contemporary medicine and psychology [reaching however] concrete, significant goals considered utopian [only 20 years earlier]".

He wanted to celebrate the event by underlining "the prospect of a progressively more human medicine and a psychology that,[would have been] better able to approach one another, in a harmonious integration between the conscious and unconscious [in order] to truly understand, and therefore adequately treat, the fundamental needs of the individual being, unrepeatable as an organism and as a person".[47]

The author, in the introduction to that celebration, hoped that his speech could constitute "at least a modest contribution to knowledge, while he claimed his Institute's dedication, from the beginning, to research and study [participating in] an original contribution to the integration of hypnosis in Italian and international culture".[48]

The author's historical reflection could not fail to consider the different international and national scientific situations. In some cases, the former lead the way over the latter. For this he courageously denounced how closed Italian academic circles were, at the time, to the innovative contributions hypnology was making – because he said – they were feared as "potentially destabilising for institutional knowledge".[49]

Guantieri therefore distinguishes between an institutional knowledge, (sometimes corporative and sectarian? Ed.) and an alternative knowledge, nevertheless deserving of serious scientific consideration.

His stance, along with that of others, helped to make a renewed interest in hypnosis begin to be felt in Italy.[50]

---

[46] Guantieri G., Angelozzi A., *A foundation and a perspective. The 'H. Bernheim' and the conceptual evolution of hypnosis)*, Edited by the 'H. Bernheim' Italian Institute of Clinical Hypnosis and Psychotherapy - Research and Training School, Verona, 1985.
[47] Idem, c.s, p. 7.
[48] Idem, pp. 11-12.
[49] Ibidem, p. 20.
[50] Guantieri recalled the use of hypnosis in obstetrics by Mosconi, in psychotherapy by Romero, in dentistry by Pavesi and in neurophysiological research by Granone.

At that time, important relationships with other Italian and foreign hypnosis study and research bodies intensified.[51]

These scientific relationships between Centres and academies, in Italy and around the world, have proved decisive contributions in creating modern history and clinical practice and the philosophical reflection of current hypnology.

These exchanges of views were fundamental for Guantieri: they were the natural consequence of the philosophical and scientific sensitivity that characterised him.

And he further elaborated: "Hypnosis [...] testifies to how the area of the exact should not be confused with [the absolute] and offers a privileged field for the investigation of factors not easily quantifiable with current tools and techniques; [it requires] a much richer background knowledge! Precisely for this reason it is important to us that there are 'concepts' of hypnosis: this allows for a comparison that can stimulate [...] growth [...] while maintaining a constant commensurability between theories that allow dialogue and exchange".[52]

2. The humanist and holistic conception of the person

What vision of man?

Guantieri's humanistic vision of man, which requires delving into the depths of his soul, integrates and overlaps with a holistic view of the humanity. He has always considered the human being through his complexity; his was a true holistic vision. Holism, from the Greek "Olos" and meaning totality, is the consideration of a whole, of the entirety, of a being that is an interconnected, inseparable set of body, mind, emotions, spirit, soul, drives, and relational needs, lived and expressed together in a given environmental context, in a specific world, natural, cultural, anthropological in which it lives.

In medicine and psychology, it refers to the person's overall state of health, that is, resulting from an inseparable union of factors that concur to create, completely, with either more or less serious difficulties, this existential condition of being and which are the mind and body interacting with a natural and social, family and public environment.

This is an epistemic inspiration, from which follows the search for improving the state of health, first of all of the person and not their illnesses, of the causes that determine them and not the symptoms they manifest, of the system and not only the single organ, of the rebalancing of the whole as a preliminary cure, stimulating the body's natural self-healing process.

---

[51] For further information on this topic, see Chapter 7 of this text.
[52] Guantieri G., Angelozzi A., *A foundation and a perspective. The 'H. Bernheim' and the conceptual evolution of hypnosis)*, Edited by the 'H. Bernheim' Italian Institute of Clinical Hypnosis and Psychotherapy - Research and Training School, Verona, 1985.

Health is not seen as the simple absence of disease, but a global well-being of body and mind that leads to the optimal functioning of an individual in every respect. Therefore, when you want to treat a pathology, you must take into consideration all aspects of the patient's life, the place where they live, the people with whom they are in relationship, the resources that their life context offers them.

This holistic vision cannot fail to project onto future scenarios supported by ideals, values, aspirations that are close to the patient, a confident predisposition to helping them by spurring them to acquire the maximum possible autonomy, empathy, involvement, and the ability to identify with themselves and their history. Guantieri argued that it was necessary to perceive man "as a psychosomatic unit in intimate contact with the environment", as happens in hypnosis, which "involves the human being in his totality, also understood as the social context, as a unit, organism and a person at the same time, in intimate contact, action and reaction with the environment, looking at him in a very particular way, that is, not paying less attention to the body, but rather more to the psyche".[53]

This consideration therefore imposes the perspective of a medicine and a psychology that become progressively more human and are better able to get closer, in harmony and integrating with one another, considering at the same time, man, the living body, his awareness and the unconscious that belongs to him in order to "truly understand, and therefore adequately deal with, the true fundamental needs of the individual being, unrepeatable as an organism and as a person".[54]

Theorising of the Self

Philosophers, psychologists and psychoanalysts of various schools and theoretical orientations have, over time, dealt with the concept of the self and complementary constructs such as Id, Ego and Superego.

Inspirations and interpretations have arisen that are not only not univocal, but often conflicting.

In this variegated framework, Guantieri conceptually elaborated a "particular Self" that bears his mark: the one that intervenes and characterises the experience of modified acts of conscience.

The Self, according to Guantieri, is an implicit individual-entity, to which he alludes several times in his work.[55]

---

[53] Guantieri G., *Fondamenti e prospettive dell'ipnologia medica*, in AA. VV., *Lezioni di apertura del Corso di Aggiornamento in Ipnologia medica*, Verona, 7-9 May 1971, Handout by the 'H. Bernheim', Verona, 1971, p. 117.
[54] Guantieri G., Angelozzi A., *Ipnosi - Un fondamento e una prospettiva - Il Centro 'H. Bernheim' e l'evoluzione concettuale dell'ipnosi*, Edited by the 'H. Bernheim' Institute for the Study of Clinical Hypnosis and Psychotherapy, Verona, 1985, p. 7.
[55] For further information, see: Guantieri G. *L'ipnosi, come oggetto di studio e mezzo di impiego in medicina*, Rizzoli, Milan, 1973, pp. 107-115.

It is about that dimension of man, conceived as an inseparable psychosomatic unit, which resonates in his intimacy and which is made up above all of emotions, sensations, sentiments and moods.

A Self that can emerge in the form of self-perception and awareness of one's own condition of being, which the ego knows how to take charge of as the "global and essential thing that concerns it".

An emergent Self in reflective phases of one's life and, in particular, in modified states of consciousness, where, as Guantieri points out, a subsystem (the Guantieri Self, therefore, Ed.), belonging to a part of the ego, is also able to emerge under conditions of hypnotic regression.[56]

This condition, of placing oneself in the dynamic dependence of a hypnologist chosen by the subject, would be assumed for clinical, pedagogical and relational reasons.

Regression at the service of the ego is achieved through sensory, motor and ideational deprivation and with the activation of adequate motivations that allow concentration and the excitation of certain areas.

All this to obtain, in addition to hypnotic expressions, psychic, psychosomatic effects, which are useful in research, prophylaxis, diagnosis and treatment of the subject.

Regression, according to the atavistic theory that Guantieri cites, would allow an archaic way of thinking (intuitive, impulsive, pre-aware? Existing already before the structuring of a sufficiently competent ego? Ed.), as occurs in the infant and in the primitive (perhaps also in some animals), where accepted suggestions would translate into hypnotic effects.[57]

A previous theory, also cited by our author, describes a primitive psychological functioning of the organism, operating from the moment of the appearance of the first consciousness of a differentiation of the individual from the environment (hence would the Self precisely take shape?).

According to Guantieri, some scholars were subsequently able to focus these themes with other multidisciplinary aspects capable of describing this entity, the Self, capable of manifesting itself well in the phenomena of regression.

They indicated neurophysiological, psychoanalytic and experimental psychology correlations and interpretations of a complex, holistic self, in which the living essence of the same would take precedent, even before the Ego, or the Superego, a Self increasingly and better integrated with them, in a positive evolution of being.

---

[56] Regression at the service of the ego, which in strictly neurophysiological terms could be explained by a partial cortical inhibition, accompanied by a concentration of excitation in certain areas, would take place, from a psychological point of view, to organise in the ego of subsystem equipped with particular functions. This subsystem would depend on the hypnologist, while the remaining part of the ego would instead continue to maintain the critical orientation that characterises it in a waking state. From the activity of this subsystem (or from the aforementioned modifications of the nervous circuits) initiated in a completely particular way by the hypnologist's voice, the multiple effects, both psychic and psychosomatic, widely and variously usable for the purposes of experimental research, prophylaxis, diagnosis and therapy (Guantieri G. *L'ipnosi, come oggetto di studio e mezzo di impiego in medicina,* Rizzoli, Milan, 1973, p. 115).

[57] Idem c.s., pp.107-115.

Humanistic philosophy, phenomenology and existentialism, were a source of inspiration for Guantieri, to outline the epistemological foundations of his own hypnological paradigm.

This is the starting cultural context on which he based his conception of mankind, in all its complexity and depth, up to spirituality and transcendence.

There were also many authors from the world of psychology who inspired him, men who showed great tenderness towards the themes of human ideality; broad, universal, not necessarily marked or limited by some religious doctrine.

Among them were Roberto Assagioli (1898-1964) — the father of psychosynthesis, that is, the psychological theorising attentive to the "care of the soul", aimed at discovering the will that is inherent in the personality of each individual and which to use as leverage in psychotherapy, in order to lead the assisted person towards the realisation of their spiritual dimension — and the psychosomatist, psychologist and humanist in reflections on life and death that was Ferruccio Antonelli (1927-2000).

If they inspired Guantieri, he himself directly manifested his transcendent dimension. He wrote, for example, quoting Gorgia di Leontini, about the power of words "which know how to calm fear, eliminate pain, invite joy and inspire pity".[58]

Thus, he considered words and thoughts, which were dear to him, of calm and serenity, of joy and mystical rapture, of pity and compassion, which are concepts of an elevated humanity, existing outside and above what is material and ordinary.

Guantieri again, with reference to his inductive modality, specifically reminds us that he had visualised – inspired in this case by Assagioli – voices evoking harmony, courage, will, vitality, faith, patience, benevolence, serenity, order, love, understanding, light and generosity.[59]

Guantieri therefore, in his own way and with his originality, was certainly able to fully experience and let his clients experience moods characterised by a contemplative, devout, ascetic, very pure, ideal, highly mystical spirit.

Ascents and dreams, abandonment and creativity, in Guantieri's soul, are universal experiences that belong to humanity.

Man is a dreamer and a mystic.[60]

---

[58] Idem c.s., p. 8.
[59] For further information on Guantieri's personal hypnotic induction method, see Chapter 6 of this text.
[60] The mystical state is not pure spirit. In these cases, the human tangle of body and psyche, which is in man, not only does not dissolve, but finds occasion for further intertwining and fusion. The psyche, the emotions, the thoughts, the soul and the raptures that occur, in these modified conditions of consciousness, involve the bodies of ascetic and mystical people and are vibrant with drive, desire, passion, which are living flesh in need of undeniable pleasures. Here are some examples: Anna Katharina Emmerick (1774-1824), was greatly devoted to the Passion of Christ. She wrote about it several times, telling of having contemplated the Nazarene in a state of scourging, made *"similar to a diaper soaked in blood"*. And she tells of a *"naked Jesus... hastened to take off his own clothes, even the last linen that encircled his back... and trembled* – adds the saint – *and twisted like a worm"*, (Anna Katharina Emmerick, *The painful passion of Our Lord Jesus Christ*, Editrice Shalom, Camerata

And for him, meditating on the meaning of existence can be a yearning for a direct, intuitive, lived encounter with highly significant, existential, valuable, wise and transcendent entities.[61]

Picena – Ancona – 2015). It is a story of blood, nudity and sadism that are mystical ecstasy, involvement and participation, troubled and sublime passion. In *The Inner Castle*, Teresa of Avila (1515-1582) describes her raptures thus: *"In an ecstasy there appeared to me a tangible angel in his carnal constitution...he was beautiful; I saw in the hand of this angel a long dart; it was of gold and bore at the end a point of fire. The angel penetrated me with the dart to my insides, and when he withdrew it, he left me all burned with love for [...] my groom, who gave me such excesses of pleasure that I was obliged to add nothing more than to say that my senses were ravished by him,"*(Teresa of Avila, The interior castle, Edizioni Paoline, Turin, 2011). Teresa's body is vibrant and a protagonist. And she is so, with her enjoyments and the fire of her flesh, while the mind, in unison, remains enraptured. Caterina Fieschi Adorno (Caterina da Genova, 1447-1510), in her compositions deals with the human condition of the deceased who end up in purgatory where she imagines being, dutifully but blissfully tormented, to atone for sinful acts resulting from irrepressible bodily stimuli consummated at the expense of a chaste soul. These tribulations assure her of an encounter with the Divine Flame – as she affirms – seized by the desire to enjoy God with an irrepressible longing. Thus she writes: *"This holy soul still in flesh, finding itself... in the Purgatory of the fiery (fiery, Ed.) Love of God who burned it all, purified it so that [...] she could reach the presence of her sweet love, God [...] loving fire"* (Caterina da Genova, *Treatise on purgatory and other writings*, Publisher Gribaudi, Milan, 2010). Jacopo dei Benedetti, known as Iacopone da Todi (1236-1306) describes a mystical embrace that he received and that made him die of desire and that he consumes, in a total fusion with God. Here is his testimony: *"Embrace me with him and for love yes claim[...] Make me die of love![...] consume me, languishing [...] I beg for you to embrace me. When you leave, yes I die living, I sigh and weep to find you again [...] so, do not delay any longer, Love [...] tied up, yes, hold me, consume my heart!"* (Iacopone da Todi, *Amor de caritate*, Publisher Laterza, Bari, 2006). Bernard of Clairvaux (1090-1153), monk, theologian, founder of various congregations, and promoter of the construction of various abbeys and monasteries, had a mystical vision that led him to an encounter with the Bridegroom – as he states – that is, with a God that nourished him with wisdom and sensations that touched his vibrant body, reminding him of a large and overflowing breast, capable of pleasurable nourishment. And he writes: *"When I feel how my senses are opened [...] or how the light of wisdom gushes from my heart [...] how the mysteries are revealed to me [...] and the sky opens up to me [...] her immeasurably large breast making my spirit overflow with rain, abundant with solicitations [...] I have no doubt that the Bridegroom is present [...] and I receive a sense of fullness [...] and I tend towards him with great desire [...] becoming compliant with him"*, (Bernardo di Chiaravalle, Sermones super Cantica Canticorum. Editiones Cistercienses, Rome, 1957). John of the Cross, (Juan de Yepes Álvarez, 1542-1591), contemporary and collaborator of Teresa of Avila, was a poet and presbyter. He is the patron saint of mystics. In the poem *Dark Night*, he gives voice to his soul and tells of a psychophysical state in which he gets lost, and tells of a visionary, transcendent, sensual falling in love, which has a fascinating and ambiguous touch of androgyny and which reaches overwhelming heights, in which then to be able to lie, lost and blessed. In a passage taken from his writings he says: *"My soul [...] from my love all inflamed, in the dark and well hidden [...] to the abandoned sleep ... without seeing what ... guided me ... there where those who knew me well were waiting for me [...] oh, more night than the complacent dawn! Oh, night that reunited the Beloved with the Beloved, Beloved into the Beloved transformed! On my flowery breast [...] he fell asleep and I caressed him [...]with his light hand my neck wounded and all my senses in ecstasy rapt. There I lie ...",* (Giovanni della Croce, Dark Night, Città Nuova, Rome, 2003.)

[61] Every healthy man can seek, through modified states of consciousness, total pacifications, awareness, further levels of human fulfilment. And one can contemplate infinities, great or infinitesimal, complex or seemingly incomprehensible, or realize contact with that which is tenebrous, untameable, desirable and vertiginous. The gentle leopardian shipwreck, where one can immerse oneself in the world of aesthetic or erotic emotions, or follow the paths that ascend to mystical levels, which attract one towards the admiration of the best humanity in the whole universe, then self-esteem, enlightenment, is possible for everyone. And this can be both spiritual and physical, above all entrancing. Love, eroticism, pleasure, the experience of a "delicious pain" are things that have to do with the mystical condition. If ecstasy can be a sufficiently satisfied sexual arousal, full amorous pleasure is also unsettling, and in some ways mystical. And these are, among many others, the oceanic sentiments of which Sigmund Freud speaks. And the loving encounter with God, for those who believe in and seek him, is the pleasure of the spirit, the culminating point of the experience with him, where the body, however, is always there and is agitated in an all-encompassing and full involvement, even with libidinal connotations, in which the pleasure of the body emerges fully. St. Francis de Sales compared mystical ecstasy to breastfeeding. If this is abandonment and regression is great and satisfying, one returns to be suckling infants. Ecstasy is a psychic state of suspension and mystical elevation of the mind, which is often perceived as estranged from the body. In fact, its etymology indicates a coming out of oneself, but, on closer inspection, it is rather a loss of one's awareness. It is the mind that loses its own rational part, but remains strongly anchored in a soma that remains involved with a modified sensoriality and

3. The historicist and anthropological consideration of hypnological phenomena

Hypnosis has an ancient and powerful link to what, from a historical point of view, can be defined as its magical phase.
This never-ending "past" exerts an enormous fascination on its followers, managing to paralyse their ability to investigate and think.
If this happens, hypnosis undergoes a fossilisation that makes it an archaeological entity, where it remains wrapped and entangled in the mysteries of the occult, where it remains the object of contemplation that dazzles and paralyses, and imposes itself with its dogmas and induces fideistic adhesions, deferential devotions, consequent passive and uncritical venerable prostrations. If we follow this path, we find ourselves in a dangerous cultural territory that fosters ignorance and stupidity and renders us orphans blind to the truth and, above all vulnerable in countless ways.
An alternative approach to the phenomena concerning hypnosis, to the characteristics that structure it, to the functional qualities it possesses and which are useful for the good of humanity, is, rather, the gnoseological one — that is, a discourse on the knowledge of hypnosis that identifies its ancient and current foundations, defines its limits, verifies the validity of what emerges from one's studies, considers the relationship that exists with the attentive and critical subject who wants to know it.
In other words, pay attention to what is used as a unifier in anthropologically very different contexts and traceable in the furthest corners of the earth.
Between past and present, and now towards the future, the continuum on which hypnosis must be thought out historiographically takes shape.
The present is relevant and full-bodied: it is that of hypnology that is currently known and studied in depth, which provides its indications and its modern methods of use.

---

in a condition of physiological intoxication; it too, like the mind, is strongly focused on exclusive entities. This enchantment hardly inhabits the left cerebral hemisphere, it does not care about rationality, it is better placed in the right brain, the recessive, passive, emotional, creative, imaginative, artistic one. And there, a state of extreme hypnotic rapture occurs at Nirvana. The mind remains stunned, focused on one point and forgets everything else. And it is bliss and inner well-being, possibly considered direct manifestations of a divine being who can also be the Dionysus adored in Bacchae of ancient Greece, revered by those women who participated in mystery and initiation cults, preferably nocturnal, open to the marginalised of society, to the slaves and metics, where the protagonists fell, dancing, singing and drinking, in states of ecstatic trances expressing instinct and libido, performing unusual actions and practicing unbridled eroticism. And they were ecstasies, which made the oracles credible as they were experienced as intermediaries between the earthly dimension and an otherworldly one. In Asian regions, usually under the guidance of shamanic masters, especially in Hinduism, Taoism, and Buddhism, the initiate is led to the sacred state of enlightenment, omniscience, supreme and perfect wisdom, the full development of potential and natural qualities present in the individual, thus arriving at Nirvana. In these states the mind becomes unlimited, no longer separated from the rest of the world, it blends, in unison, the microcosm of the person with the macrocosm of the universe.

But there is a continuous evolution, current and future, of hypnology, the path of which can already be traced, specifying a whole series of scientific questions that remain open, of subliminal perceptions, a series of parapsychological phenomena, the deepening of knowledge of the peculiarity of this interpersonal relationship that is created between hypnotists and their experiential subjects; but the past cannot be ignored. It represents the robust roots of a hypnological tree which by now has a powerful structure, and which produces the seeds necessary for a future in which it can and will have to replicate itself, in a new way.

The history of hypnosis, its subdivision into the phases that Guantieri has defined and described, with an abundance of information, distinguishing them into pre-scientific, scientific and current, are topics summarised in the first part of his book 'Hypnosis as an object of study and a means of use in medicine' (1973), which we find summarised in the sixth chapter of this text.

This history of hypnosis, as old as mankind, deserves to be further explored, it has been and must be investigated with a historical scientific procedure, supplemented by the contribution of cultural anthropological research.

These lines of study have indeed further explored hypnosis and made it more known, but it is not enough.

Today we know that hypnosis has been traced in every page of human history and in every corner of the world and that it has different connotations in various cases, and thus that it has been and is influenced by a thousand factors, which are themselves historical, ethnic, environmental and cultural.

4. The multidisciplinary approach to the study of hypnosis

Guantieri, a scientist, had an eclectic and multidisciplinary inclination in his hypnological reflections.

Many doctors, neurophysiologists, psychologists, psychotherapists, sociologists and scholars of systems theory, were interesting for Guantieri as hypnologists or hypnotists, even if they could be criticised in terms of their knowledge.

What mattered to him was their contribution to understanding the complex nature of hypnosis.

Therefore, he accepted the neurophysiological interpretations proposed by scholars such as, for example, Ivan Pavlov (1849-1936) who elaborated the theories of cortical inhibition and the inferences relating to the sleep-hypnosis comparison.

Guantieri then considered important the remarks put forward by general psychology, [Ernest Hilgard, (1904-2001) is an example: with his psychology of hypnosis, he underlined the importance of the history, motivations and personality of the individual subjects involved in hypnotic experiences].

Another contribution to the study of hypnosis has been acknowledged in the psychology of learning [Guantieri cites the "Learning-Theory", by Clark Hull (1884-1936) relating to repeated stimulus-response experiences]; of other authors of this school, he considered their descriptions of homoation and heteroation, as well as the correlations between learning, cortical inhibition and the state of widespread emotional reactivity.

Guantieri appreciated the socio-psychological contributions concerning themes of suggestibility, "attitudes" and "role theory".

Anthropology and sociology were not lacking in his studies, precisely because the person he conceived could not ignore the roots on which his evolution was based. On this point of sociology, Guantieri's reflections "were of acceptance, subject to [some contributions] as it was important that, in hypnotic behavior, the aspect of an act that has to do with the expectations of the society to which the hypnotised subject belongs, also comes into play".

He specified that there are particular phenomena, worthy of further specification, which require psychological insights such as: "post-hypnotic amnesia, age regression, free expression of unconscious content, automatic writing, certain perceptual distortions, the way in which extrasensory perceptions, catalepsy and hypnotic imagination are realize".[62]

Our author then accepted, widely and completely, the contributions inherent to the study of hypnosis by dynamic psychology in the first half of the twentieth century (in particular, the themes of transference and regression at the service of the ego in psychoanalysis).[63]

This did absolutely not mean – let it be clearly stated – any adhesion by Guantieri to any psychoanalytic school.

Rather, he understood, with other authors, "the importance of innovative contributions, in a panorama of precariousness of the various theoretical structures, of the renewed conception of the pathology of the symptom that demanded the need for an integration between physiology and psychology, with new hypotheses that better grasp the relationship between symptoms and personality".[64]

Inherent in the relationship between hypnology and psychoanalysis, the theme of the need to structure modalities of short psychotherapy did not escape Guantieri's attention.

This means, therefore, that the research he did, even within psychoanalytic knowledge, did not betray the intent that he always kept firm, to isolate the

---

[62] Guantieri G., *L'ipnosi, come oggetto di studio e mezzo di impiego in medicina*, Rizzoli, Milan, 1973, pp. 105-106.

[63] *"Psychoanalysis"*, Guantieri reminds us, *"interpreted the hypnotic intervention as a partial modality, easily explained in analytical terms: an exclusively temporary and symptomatic intervention, which had to be overcome"*, (Guantieri G., Angelozzi A., *Ipnosi. Un fondamento e una prospettiva. Il Centro 'H. Bernheim' e l'evoluzione concettuale dell'ipnosi*, Edited by 'H. Bernheim' Italian Institute for the Study of Clinical Hypnosis and Psychotherapy -- Research and Training School, Verona, 1985, p. 15).

[64] Guantieri G., Angelozzi A., *Ipnosi - Un fondamento e una prospettiva. Il Centro 'H. Bernheim' e l'evoluzione concettuale dell'ipnosi*, Edited by 'H. Bernheim' Italian Institute for the Study of Clinical Hypnosis and Psychotherapy -- Research and Training School, Verona, 1985, p. 16)

aspects inherent to the phenomenology of hypnosis, so that useful knowledge could be achieved for a better and more complete definition of the object of study that he investigated.

On the other hand, a generalised adherence to psychoanalysis, in the coherent setting of the scientific foundations of hypnology, entails the risk of a distortion and confusion in which his hypnology ended up reduced to a complementary technique of other disciplines.

He – we reiterate – never gave up on the idea of a particularity of hypnosis that only a strict, attentive and consistent hypnology can preserve.

Sigmund Freud (1856-1939), in this epistemological framework, was important for Guantieri precisely in order to explore in greater depth the theme of the interpersonal relationship, but he could not accept the idea that everything would be resolved simply in terms of transference and countertransference because these dynamic elements do not, according to Guantieri, capture the peculiarity of a relationship that still remains mysterious in certain respects today.[65]

Many other psychoanalysts, whether or not they are orthodox, were interesting to Guantieri only in so far as they dealt with hypnosis.

The other things that they dealt with were outside the paradigm that he was defining and did not interest him much.

In any case, he always remained set on the idea of a multidisciplinary hypnology.

If he also had a psychodynamic orientation, this was always complementary, very free, disenchanted and critical, not necessarily psychoanalytic, but also, as we have seen, psychosynthetic, transactional, Gestalt, etc.

What was most important to him was the thesis - as we mentioned before - of the specificity of a paradigmatic construction that had to emerge as an authentic evolution, starting from the totality of human knowledge.

---

[65] Regarding the characteristics of this relationship, Carlo Piazza offers us a contribution. He talks about clinical relationships that take place in a special context: that of a "borderland [...] a common field [...] a grey area [...] a place where the sufferer and the therapist meet [...] where books whiten [...] where [it is possible to] perceive, feel, hope and despair, where [one tries to] understand [...] where [one tries to] get out of time and causality, where [one can] think, reflect, participate, gather and grow [...] understand each other [...] provoke and stimulate, listen, sharing, pitying (in the sense of compassion, of feeling together, as of understanding, of taking charge [...] in providing care) [... where] the passion of feeling [is] emotion [and] asking oneself, exposing oneself [a] lived commitment and [a] shared participation". Piazza C., Il dolore esistenziale, terra di confine tra corpo, mente e spirito; tecniche immaginative di rilassamento in gruppo per l'approccio al dolore e alla malattia, in the journal Acta Hypnologica, Edited by 'H. Bernheim' Italian Institute for the Study of Clinical Hypnosis and Psychotherapy -- Research and Training School, S. Martino B.A. (Verona), Year XIII, n.2, May 2010.

5. The Psychosomatic inspiration

If the definition of hypnosis cannot be separated from a multidisciplinary approach, this study can "be made feasible with a psychosomatic orientation [...]. In order for such a study to be successful," concluded Guantieri, "a multidimensional approach to hypnosis is appropriate which can be made feasible with a psychosomatic orientation".[66]

This orientation must align with a global vision of man.

Psychosomatics itself is a holistic approach to the healthy or sick person that takes into account the living body, the emotions of the individual and the environment in which they live.

It is therefore a discipline that studies the reactions of healthy or sick people that manifest in the soma as an expression of movements and disturbances in the psychic sphere.

For example: shame is a psychosomatic condition that is expressed in a body that lowers its head and blushes, while on the psychic level there is a profound discomfort that makes the person feel unworthy and stimulates the urge to hide and not be seen anymore.

Fear of danger induces the same reactions, whether it is a real or imaginary event. In this case, the subject with the body may run away, while fearing the worst on a psychic level.

Hypnosis and psychosomatics go well together.

The psychosomatic consideration of hypnosis is the foundation of the scientific paradigm that constitutes it.

Hypnosis, in turn, is a very effective tool in the treatment of psychosomatic diseases.

6. The need for a competent hypnological community [67]

Guantieri and his Institute were hypnological communities, comprised of scientists, researchers, and pioneering educator mentors. They were an association

---

[66] Guantieri G., Fondamenti e prospettive dell'ipnologia medica, in AA. VV., Lezioni di apertura del Corso di Aggiornamento in Ipnologia medica, Verona, 7-9 maggio 1971, Handout edited by the 'H. Bernheim' Institute, Verona, 1971, p. 116.

[67] The following paragraph takes up various articles (from which quotations are often omitted), which we have published on this subject. We recall only the original sources:
Guantieri G., *Fondamenti e prospettive dell'ipnologia medica*, in AA. VV., *Opening lectures of the refresher course in medical hypnology*, Verona, 7-9 May 1971, handout edited by the 'H. Bernheim' Institute, Verona, 1971;
Guantieri G., *L'Ipnosi*, Rizzoli, Milan, 1973;
Guantieri G., *Il setting ipnotico in prospettiva psicodinamica*, in *Il linguaggio del corpo in ipnosi*, (edited by Guantieri G.), Editions Il Segno, Negrar, (Verona), 1985;
Guantieri G., Angelozzi A., *Ipnosi. Un fondamento ed una prospettiva. Il Centro 'H. Bernheim'e l'evoluzione concettuale dell'ipnosi*, Edited by 'H. Bernheim' Italian Institute for the Study of Clinical Hypnosis and Psychotherapy -- Research and Training School, Verona, 1985.

and congregation that provided vital and cognitive momentum to a significant and highly articulated body of knowledge, increasingly becoming common cultural heritage, purified and freed from unconscious concessions to a hypnosis still capable of dangerously suggesting, due to its esoteric and magical components, even to the scholar who engages with it.

Guantieri considered the study of hypnosis, the inherent scientific research, hypnological knowledge and the training of the hypnologist as partial aspects of his discipline, inseparable, if not for the need for academic learning.

He supported the idea of a "foundation of the study of hypnosis that could not ignore the focus on reflection of the subject-hypnologist, for their training in the field of research on the phenomena of hypnosis".

In fact, the 'Bernheim' Centre-Institute, an inseparable and equal combination of study seminars, research, and training, has been a laboratory for investigation and hypnological application since its foundation (1965), where educational value has always been central.

It has been a place of human relationships, strongly characterised by its human-oriented master-hypnologist, clinician and well-known charismatic healer and particularly sensitive educator-trainer.

The knowledge of a hypnology that was deepening and progressively accumulating, acquired also through a strong interaction between teachers and students, was in any case transmitted to the students, who were present and engaged in a pioneering field of this discipline.

Guantieri felt, alongside the need for research, the parallel need to consistently disseminate the knowledge that was being acquired (and to which his Centre was contributing), not only to his students, but to the whole academic world.

He argued that it was necessary to "constantly adjust the applicative needs of particular specialised fields to the necessity of education that cannot ignore a personal, relationally oriented preparation within a vision of hypnosis that can enlighten, even in the future, our progress along the path we have laid out."

As a teacher of future adept educators or hypnotherapists, he loved to underline the procedural aspect of that effective learning which he preferred, and that is built through training in the realm of study and life experience, lived in the first person, of the hypnotic condition.

He was not interested in simply training "mere hypnotists or, worse still, hypnotisers", but, representing a model hypnological scholar; he required great levels of involvement and a strong, new, incisive and pressing in-depth analysis of the fundamental and constitutive aspect represented by the theme of interpersonal relationships. "The vision of hypnosis identified not only as a psycho-physical state", he suggested, "but also as a relationship between operator and subject, certainly could not be seen purely as a set of techniques that are mechanically learnable and applicable. Instead, it placed itself as a constant dialectic between these and the complexity of hypnotic being together, on the understanding and mastery of which an effective and correct application of hypnosis depends.

Therefore, teaching could not ignore the focus on aspects and characteristics of the hypnotic relationship, closely related to the previous and post-hypnotic ones, which could only be highlighted and materialised through a training centred on the individual and relational dynamics of the students. For them - along with the teachers - it was an immersion and meditation within repeatedly lived hypnotic experiences, characterised by intense involvement and strong, new, incisive, and pressing analysis, especially of that peculiar aspect of the interpersonal relationship that is built in the complexity of a close and intentional togetherness, to promote unusual, non-ordinary psycho-physical states, open to the depth of the psychologies and the unconscious of all participants".[68]

On hypnological teaching, Guantieri also wrote: "The preparation of the hypnologist must consist of particular education, acquired through an appropriate didactic-therapeutic training. A complex problem," he added, "because today the preparation of the doctor from a psychological point of view is very lacking, while completely new notions are indispensable and which, in order to be accepted and become productive, must find adequate orientation and certain tendencies, attitudes and abilities must be developed and others reduced or eliminated, as the induction of hypnosis and the use of hypnotherapy involves an almost always great emotional commitment, at least initially. The knowledge of one's own possibilities and limits is acquired", he specified, "not necessarily through analysis (especially for those who do not practice psychosomatic medicine or psychiatry), but through other dynamics such as group activities, namely Balint, psychodrama, or through the experiences that can derive from a gradual, prudent manipulation of one's own unconscious and that of others".

At the basis of this was the need, outlined to the future practitioner, for a training that would allow them an "approach to the patient based on recognition, respect, the acceptance of their needs, the confident expectation of the realisation of their desire to change, knowing how to allow them to draw on past experiences, creating new life experiences in therapeutic situations.

In this setting, a context of particular protection and nourishment for them takes place, in which the relational component [favours] the integration between the conscious and the unconscious, the regression in the service of the Ego, experiencing the body no longer as a problem but as the target of problems in a vision that is as unified as possible".

---

[68] Piero Parietti, founding member of the 'Bernheim' and teacher of its training courses, reiterated that *"The preparation of the hypnologist [...] cannot be limited to a cultural study, [but must] be realised through a personal transference experience",* (See Guantieri G., *L'ipnosi, come oggetto di studio e mezzo di impiego in medicina*, Rizzoli, Milan, 1973, pp. 212-231). He also specified that it was necessary for the followers to whom he dedicated himself, *to* acquire *"new skills [...] purely psychological, fundamental for a correct attitude towards [...] sexuality, love, human relationships, life"* (Idem cs, p.326. See also Faretta E., Parietti P., *Ben Essere e Sviluppo delle Risorse Personali. Tecniche dal Mal Essere al Ben Essere Consapevole*, Alpes Italia, Rome, 2012).

Guantieri then commented on this point: "It is in this way of operating – we believe – that hypnosis can undoubtedly offer other valuable fruits in the field of human sciences".
The study of hypnosis could therefore not overlook the focus of reflection on the subject-hypnologist.
He also highlighted how the following study topics, to which he referred, had a significant influence on his conduct:

1) The attitudes that lead him to the decision to use hypnosis;
2) The induction methods he used;
3) The method and the goals that he aimed for;
4) The ability to achieve various manifestations;
5) The structure he gave to the interpersonal relationship;
6) The hypnotic manifestations that derive from this modulation;
7) The effects that the hypnologist, with their aptitudes, abilities and limitations, has on the subject's conduct and on what the latter reports.

Guantieri's training project specified the qualities and skills that the student must acquire during training.
" First of all ", he argued, "the following should be considered: the safety of one's own means, the ability to identify, the understanding and control of the emotions that underlie the reactions of the subject, as well as one's own favourable expectations, which are not difficult to establish if they do not exist, marked endogenous depressive components or feelings of guilt, the 'vis medicatrix naturae', certainly activated to a great extent and widely employable in hypnosis and by means of hypnosis, the ability, as well as phonetics, to express various concepts with clarity, simplicity, gradual exposure, the ability to initiate or strengthen motivations and the ability to analyse the subject's responses".
Personal training, both theoretical and practical, to be understood fully as continuous, never-ending, for one's entire professional career: "Another problem connected with teaching is that of continuous updating of practitioners who have completed their training and the mastery of the latest acquisitions on the subject and their harmonisation with the pre-existing conceptual heritage".
However, we were discussing that very special interpersonal relationship that is so central to the thinking of Guantieri, as scientist and educator-trainer.
It was precisely in the field of teaching that he measured the fundamental value of this issue, explored its most hidden implications, formulated its conception and tested its resistance.
And it was precisely, emphasising the peculiarity of the hypnotic relationship, that the natural and resulting attention of the teacher could not ignore the specificity of each of his pupils.
And this originated from the appreciation of the uniqueness of each person and from the consideration of the pedagogical and clinical power of the hypnosis

object the idea of proposing to his students his own method, not only clinically, of close, empathic, convincing, welcoming,"maternal" teaching of hypnosis, which made him a much-appreciated therapist who greatly enhanced his students.

He believed, albeit on the basis of an inextricable formation-initiation, in the ability of every person, whether his student or not, to draw personal formation resources from within themselves.

As such, his training method was original, a gradual and convincing approach to the profound and delicate phenomena of hypnosis. In this sense he was welcoming, to all those who solicited him for therapeutic treatment, or wanted to and knew how to approach him for a particular scientific and human interaction, within his school.

We would like to reiterate an idea already touched upon previously: at the 'Bernheim' Institute there was a "Great 'Gualtiero Guantieri' School of Hypnology". Why?

In the manner of the greatest pedagogical traditions from the distant past to modern times, it brought together, in a singular context, teachers, researchers and students who shared, certainly carried out cultural events, didactic and experimental activities, but with a relational climate and an formative intent, of individual and collective growth that involved everyone, from the lowest-graded pupil to the supreme luminary whose charisma made its mark on the school.

Guantieri – we argued, and we maintain – was a master of dialogue (from the Greek dià, "through" and logos, "speech"), of verbal, logical and rational, but also non-verbal confrontation, so as to foresee emotional and affective manifestations, with a relationship and teaching style that was lively, colloquial and confidential.

He sought the souls of his interlocutors to whom he opened up, with a welcoming and reassuring attitude.

He based learning mainly on experience, to which, in an undeniably complementary way, he gave a methodological role.

And it was in this way that the experience lived by the student-disciple, in close and cohesive participation with the teacher, gradually gained true wisdom.

Thus those thoughts that were constructed, with creativity and intuition, gradually integrated with each other, until they took the shape of a corpus that was outlined in his hypnology.

Guantieri thought of a hypnologist as someone who, with their own personality and behavior, was a therapeutic agent, and that hypnotic therapy should always be considered curative, even when the disease originated and evolved in the body.

He also warned that psychotherapy implies training the hypnologist so as to avoid possible pathological inclinations, both conscious and unconscious.

He generously encouraged an attitude that was conducive to training experiences, informing, motivating, guiding the development of particular psychophysical states and a different state of consciousness (technically achievable by simply directing attention to the hypnotist's voice).

A particular interest of his was to facilitate collaboration among students (but also among his patients), in order to avoid issues of dependency from the outset.

The goal he pursued was to achieve (through hypnotic experiences possibly lived in a state of well-being, safety, efficiency) their personal growth, their autonomy, further self-understanding of their personalities.

The original teaching style of Guantieri and his loyal collaborators, therefore remained systematically attentive to the specificity of each student.

Their relationship with students was close, empathetic, convincing, welcoming, caring, of those who knew and know how to value talents.

These teaching methods were thus a stimulus for the study and in-depth understanding of hypnology; a propellant to a strong desire, rather than a need, for further involvement, a natural push to gaining shared, convinced knowledge.

The hypnologist between omnipotence and impotence

Guantieri warned his students of the danger of "pathological needs for omnipotence or sadism or narcissism, which can often be the basis of systematically very authoritarian methods of induction and treatment, and that motivations for an indiscriminate use of hypnosis can be rooted in a strong sense of frustration, or the need to feel good, or feelings of inferiority or guilt, difficulties and fears, to establish a particularly intimate interpersonal relationship and then use it profitably".

The expert hypnologist who studies and practices hypnosis, and talks about it and disseminates it, is not free of fears regarding the object of study that involves him or her, but is sensitive to their charm, just as may happen with anything magical and mysterious.

This professional, who values and appreciates the masters of hypnology, especially those who have great charisma, and admires them, should usually have a critical sense, avoiding mystifying idealisation.

There are many shamans of all kinds, many healers revered by the public, and there are South American "curanderos", Indian gurus, psychics, palmists, pranotherapists, and then magicians and sorcerers who can distract and dazzle even modern hypnologists.

Milton Erickson (1901-1980), for example, undoubtedly also a master of world hypnology, is easily – exaggeratedly – widely deified as an absolute mentor.

This – let us not forget – could also be a risk with many other characters from the world of hypnology, including Gualtiero Guantieri.

In short, it is easy for the devotees of this knowledge to feel, more or less, "priests" of sectarian, esoteric, exalted and diabolical "churches".

The hypnologist-in-training should therefore ask themselves how fascinated they are in general by what is magical and mysterious, to the point of making it their own, coddling it, holding on to it as it is, to carefully avoid unveiling it, dissecting it, understanding it, as far as possible with total intelligence, because of an underlying fear of losing that captivating enchantment it holds for them, as well as for the patients they care for.

This would be a case of plagiarising one's own soul, that unconscious part that belongs to us all, otherwise anxious of losing an attraction, an energy, but also a feeling of greatness and power.

A useful question that the hypnologist-hypnotist could ask themselves is the following: "Will the hypnosis that I practice not be a halo that makes me holy in my own self-perception, even if I also know that I am a little foolish, so sometimes I also assume a modest attitude - even if that sacred halo on my head must remain there, without my carrying out any true and profound scientific analysis?".

In short, as if the hypnologist-hypnotist did not want to remove that luminous circle that could have been placed around their head, to be special.

Another pressing question could be: "In short, can we tolerate the fact that reason reduces our hypnosis to a simple, understandable, earthly, absolutely human entity?".

Contrary to these feelings, the hypnosis practitioner can also feel bad, become caught up in some qualms, feel that their head is in the clouds, feel the need for clarity regarding their own conception of hypnosis, its validity, and have doubts about themselves, as a scholar and hypnological practitioner.

Hence the need for transparency and clarity with respect to the training programs inherent in modern hypnosis, which can be defined with precision.

A linearity that can be clouded by those affective and unconscious implications already mentioned.

Reason would have it that hypnosis, scientifically considered, is today cleansed of spells and occult aspects, but the heart of its practitioner can be an obstacle to this vision, where great resistance is unleashed, to still retain (perhaps forever?) a magical aspect that makes them histrionic, even in this advanced phase of the history of hypnological science - of which the hypnologist-hypnotist must be an epigone anyway.

Many people are attracted to the subject of hypnosis, both on the side of the scholar and those who seek hypnosis. They have particular inclinations, certain personality traits, common sensitivities that push towards this "hypnotic cosmos". This group of individuals is "insane" in its own way.

The hypnologist-hypnotist might then recognize that they also have dimensions that are somewhat strange, even creative, very elevated, perhaps not of a very canonical spirituality, and a curiosity to understand and find answers to pressing questions that man always asks himself, but which are perhaps not fully satisfying. They must make their own ideologies explicit, the things they believe in and would like to be universally shared. Otherwise it ends up that they are then proposed obtusely, unconsciously, with great fascinating suggestion, which is also – mind you – egoic nourishment for themselves.

Were it so, it might happen, even if in good faith, even if innocent, that the protagonist turns out to be even a little bit naive.

Rationally, adequate reflections are necessary so that one can, with courage and effort, devote oneself to one's profession, other already acquired or in the making. The training of the hypnologist must certainly pay harmoniously relevant attention to theory, to the acquisition of professional technical tools, that is to the various inductive methods and techniques, but above all to their own, continuous, responsible, introspection of his way of placing themselves in the world and at a professional level.

All this must be concretely and actively experienced: not only the acquisition and accumulation of knowledge and operational skills, but also an innovation of oneself, sometimes a metamorphosis of one's own identity, should take place.

7. The future prospects of hypnological science

A conception of hypnology anchored in the past, but highly evolutionary and in progress, cannot neglect its future prospects for study and research.

Guantieri, in the 1970s - let us remark, once more - outlined some points on these issues, to his followers, writing that, having defined the foundations of hypnology, there was undoubtedly the need to seek new acquisitions, noting cognitive shortcomings, many questions open on various levels and from multiple origins, "so as to allow, on the one hand, an action that is no longer empirical but increasingly rational, on the other the opening of multiple perspectives, both experimental and clinical".[69]

This was the basic guideline on the basis of which he proposed research:
1st) relating to hypnotic phenomena that are connected to psychologies, both general and dynamic; 2nd) studies on the correlations and interactions that can occur between psychosomatics, psychopathology and hypnosis;
3rd) on observations and analysis specifically aimed at a deeper hypnological knowledge.

In the first case, the indications were those of amplifying psychological knowledge on dreams, whether spontaneous or induced, on symbolism, on responses to intelligence, personality and projective tests (Rorschach and others); in the second case, Guantieri pointing out the themes of investigation on somatisation, the 'organ language', conversions, paramnesias, the differential diagnosis between organic and functional syndromes and the consequent modifications of the body scheme and the image of the Self; in the third case, proposing an observation of concepts such as visualisations, the vivification of emotions, the activation of conflicts in the hypnotic and post-hypnotic state, automatic writing, age regression, and again – a central question – the need of

---

[69] Guantieri G., *Fondamenti e prospettive dell'ipnologia medica*, in AA. VV., *Lezioni di apertura del Corso di Aggiornamento in Ipnologia medica, Verona, 7-9 maggio 1971*, dossier by the 'H. Bernheim' Institute, Verona, 1971, pp. 134-136.

further investigation into transference and counter-transference within that particular, specific, extraordinary hypnotic relationship that is established between the hypnologist and the subject experiencing hypnosis, in both intra-hypnotic and extra-hypnotic moments.

Evidently, this was a manifesto-program for the development of hypnology, so that it would acquire "true value in the human sciences, through research, the careful study of serious works, congresses on hypnology, teaching activities, gradual internship".[70]

8. Conclusive comments

Guantierian Hypnology proves to have valid and modern foundations of the philosophy of science, a flexible, trans-cultural structure, and therefore a very clear and sure universal scientific value and unmistakable originality.[71]

This hypnology tends to promote the enlightenment of learners and the health of patients by preserving them all from possible damage and probable manipulation.

Guantieri's science has the harmonious connotations of a powerful paradigm that he himself essentially built; it possesses its own unmistakable style and language, proper rhetorical, ontological, moral modulations and a wisdom that is the quintessential to intense, lucidly and profoundly understood and prosecuted experiences.

Guantieri left, in those and through those who knew him, a tangible sign of an unprecedented human and scientific interaction, a seed that must not be lost.

This cultural heritage must be carefully guarded and defended by the entire national and international hypnological scientific community with seriousness, honesty, sincerity and gratitude.

---

[70] Idem c.s., p. 137.

[71] The importance of a multidisciplinary perspective in the study of human behaviour characterises the need for a psychosomatic orientation and an essential overall vision of man in his physical, psychic and relational components is exemplified by a 1989 paper, where Guantieri indicates the close, dual-track relationship , which exists between hypnology and algology and describes the experience of pain as " characterised by a series of neuromuscular, neurovegetative, biochemical, regressive phenomena [... which] has various meanings: temporal, psychological, somatic, emotional [and affective, such as] attributes responsible for the development of ideas and associations, exquisitely individual, that through sensations and emotions and experiences [...] are declined [...] in the most varied behaviours [that] involve the whole person in t heir verbalisations, gestures, postural attitudes [...] and expectations, motivations, vigilance, attention, memory, unconscious learning are involved". In the same work he adds "that there are not only somatic pains, but also psychosomatic pains, which being very different in their genesis and dynamics, imply different approaches particularly in the hypnotherapy field"; because the pain that a person registers on the sensory level at a given moment inevitably recalls previous painful situations, which are therefore immediately relived, but also interpreted and projected into the future, thus made a harbinger of subjective expectations, more or less feared and of a certain degree of severity, considered easily real, indisputable, inevitable, often considered invincible and therefore alienating and depressing (Guantieri G., Ipnosi e terapia del dolore, (Hypnosis and pain therapy), in Newsletter magazine, Edited by 'H. Bernheim' Italian Institute for the Study of Clinical Hypnosis and Psychotherapy -- Research and Training School, Verona, Vol. II , n. 2, October 1989, pp. 7-8).

CHAPTER 4

The Guantierian definition of hypnosis

Hypnosis is the object of study and the means of clinical use with which hypnology is concerned.
The hypnological definition of hypnosis, of the fundamental concepts on which it is based, and its overall consideration, therefore claim a priori, to define boundaries that are modern and scientific and consider precise purposes as opposed to a galaxy of fictitious, fallacious, implausible, very broad, delicate, very confused, magical and occult matter, often proposed by presumptuous and ignorant charlatans and swindlers, who practice – and in acting thus, render – hypnosis a feared and dangerous entity.
It must therefore be implied that hypnosis promoted by hypnology is to be understood as clinical, therapeutic or pedagogical hypnosis.
The hypnotic state that it brings about, when applied in these areas, consists of a collection of neuro-psycho-physiological conditions that the person achieves when hypnotic induction has taken place.
It is a Fourth Organismic State, different from the state of wakefulness, from that of non-REM sleep (in which one sleeps but does not dream) and from REM sleep, which is typical of dream activity.
Guantieri and the 'Bernheim' Institute of Clinical Hypnosis considered and conceived of this hypnosis as the means to respond positively to the requests for support or help that the person may address to pedagogy (hypnology is undoubtedly pedagogical, at least if taught to hypnological students), psychosomatic medicine and therefore to devotees thereof: conscious and responsible doctors, psychologists, educators or psychotherapists.
These specialists in the subject first consider mankind in its holistic complexity, that is somatic, psychological, relational, placed in a context in which the person has grown up and lives and to whom to turn with a spirit of service.

Guantieri specified that one should "consider and, above all, feel man [...] as a psychosomatic unit, organism and person at the same time, in intimate contact, action and reaction with their environment [...] and to look at him in a very particular way [...] that is, not paying less attention to the body, but rather more to the psyche".[72]
He and his collaborators highlighted that hypnosis is inherent in the mental and affective sphere and acts in that psychological space of free Levinian movement

---

[72] Guantieri G., *Fondamenti e prospettive dell'ipnologia medica*, in AA. VV., *Lezioni di apertura del Corso di Aggiornamento in Ipnologia medica*, Verona, 7-9 maggio 1971, dossier by the 'H. Bernheim' Institute, Verona, 1971, p. 117.

as Kurt Levin (1890-1982) would say, where emotions and thoughts can be expanded beyond the limits of the usual.

Thus, an area is defined where the person can find full freedom to be present and to interact, to open up to introspective experiences, to rediscover noble and sublime feelings that arise in the presence of the grandiose, the fascinating, ecstasy, the sacred, or even horror, but to acquire awareness and necessarily recognize every human emotion, even if considered negative, such as fear or anger, disgust or sadness, so that all this translates into a more precise awareness and allows realistic consideration, open to the contemplation of oneself and the world.

Clinically speaking, sometimes the hypnotic experience materialises in the search for wounds due to old traumas, suffered and erased in the memory so that they can be brought back to awareness and healed. This is neither easy nor fun, but it is important for these events to be integrated into the patient's personal history.

We come therefore to the definition of hypnosis, hypnologically framed by Guantieri's academy.

"Hypnosis is a process of learning to develop, in accordance with certain principles and by means of adequate stimuli, multiple skills which, expanding the dimensions of man conceived as an inseparable psychosomatic unit, in conditions of health or illness, are variously and widely usable for experimental, prophylactic, diagnostic and therapeutic purposes". [73]

Some have proposed additions to Guantieri's explanation of hypnosis, pointing to a corollary assumption that would find synthesis in the expression "passing through the body, that is, involving multiple Self-and hetero-induced bodily responses".

This subsequent elaboration of the thought of the 'Bernheim' Institute founders, however, appears to be a redundant and misleading addition in that, where it is said to underline the somatic element – in the light of that vision of the holistic man mentioned above – it is not only an addition, but it places the same as a pre-eminent factor of imbalance with respect to that unitary whole that Guantieri indicated as necessary to recognize.

On the other hand, the enrichment of the definition of hypnosis derives from an integration of considerations, elaborated by the same author, about a fundamental aspect of the hypnotic state: the special, peculiar relationship, in many respects still in need of study and research, which is the interpersonal relationship.

The psycho-physical state that is established in hypnosis cannot be separated from the dynamics that develop in the interpersonal relationship.

These two cornerstones – state and relationship – on which hypnosis is articulated are quite peculiar and are intimately related to each other. Together they contribute to the establishment of multiple psycho-dynamic phenomena that

---

[73] Guantieri G., *L'ipnosi, come oggetto di studio e mezzo di impiego in medicina*, Rizzoli, Milan, 1973, p. IV on the front cover.

involve the person and their way of being, in expression and affections, which are progressively, increasingly totalising.

In this special state of being, a regressive, dynamic and reversible Self of the protagonists' being in hypnosis would be established, according to Guantieri. This is true, albeit in different ways, because the roles cannot be confused, for either hypnotist or experiential subject.

This regressive Self would prevail, for the subjects who live it, over an "I" which, in a condition of modified consciousness, concedes to it, regressing, letting go, trusting trustfully, for a perceived, proper, beneficial and healthy interest of those who offer and those who receive help, to an extraordinary interaction, very free from patterns and norms, where affections, emotions, desires, feelings and full self-expression prevail.[74]

---

[74] There are many states of consciousness. The typically ordinary one is experienced when one is awake and alert. William James, (1842-1910), American psychologist and philosopher, one of the fathers of modern psychology, explored the theme of states of consciousness in great depth. *"Our ordinary waking consciousness"*, he wrote, *"is only a special type of consciousness, while all around, separated by the thinnest partitions, stand entirely different potential forms of consciousness. We can live a whole life without suspecting their existence; but as soon as the necessary stimulus is applied, all of a sudden they appear in their full completeness"*, (James W., *The force of character*, Società Editrice Libraria, Milan, 1901). Listening to our body which is hot or cold, wet or dry, hungry or thirsty, or sleepy, considering the signs we write or read and understand, make comparisons with past experiences, experience emotions, know where to go, what day it is, what time it is, eventually deciding to turn on the radio to listen to music or go somewhere: these are ordinary conditions of consciousness. They have to do with adaptation and survival, with consensual realities of cultural sharing of languages and tools, values, institutions, authorities, etc., while at the same time being beneficiaries and victims of this consciousness with which, at the same time, understandings and compromises are created, but at the same time limits are built on the perception and consideration of what is outside these schemes, thus ceasing to look, feel, perceive, think. In these contexts, some experiences are encouraged, while others are discouraged or repressed in order to build ordinary and collective culture. Similar or analogous forms are easily received and understood on the basis of past experiences, but conclusions are determined that can be deceiving, as the idea that they can sometimes be different from usual is neglected. We 'see' what is expected, even if this is not true. There is a rigid use of functions and procedures in ordinary consciousness, one acquires familiarity with some things of the world, but many others remain foreign. Thus the body, emotions, thought itself, and decisions and decision-making methods, and the use of memory, concepts of time and space acquire a stable structure and conform to what common thought proposes. Different cultures easily express different, often opposite states of ordinary consciousness. For example, people who belong to ethnic groups in which black magic is normally practiced have no difficulty in relating to benevolent or malevolent spirits, while in other anthropological contexts these things are not even conceived, or simply, considered silly. Furthermore, in the complexity of the picture, the individual variables (mainly emotional), can lead people, even if belonging to the same culture, to perceive and understand the same events in absolutely irreconcilable ways. An example might be that of the consideration of the phenomenon of immigration in Europe. On the other hand, there are non-ordinary states of consciousness in conditions of extraordinary happiness, of mystical raptures, of paroxysmal excitations, in moments of sexual climax, when one has a fever, in psychopathological states of delirium or hallucination, when the mind is in the capacity to produce sudden and exhilarating causal intuitions, when subtle cognitive or overwhelming parapsychological experiences are operated. A singular case is that of the dream. It involves perceptions, memories, thoughts, emotions, according to very particular modes of functioning. In this case, what is hidden in the depths of the human soul, repressed desires, the subconscious, the unconscious all tend to reveal themselves, while reflective thinking and logical intelligence fall asleep and fail. Hypnotic immersion is also a modified state of consciousness. It enhances the ability to concentrate on the hypnotist's suggestions to which particularly vivid attention is directed. In this case, the hypnotised person can have unusual, out-of-the-ordinary experiences. They may perceive themselves, for example, as smaller or taller, heavier or lighter, regress to an earlier age, younger or infantile, they may experience suggested emotions, remember forgotten things, buried over time by a psychological need for self-protection from painful trauma suffered. Hypnosis can promote better and more incisive intentionality, or even very introspective centring on one's self, thus improving self-awareness and self-image.

Of course, the regressive nature of the hypnotic condition is not exclusive; it also belongs to sleep, to disease, to many other modified states of consciousness. It is not always desirable. In clinical or pedagogical hypnosis, this regression manifests itself in primitive, infantile, simple and genuine modes of behavior that enhance the interpersonal relationship.

Hypnosis is therefore a tool capable of innovating the traditional doctor-patient relationship, making it more stringent, thorough, effective, and even faster.

CHAPTER 5

Self-hypnosis and relaxation techniques

Hypnology, psychosomatic medicine, dynamic psychology and pedagogy offer multiple methods of relaxation. Hypnology considers them one of the areas of its expertise; it can give them theoretical support, consider their validity and limits, and knows how to specify their indications and contraindications.

They are useful for achieving deep rest, recovering energy, reaching a state of calm, and therefore the search for a parasympathetic neurophysiological condition, but they can be very introspective and are thus of important psychological importance.

In any case, if well employed, they are useful for promoting the health of the person, who wants to actively take charge of this emotional investment in themselves.

Sometimes they focus on more somatic and neuromuscular aspects, in other cases on relaxing themes that can nurture calm, serenity and positive thinking.[75]

When you want to dynamically consult the deep, unknown and mysterious psyche of the Self, the methods pre-eminently assume a psychoanalytic character.

1. Self-hypnosis as a singular hypnotic modality

Many relaxation methods are self-hypnotic.

We could say otherwise that self-hypnosis can be achieved through different procedures.

How can it be known, how can it be learned?

The shortcuts that lead to the knowledge of self-hypnosis by avoiding and neglecting the study of the basics of hypnology are absolutely inadvisable.

Progressive muscle relaxation, autogenic training, transcendental meditation, yoga and other relaxation techniques, many of which are of Eastern origin, can

---

[75] Positive psychology deals, among other issues, with the methods that allow for the promotion of subjective well-being and the enhancement of a person's potential. In this way, it implements interventions aimed at mobilising skills and resources that open one up to the prospect of prevention, personal growth, strengthening resilience and, consequently, a better quality of life. It promotes research that uses meditative and relaxation techniques aimed at increasing the level of pleasurable activities, teaching an optimistic explanatory style and coping strategies, characterised by the discovery of positive meanings even in adversity. The results show that, by cultivating positive emotions, in addition to preventing and relieving problematic negative emotions, health and well-being are optimised and states of the organism are produced in which the regulation of vital processes become efficient and optimal, easy and freely flowing, associated with positive feelings that in the long run, from occasional experiences, can become concrete brain engrams, connections, synaptic connections that strengthen between neurones, i.e. brain structures, as well as distinctive psychological personality traits (for further information see also Meneghini AM, *Meditation and broaden-and-build theory*, ReS magazine, CISERPP, Verona, Year XXI, n.1, 2013)

constitute in the modern age, as we said, partial chapters of the science of hypnosis, even if many of them were conceived by authors unaware of any hypnological principle and now have practitioners who proceed blindly, ignorant of what really characterises their instruments.

Any method of relaxation today cannot disregard the in-depth study of the scientific principles behind it and the clinical and pedagogical implications it has, in order to avoid the risk of inexperience and major contraindications.

Self-hypnosis, thus a branch of hypnology, can be an important skill that in general anyone can acquire, through brief training courses.

It allows one to create states of relaxation and conditions of reflection to better forge in oneself, gradually and progressively, personal skills of concentration and physical and psychic self-control, to gain decent control over anxiety, to better master one's of emotions and see even more significant enhancements in physical, cognitive and relational performance.

But moreover, with this tool one can carry out relevant self-analysis,[76] going as far as immersion in profound existential meditation, contemplate spiritual aspects of one's existence, reach a state of trance or true contemplative, religious or secular rapture.

So this is the path, then, to self-hypnosis: start with hypnology!

Hypnosis has always belonged to man; it is inherent in our essence; it would be unthinkable to conceive and understand one without the other and vice versa.

Angelico Brugnoli defines self-hypnosis as "a modified state of consciousness obtained through long and motivated training [...] with the use of various methods of relaxation, practicing introspection [...] and reaching degrees [...] of total involvement of our deepest personality".

Training is therefore the key that, in a slow and constant way, allows for, the "journey [...that is] never completely finished, because once a goal has been reached [...] others appear on the horizon of the mind [...] open to a kaleidoscope of sensations, of visualisation of colours, environments, situations, always new and fascinating experiences".[77]

2. Differences between hypnosis and self-hypnosis

In his historical reflection on the phenomena of hypnosis, Gualtiero Guantieri identifies three fundamental elements necessary for the realisation of these extraordinary human experiences.

---

[76] A concrete example of self-analysis can be the production, in a self-hypnotic state, of free whispered abreactions, of emotions, feelings, desires, the most secret and unspeakable, to be recorded through a tape recorder, for a subsequent transcription and meditation, (See Malesani P.G., *Self -hypnosis and abreaction: exposition and a case discussion,* in AA. VV. (edited by Guarneri G.), *Hypnosis in Psychotherapy and Psychosomatic Medicine,* (Proceedings of the III European Congress on *Hypnosis in Psychotherapy and Psychosomatic Medicine,* Abano Terme (Padua), Il Segno, Negrar, (Verona), 1985).

[77] Brugnoli A., *Stati di coscienza modificati,* self-printed, Verona, 2000

The first factor is the "person endowed with particular attributes, always a source of original information", the second is a complement represented by the subjects "who must develop certain effects", the third is supported "by the environment from which stimuli come, aimed at contributing to the initiation and evolution of the phenomena that we intend to achieve, which differ according to the purpose".[78] The author emphasises the relevance of the context in which these experiences take place (for example the temple and its rituals, the night, dances, songs, libations or otherwise the hypnoanalyst's couch).

He has always indicated the hypnotic relationship as a "conditio sine qua non" to bring about the change in the psycho-physical state as a corresponding situation of modified consciousness; the two polarities in relation mutually influence each other, so that the closer the first is, the more profound effects the second achieves, which in turn gives energy to this singular sharing, of a regressive nature, which manifests itself in often primitive ways and with sometimes primordial behaviours.[79]

Here, however, an apparent paradox opens up: considering the above, hypnosis and self-hypnosis would differ in a radically different, irreconcilable way, due to the lack, in the second case, of one of the three constitutive pillars of hypnosis: that of the interpersonal relationship.[80]

At this point, the same thesis that self-hypnosis is a chapter of hypnological science would fall.

However, self-hypnosis is able to promote psychophysical experiences that deeply involve the unity and complexity of the person.

In addition to relaxation, one can reach the heart of one's self, get a glimpse into the preconscious and the unconscious, thus encountering very deep or otherwise transcendent aspects of one's personality, where one can open up to contemplative gazes on those constitutive aspects that are rooted in the tonic-emotional body, that is, in that individual essence from which every vital and existential expression emanates.

There is no doubt, therefore, that very significant changes in the typically hypnotic ordinary condition can be achieved with self-hypnosis.

The question that remains open, then, is the following: how is an interpersonal relationship configured in self-hypnosis?

The first consideration we could make concerns the instructor from whom the learning of self-hypnosis cannot be separated.

They are undoubtedly a kind of care provider, as clinician, doctor, psychologist, psychotherapist or psycho-pedagogist.

---

[78] Guantieri G., *L'ipnosi, come oggetto di studio e mezzo di impiego in medicina*, Rizzoli, Milan, 1973, p. 115.
[79] Idem c.s., p. 50.
[80] Undoubtedly, on a dynamic and psychoanalytic level, without the hypnologist, neither transference nor countertransference, relational aspects that are not exhaustive but essential to the hypnotic condition, can take place. The result would then be to obtain a modified state of consciousness, but as a set of conditions similar to those obtained through the hypnotic relationship, but not coincidental.

They intend to use hypnological tools according to precise regulatory and technical prescriptions that they must respectfully comply with.

This, of course, without forgetting the possibility of infiltrating the world of clinical and pedagogical hypnosis by self-styled hypnotists, who are ignorant, presumptuous charlatans from to stay away from.

It is evident that if one follows this instructor, one proceeds to build a relationship of mutual trust, while forming a bond that strengthens over time.

In fact, the instructions that they give have bodily and psychic relevance, must be accepted and shared, involve completely unique involvements, involve verbalisations on the part of the subject which are communications relating to the latter's own intimacy.

It may also happen that the subject arrives at self-hypnosis and implements an initiation simply by consulting a few (practical) handbooks, among the many available on the market: there are all types, many of which are very serious and scientifically valid.

This is a path that leads to an arduous journey, where one can easily give up, but if it works, we might imagine the level of sharing that can exist between those who wrote the book and those who read it.

Is it possible, then, to hypnotise oneself? The answer is yes, however, on the condition of the previous considerations.

Everyone has an inclination to and capacity for introspection.

However, there are self-hypnotic techniques in which the principle of self-control is deliberately activated and can be organised continuously, thus paving the way to invest in one's self.

Using these easy-to-learn specific techniques on one's own,, it will thus be possible to enter into modified states of consciousness that simply consist of a withdrawal from the world and from one's ordinary relationship with time and space, to the benefit of a gradual deep concentration on one's own psychophysical perceptions, representations and images concerning oneself.

The achievable goals will be, progressively, to simply rest (in a state of pleasant calm), to release tensions, to lower the levels of one's psycho-physical attrition, to recharge energy, but also to expand one's psychological, existential and spiritual freedom.

CHAPTER 6

The Guantierian hypnotic induction method

"Our method," writes Guantieri,[81] "is based on the conception that hypnosis can be considered as a learning process to de-automate the ego systems (inductive phase) and subsequently re-automate them ("deepening" phase), resulting in the activation function of a subsystem of the ego, (the Guantierian Self, see Chapter 3), endowed with particular properties, while the realistically oriented ego persists at the same time. The method tends to facilitate these processes as much as possible. Progressive de-automation is favored by us by initiating expectations in the subject that conform to the concept we have today of hypnosis, even before starting induction. We therefore distinguish two precise phases in the hypnotic approach: pre-inductive and inductive".

1. The pre-inductive phase

In the first stage, an interview is initiated aimed, in addition to collecting anamnestic data, at bringing out elements that lead to the discovery of distress or a diagnosis of illness and an orientation of the patient's personality, while establishing an appropriate interpersonal relationship.

It is thus explained, with the frequent use of analogies, that hypnosis is nothing more than a learning process to develop a particular psychophysical state, different from both sleep and wakefulness, which allows a new, very productive way of functioning of the organism and a different state of consciousness. That is, it is a succession of mental processes, of particular psychic activities that also lead to somatic effects, which initiates latent functions in each of us or improves them, if already manifested, as happens when we play certain games, such as chess for instance, which can therefore be recommended as real therapies. Like any learning process, for example that of learning a language, a sport or a hobby, developing hypnosis implies particular knowledge and attitudes (the latter present in a latent state in each of us) and a training method to be followed with interest and constancy, which proceed gradually.

However, this learning does not imply any commitment, since the initiation and proceeding of certain mechanisms by the action of precise stimuli are completely spontaneous. In fact, it is sufficient to direct attention to the voice of the hypnologist-hypnotist: this will act on certain nerve Centres, both as a physical stimulus, like music or a sound, and as a psychological stimulus, favored by

---

[81] Guantieri G. *L'ipnosi, come oggetto di studio e mezzo di impiego in medicina*, Rizzoli, Milan 1973, summary, also compiled by the author, pp. 157-167.

environmental conditions, the passage of time, one's mental orientation or the position assumed.

The position best suited to allow hypnosis to develop is that which is consistent with muscle relaxation. We therefore invite the patient to assume a comfortable position in an armchair, with an adjustable backrest. In fact, the horizontal position may be experienced as a state of succumbing and therefore may be undesirable or unsuccessful. We then invite the subject to again turn their gaze to wherever they so choose and pay attention to our words. We also note that this fixing of the gaze together with the action of the timbre, tone and volume of voice, will determine responses that will be perceived, in a more or less subjective way, as psychophysical changes, such as inertia or numbness or relaxation or distension, while the point where the gaze is fixed will oscillate or blur and may present other variations due to fatigue of the eyeballs. These changes, which become progressively more and more evident, may be followed gradually, initially by the desire to lower the eyelids, then their closing, however this is not essential. Parallel to the aforementioned changes, others will be established in the brain structures, which are responsible for a special kind of rest, that is increasingly complete, widespread and profound.

This rest will extend until it permeates every mental, nervous and muscular structure, causing even further modifications that are also very beneficial. The attention constantly directed by our voice towards these changes will be able to perceive and appreciate them more and more.

The subject will thus learn to enter a very pleasant, entirely new, state, thanks to the stimuli used, just as they have already learned to enter, in a completely spontaneous way, into wakefulness from sleep. From the hypnotic state then developed, they will be able to distract themselves with equal ease, following certain suggestions, given at the right moment. In this way, at each session, what was learned in the previous session will be enacted, while new skills will also be refined from time to time.

The experiences will feel more and more pleasant and become a source of satisfaction, as is always the case, after all, when one proceeds successfully in a new activity of particular interest.

2. The induction phase

In the induction phase, the key is essentially spoken word, properly employed. It is in fact the most powerful activator of the hypnotic process, both in physiological and psychological terms, since, by expressing emotions, sounds and concepts at the same time, it contains within it stimuli that act, simultaneously and at different times, on each of the mechanisms that can be considered the onset of hypnosis.

Initially, the same tone, timbre and volume of voice should be maintained used during the informative interview, immediately preceding the induction; at the same time, however, between one word and another, we insert progressively longer pauses of silence. That is, first of all, slowly and gradually, a stimulation that meets the requirements of monotony and rhythmicity should be realised. Subsequently, when the prodromes of relaxation appear, the characteristics of the voice change, differently from individual to individual, so that specific individual affective needs are satisfied and the most appropriate hypnotic interpersonal relationship develops spontaneously. In fact, those who want to be guided gently need different verbal stimuli, not only for the concepts they express but also for the way in which they are given, from those needed by those who instead want to be led authoritatively, or to those who prefer to be simply directed and therefore left free to perform their tasks. In other words, verbal stimuli — essentially mechanical in origin -- should be strengthened, that is, aimed at inducing above all a narrowed field of perception, making them capable of also acting psychologically, parallel to the concepts that they are progressively communicating.

The concepts suggested are as generic as possible (inertia, numbness, relaxation, rest). The patient can thus translate them into concrete realities in a completely subjective way and more freely than when specific suggestions such as lightness or sleep are given, which in the initial phase of induction may be rejected as unlikely, at that point.

Such realities end up being identified, thanks in part to the expectations initiated in the pre-induction phase, in the inhibition of voluntary movements, which paves the way for the "deepening" of hypnosis. This neuromotor phenomenon, even if not suggested in any way, usually results spontaneously from the sense of inertia or numbness, subjectively developed as lightness or heaviness or as another sensation. In fact, with considerable frequency, once the induction is over, the subject reports an inability to move their hands or upper limbs, or an alteration in relation to these body parts and the space around them.

Any resistance is thus reduced or eliminated, through the aforementioned pre-inductive and inductive methods, motivation is more easily activated or strengthened, the collection of information and its integration with previous information are facilitated; in turn thus facilitating the collaboration of the subject.

Even particular problems of dependency are avoided from the outset, as the interpersonal relationship that the method tends to establish is similar to that between a person who wishes to acquire certain skills, who is aware of having the means, and another, who, by means of certain instructions and stimuli, is progressively led to such an acquisition, which they naturally consider possible.

At the end of the session, the subject is invited to report on what they have experienced: their responses and judgments are taken into careful consideration, in order to better understand their personality, possibly improve the induction method and further orient themselves on how to follow the treatment or finally enhance certain therapeutic effects, already initiated spontaneously.

If no effect develops during the first induction, the procedure is repeated unchanged, if there are no reasons to suggest a modification, after several days, in a second or possibly third session, at the same time   at the same time initiating the subject into a relaxing technique of psychic self-concentration, known as Schultz Autogenic Training.[82]

3. The intensification of hypnosis

A "deepening" of hypnosis can be reached, once the inhibition of voluntary movements has begun, by activating the hypnotic imagination.

In other words, certain figurative representations, at first simple and then more complex, are induced, with an appropriate procedure, slowly and gradually, usually throughout several sessions, aimed at arousing specific progressive effects; the hypnosis then intensifies.

That is to say, at first the subject is led to "visualise" the various elements of a scene of which they are a spectator; subsequently, to project themselves and to identify with the scene itself, experiencing it in such a way as to feel particular effects, including of a sensory nature.[83]

The production of hypnotic images may initially be either slow or quick, clear or confused; in subsequent sessions this usually happens, from time to time, increasingly faster and clearer. The suggested images are shaped more or less subjectively, also depending on the induction method used (permissive or authoritarian).

---

[82] Schultz J.H., *Il training autogeno: esercizi inferiori*, vol. I, Feltrinelli, Milano, 1968; Schultz J.H., *Il training autogeno: esercizi superiori*, vol. II, Feltrinelli, Milano, 1971.

[83] It seems to be correctly deduced that, in the Guantierian vision of hypnosis, in its hypnology, visualisations are appropriate above all from a perspective of involvement that never deviates from a global consideration in which the body always remains, with its physiology and its sensations, anchored to the psychic, emotional, experienced facts, contemplating, in this way, the hypnotic state, strongly integrated by a peculiar interpersonal relationship that is essential to the realisation of the hypnotic clinical condition and to the production of powerful effects of treatment, of healing the patient or trainee. Guantierian clinical hypnology, well grounded in epistemological assumptions, strongly structured on solid principles, has its own original trait with regard to the theme of visualisations that are so often proposed in hypno-therapeutic sessions to the subjects of the hypnotic experience. On this basis, pindaric pursuing of the sublime is to be avoided, nostalgically pursuing timeless worlds, being fanatics of myth and heroic action, rhetorical singers of pure poetic praise, men eager to intensely express peaks of exaltation of civil and cultural ideals; simply: it is good to be concrete hypnologist-hypnotists. Psychosomatic realism does not mean that creative space is excluded. Rather, what should be feared are the self-centred affective dynamics of practitioners inadvertently led to the manipulation of their clients. Guantieri, in order to achieve analgesia, proposed, for example, to the subject, to visualise various elements of a scene in which they were, at first, a spectator and, subsequently, a protagonist projected and identified with it, experiencing certain — even sensory -- effects in an experimental way, for instance in the phase during which a snowy expanse is suggested,, with a pile of snow into which to place their bare hand, to feel a sensation of intense cold, as they had presumably already experienced concretely in previous real-life situations.

4. The de-hypnotisation phase

De-hypnotisation is achieved in a much simpler way than those necessary to carry out the induction: the subject is usually informed that hypnosis will cease when they sense a certain signal.

It may be suggested for instance that "hypnosis will wear off soon", and will cease completely when the subject opens their eyes — in doing so, however, leaving behind all its beneficial effects.

Instead, in saying that it is time to slowly move away from this particular state of concentration and gradually return to reconnect with external reality, and in reiterating that hypnosis will thus begin to become less intense, it will nevertheless retain all its beneficial effects, be they general or local, superficial or profound. The hypnologist will continue to tell the subject that they will continue to remove themselves and that hypnosis will lessen in intensity with each passing moment, more and more. The subject will then be told that the hypnosis is now light, or superficial. However, the hypnologist emphasised that its beneficial effects remain unchanged, that everything is perfectly normal and self-regulated.

At that point, the subject will be invited to open their eyes, with the hypnologist pointing out that hypnosis has now ceased, that the person who has experienced it is in perfect shape, is perfectly efficient in every aspect, from spiritual, to mental, and physical, once again returning to that relationship, in a very satisfactory manner, with their entire external reality.

After a few sessions, when the patient has fully experienced all that is suggested, they will be told that the procedure is much faster: they will simply be informed that they will gradually come out of the hypnotic state, in the way they have by now become familiar with.

With the aforementioned modes of de-hypnotisation, the subject will be allowed time to gradually reorganise their being in the most suitable way for resuming contact with their external environment. This recovery also occurs completely rationally; equally rational are the persistence of well-being, safety and efficiency developed in hypnosis.

As soon as the de-hypnotisation procedure has been completed, the subject generally presents an appearance similar to that of a person awakened from physiological sleep; they usually continue to feel the same sense of well-being and calm perceived during the state of hypnosis, while it was wearing off. Sometimes, very rarely, the subject may complain of minor symptoms although these are usually completely transient, referable to unconscious resistance or to excessive mental concentration or finally to a too rapid de-hypnotisation.

It is also possible to observe, albeit very rarely, that the subject, despite the suggestions that hypnosis is about to wear off, does not immediately withdraw from the hypnotic state. This may be down to the subject experiencing hypnosis as a situation so gratifying that it would be undesirable to abandon it, to not having exactly understood the instructions or even to having fallen into a state of physiological sleep. The latter can sometimes occur when the pauses of silence between one suggestion and another have been too long, so that the relationship with the hypnologist has been lost. It is therefore advisable, in the event that prolonged moments of silence are interspersed, to inform the subject that there will be pauses, despite which, when the hypnologist resumes speaking, the subject will return to perfectly following instructions.

In each of the aforementioned cases, it is possible to insist the cessation of hypnosis either by communicating to the subject that they will be able to come out of hypnosis when they deem it most appropriate or are completely disinterested in the event.

In any case, hypnosis nevertheless ends spontaneously; the person who has been asked about the reason for their conduct is often also able to answer why.

Just as suggestions directed toward bringing hypnosis to an end may not be followed, so may one come out of hypnosis contrary to the directions given. This may be due to disturbing intra-hypnotic sensations (spontaneous or indirectly suggested) or to the fact that a given task is too unpleasant or difficult to perform, or to the onset of resistance, for which the subject, not wishing to follow a certain suggestion or, more simply, if the way in which it is given to them is very unwelcome, they defend themselves by coming out of hypnosis.

Prudence is also necessary in dismissing the subject: they must be left alone, when one is sure that the hypnotic state is completely over.

CHAPTER 7

Compendium of Guantieri's 'L'ipnosi' ("Hypnosis")

The text opens with a quote from Gorgias of Leontini's Encomium on Helen, with a clever and futuristic choice that is truly "evergreen" because it seems to be written by modern holistic and neuroplastic scientists:

"Speech is a powerful ruler, which with a very little and invisible body accomplishes divine deeds; for it is able to stop fear and to remove sorrow and to create joy and to augment pity."

A preamble then follows, relating to the field of medicine in the 1970s , deeply shaken by the need for renewal and interest in a comparison with various disciplines in order to make progress in the overall knowledge of man.
Among these sciences is hypnology. By dealing with the study of hypnosis, it allows the critical investigation of the phenomena that constitutes its essence, allows its onset, its stabilisation, its expressions, its somatic and psychic effects.
The opening passage concludes by outlining the various parts of the book: the remote origins of hypnosis, its phenomenology, its nature, the modalities of its induction, the experimental and clinical aspects, the treatment of somatic and psychosomatic disorders, and attention to its applications in obstetrics, surgery and dentistry.

1. Development of hypnosis studies

The pre-scientific phase

The pre-scientific phase of hypnology, founded exclusively on empiricism and observation of phenomena, originates in the mists of time.
Archaeological finds, discovered in prehistoric tombs and temples, lead us to believe that, as far back as the earliest times, phenomena of hypnosis or manifestations related to it were known, as were methods practiced by shamans, sorcerers or priests, through ceremonies or rites tending to induce non-ordinary states of conscience propitiatory of divinatory faculties or therapeutic effects, were known.

There is no shortage of a biblical references to hypnotic episodes: the prophet Elijah's sleep in the cave of Haifa[84]; reports that in ancient Greece[85] Asclepius

---

[84] Elijah experienced extraordinary moments in the desert. In the Bible we read: *"Then a great and powerful wind tore the mountains apart and shattered the rocks before the Lord, but the Lord was not in the wind. After the wind there was an earthquake, but the Lord was not in the earthquake. After the earthquake came a fire, but the Lord was not in the fire.*

healed his patients in ways that were certainly hypnotic, as is found in accounts of the Dionysian or Bacchic mysteries, e.g., of the "Magna Mater" described in "Attis" by Gaius Valerius Catullus (84 B.C.-54 B.C.).

The 6th century BC fire ritual of Persian medicine is mentioned, as well as Indian practices of the time, inspired by Brahmanism[86] and Buddhism,[87] the rites of the

---

And after the fire came a gentle whisper. [...] Then a voice said to him, 'What are you doing here, Elijah?' He replied, 'I have been very zealous for the Lord God Almighty. The Israelites have rejected your covenant, [...].' The Lord said to him, 'Go back the way you came, and go to the Desert of Damascus. When you get there, anoint Hazael [...] Also, anoint Jehu [...] and anoint Elisha...'" (2 Kings 19:21). Non-ordinary conditions of awareness are repeatedly found in the Bible. Remember, for example, the patriarch Joseph son of Jacob who had knowledge and ability to interpret his own dreams and that of others. Among others, he managed to impress the king of Egypt himself with his dream interpretations. Religious and Christian literature is very rich in texts that allude to hypnotic states. Francisco of Osuna, in the *Third Spiritual Alphabet*, illustrates an exegesis of contemplation performed in a state of deep psychophysical relaxation and based on the repetition of words of prayer or the monosyllable *"no"* to detach the mind from thoughts that are not addressed to the Lord. In a medieval religious 15th-century text, *The Cloud of the Unknown* it is suggested to exclude sensory distraction and physical activity to obtain a different state of consciousness of union with God through the continuous repetition of words of religious content.

[85] In ancient Greece, Asclepius was the God of medicine. Son of Apollo and Coronis, he was entrusted by his father to the centaur Chiron who taught him the art of medicine. Having then dared to bring the dead back to life, he was electrocuted by Zeus. His attributes were the staff, the book scroll, the bundle of poppies, but above all it was the snake which had brought him the miraculous herb that was used to resurrect Hippolytus, the son of Theseus. After his death, Asclepius and the serpent were placed in the sky in the constellation of Ophiuchus or Serpent-Bearer. Asclepius' wife was Epione and their daughter was Panacea, *she who heals everything*. Sticks and poppies, snakes and divine elements come together in an ideology of creative medicine, capable however of producing marvellous transcendences able to soothe suffering and healing.

[86] In the Vedas and Upanishads we come across a sort of Castanedian *peyote* (ally) (Castaneda C., *The Teachings Of Don Juan*, Edizioni Astrolabio, Rome, 1968) which is Soma. According to some hymns Rigveda (from about the 11th century BC), it is the juice squeezed from a plant, which is exciting and hallucinogenic, and a source of health and immortality. In Vedic rituals, it is also God, honored as a source of creative power from which to draw inspiration. By taking potions, one imagines visionary and kinetic ecstasy. Vedic rites foresee the passage of *The Consecration of the King, The Sacrifice of the Horse, The Rite of the Drink of Pleasure*, sacred acts such as *The Fire Ceremony*. Pleased the gods with the offerings of Soma, priest-poets and worshippers take the drink with extraordinary results whereby the blind can see and the lame can walk. And there are ecstasies that grant exclamations such as *"I, with my immense power, have overcome the sky and this immense earth"* or *"I am great! Powerful! Able to fly up to the sky! Haven't I drunk the soma?"*. Soma is similar to the *Haoma* of pre-Islamic Iranian Zoroastrianism. It is not only an entity worthy of veneration but the personification of divinity. Obtained from Ephedra, *Haoma* is stimulating hallucinogenic juice. Ancient texts conquest that *Haoma*, taken during certain rites from the recitation of lyrical hymns, bestows strength, victory and wisdom and induce an ecstatic state. With great differences and yet many similarities, Taoism was established in ancient China around the first century BC.. *Tao* is the vital flow that is the origin of everything and flows ceaselessly, always changing and always remaining the same. It is represented in the *Yin-yang* which is Spirit, Soul, Genius, with the body of coiled and intertwined serpents, which produces and brings to life in itself the two complementary principles, concentric and coincident, inseparable and opposite, in which the Unity has differentiated   into existence. Immortal   are those who comes to purify their own flesh from decay through specific practices. These are techniques of mental concentration and meditation, connected with breathing exercises for the circulation of *Chi Kung*, taught by Taoist monks. They are shamans, evokers of the spirits of the dead, doctors, magicians, astrologers, fortune-tellers. They aim for the realisation of the *"Immortal, Holy Man, who obtains Long Life since nothing has a hold on the body when the spirit is not disturbed. Nothing can harm the Sage, wrapped in the integrity of his nature, protected by the freedom of his Spirit"*, (Lieh-tzu II). These monks preside over *Rites of Reintegration* (death and mystical resurrections), *Ecstatic* (new knowledge that subtracts death and pain), *Ascetics* (cancellation of the personality for a longer or shorter time), with a sexual, sacralising and cosmic background. They also develop alchemies to make drugs, elixirs and medicines, mainly intended to prolong life. Their intent is that the energies circulating in the body (sexual and digestive), are refined and transformed, through breathing, into a special, life-saving Internal Energy.

[87] A defining aspect of Buddhism is the orientation towards meditation for a renunciation of the world and a detachment from it, which will be rewarded with *Nirvana*. We find a similar point of view in Zen aimed at

Mayans, Aztecs and Incas of Central and South America.[88]

We recall famous ancient Egyptian papyri, such as that of Edwin Smith, which represents medicine practiced in a highly suggestive way among those peoples, around the 30th century BC.[89]

Initiation rites still practiced among ethnic groups linked to millennia-old traditions are also mentioned, together with the cases of the Tari in New Guinea and the Arunta in Australia:

the former celebrate initiation ceremonies and barefoot, frenetic dancing around fires that end over lit coals to demonstrate the initiates' ability to tolerate pain; the latter involve monotonous sounds that stun young people capable, at the ritual, of showing, without the slightest complaint, very high tolerance of pain caused by the removal of their incisors.

The Pompeian remains of the Villa of the Mysteries with murals depicting Silenus are cited, where the initiation phases of a small satyr, follower of the mythical ancestor of Dionysus, are illustrated.

Therefore, the constant presence of three fundamental factors can be noted in all of the above examples:

1) The presence of a character endowed with particular attributes and abilities: a sorcerer, a shaman, etc.;
2) The participation of people motivated to develop effects;
3) A comfortable, enticing environment, favouring the concentration and hypnotic involvement of the subjects present.

It is a magical phase that hypnology would only be able to dispel, through patient progression, from the second half of the 18th century onwards.

This considerable length of time can be explained by universal associations between the magical, occult and spectacular, which are linked to hypnosis as they

---

reaching, through meditation, *Satori*, that is, an illumination that leads to a higher level of consciousness that allows an active and conscious participation in the world and not an escape from it.

[88] The Incas' sacrifices in honor of the *Pachamama*, a fertility deity, often consisted of the spilling of the blood of llama foetuses on the ground. In the often dark, sacrificial rites of human children practiced by the Maya, the moods of the participants could not fail to be extra-ordinary. Their divinities were, *Itzamà*, the supreme solar god, inventor of writing and protector of agriculture, *Kukulkàn*, the two-headed feathered serpent, identified with the heavens, *Ixchel*, lunar goddess, protector of women in childbirth and female practices, *Yum Kaa*, God of corn and *Ahpuch*, God of death. Religion and ceremonials were directed by *Ahaucan* (prince of snakes), holder of astronomical knowledge, and the complex calendar of festivals that took place with propitiatory rites, human sacrifices, prayers and banquets.

[89] In the Chester Beatty Medical papyrus, dating from 1200 BC., there are examples of inductive mottos used in various therapies. One of these is related to the treatment of migraines which reads as follows: "*The head of a man, the son of a woman, is the head of Osiris Onnofri on which three hundred and sixty-seven divine serpents were placed that spat flames to force them to abandon the head of a man, son of a woman, like the head of Osiris Onnofri*". There are also expressions designed to immunise the doctor against the disease of the patient he was to treat. Here is one: "*I left Heliopolis with the Great of the temples, holders of protections, Lords of eternity. Likewise, I went out of Sais with the Mother of the Gods. They assured me of their protection; I have formulas prepared by the Universal Lord to eliminate the pain caused by a God or a Goddess, a deceased man or a deceased woman. I belong to Ra. He said: 'I myself will protect him from his enemies. Thoth will be his guide, the one who divulged the scriptures and is their author and bestows powers on the scholars, doctors, his disciples, to free from illness the one whom God wishes to keep alive*", (www.egittologia.net).

determine emotions and fear of a process that, however, involves the whole person.

Other difficulties are also due to an understanding of science that is characterised by some fundamental principles that are objectivity, rationality, controversiality and autonomy, thus creating an inadequate paradigm for the study of hypnosis, that is, of acquired phenomena that are difficult to objectify and measure in laboratories by common means of investigation.[90]

A breakaway from this magical phase was first attempted, after an interpretation of the philosophy of science, by the Viennese doctor Franz Anton Mesmer (1734-1815) who was the first to propose a physio-naturalistic of hypnosis (Mesmerism).

His theory presupposes a natural magnetism, a vital fluid, present in matter at a universal level in different concentrations and determining, by its modifications, the properties of bodies. The disturbance of these levels of concentration would explain the disease, requiring the doctor-magnetiser", that is, abundantly equipped with special vital fluids, to transmit them to his patients so that the necessary harmony would be restored.

Steps towards a scientific hypnology were progressively made by various authors.

Jacques de Chastenet (1751-1825), was able to formulate hypnotic inductions of mental calm, considering and respecting the psychological connotations and ethical principles of the subject being assisted.

Abbot Faria (1775-1819), emphasised the subject's psychic impressionability and the ability to concentrate, experiencing hypnosis as a determining factor of the hypnotic result. He then, proposing paternal, i.e. authoritarian, modes of induction, underlined the importance of monotonous and repetitive music in "lucid sleep", that is, a state of deep relaxation without restriction of the will and inner freedom of the person being hypnotised.

James Braid (1795-1860), first spoke of hypnotism, fatigue resulting from the fixation of shiny objects, concentration on a single idea (ideoplasia, that is the capacity that the suitably oriented mind has to act on the body), an imagination capable of taking on the value of real experience, and hypnosis which, when repeated several times, reappears more and more quickly.

Ambroise-Auguste Liébeault (1823-1904), theorised how the hypnotic state was the result of a concentration on a single idea, facilitated by fixating on one point, and making suggestions to the person who is isolated from the external world and is in close relation with the hypnotist.

---

[90] It is a theme that we might define, with Thomas Samuel Kuhn (1923-1996), of *The structure of scientific revolutions,* (Kuhn T.S., *The structure of scientific revolutions,* Piccola Biblioteca Einaudi, Turin, 1962), as necessary upheaval- as the construction of new paradigms - where obsolete scientific models prove over time to be insufficient in understanding the phenomena to be investigated.

The scientific phase

Various authors have traced the passage from the prescientific to the scientific phase. Mesmer, for example, placed himself in the former phase, but laid the foundations for the opening of the latter.

The most prominent figure in the shift to the latter is that of Hippolyte Bernheim (1837-1919) who, nevertheless, owes much to others and especially to Liébeault. The two collaborated in the opening of the School of Clinical Hypnosis in Nancy.

Bernheim was the author of two seminal hypnological texts, 'De la suggestion hypnotique dans l'état hypnotiqe et dans l'état de veille'[91] and 'De la suggestion et de ses applications à la thérapeutique', both to a large extent still valid today and which contributed to the further development of the discipline.

He defined hypnosis as a peculiar psychic condition that enhances susceptibility to suggestion, understood as the influence of an idea suggested to the mind, inducible in every individual, and therapeutically useful, which does not involve true loss of consciousness. This susceptibility to suggestions given in hypnosis determines the development of various hypnotic phenomena and depends in part on the constitution of the subject and in part on the psychic influence exerted by the hypnologist.

The Nancy school was dialectically opposed to that of Paris, embodied by the neurologist and lecturer at the Salpetrière, Jean-Martin Charcot (1825-1893).

Charcot, erroneously, misdefined hypnosis, considering it a recognisable neurosis in the three stages that he hypothesised: lethargic, cataleptic and somnambular.

However, he remained victorious in the clash with the Nancy group for a long time, due to his fame, not only in France.

Sigmund Freud (1856-1939), met and attended the two schools across the Alps.

He, too, had a very questionable regard for hypnosis, considering it an erotic type of transference (perhaps forgetting what his countertransference was), determining fleeting therapeutic effects and inducible only on a few people.

Many psychoanalytic hypnologists challenged him, with good reason, for his authoritarian and hasty ways of inducing hypnosis; some more precisely attributed to him an attitude of devaluation of hypnology, in the form of considerations relating to hypnotic phenomena, as an expression of his conflicting reaction to a powerful attraction he felt towards this medium, while the technical failures he encountered were frustrating.

Obviously, such serious scientific errors, committed by well-known and prestigious personalities, slowed down the evolution of hypnology considerably.

---

[91] Here is a recent editorial revival of this work curated by Giancarlo Odini and translated into Italian: Odini G., (edited by) *Hippolyte Bernheim, Della suggestione nella stato ipnotico e nello stato di veglia*. Translated into Italian by Biondelli A., Sometti, Mantua, 2017.

Bernheim reduced Charcot's magnet to a simple, suggestive and somewhat misleading idea, making it clearer that hypnotic images are entirely generated in the subject's imagination, as they are totally disjointed from the laws of optics. Furthermore, the author from Nancy was able to dispute the existence of the phases connected to sleepwalking.

Ivan Pavlov (1849-1936), a Russian physiologist and ethologist, considered hypnosis as a psychotherapeutic means, in the light of his studies on conditioned reflexes. He defined it as a process of prevalent cortical inhibition which is accompanied by concentrated arousal, achieved through rhythmic stimuli, whether weak and monotonous, or violent and sudden.

During these procedures the subject becomes insensitive to impulses that come from their external environment, other than those of the hypnologist, in relation to their communication and the overall relationship that is established with them. They use the signals they receive to fuel, if they so believe, said arousal, producing profound hypnotic effects.

Through this activity, the nerve circuits underlying each of the subject's previously lived experiences are put into operation, resulting in associative enhancements between stimuli and responses and real effects on a neurovegetative, motor and psychic level.

Clark Hull (1884-1952) foresaw hypnosis as a particular type of learning, that is, a process of acquiring the ability to respond more appropriately to a given situation, consequently to experience.

Other authors identified in hypnosis the unfolding of mechanisms of homo-action, hetero-action, dissociation and the partial inhibition of cerebral cortex activity, emphasising the importance of the subject's history and motivations.

Some argued how there may be, subjectively, special hypnotic abilities, or that sometimes people in hypnosis lend themselves to the performance of a hypnotic role, that they have a certain emotional reactivity, or are prompted by gregarious instinct.

According to various psychoanalytic schools, hypnosis could be the expression of regression or gratification of unconscious Oedipal, masochistic or narcissistic needs.

The current state of hypnosis studies

In in the 1950s-1970s, a number of national hypnological scientific associations were organised around the world.

In Latin America, the Latin American Federation of Clinical Hypnosis was established, with various sites in Argentina, Brazil, Uruguay, Colombia, Venezuela and Peru, while various national societies were active at the time, such as the 'Sociedad Española de Hipnosis y Experimental', the American Society of Clinical

Hypnosis, the Japanese Society of Hypnosis, the British Society of Medical and Dental Hypnosis, the Osteirreichische Gesellschaft für Ärtzliche Hypnose und Autogenes Training, the CesksIovensKa Gipnose Society and others.

These societies in turn formed international organizations, divided into national departments or branches in Europe, South Africa, the United States, Canada, Australia and Japan. They gave rise to congresses such as those in Paris in 1963, in Kyoto in 1966, in Mainz in 1970 and in Uppsala in 1973.

Much of the research at the time related to hypnosis was carried out at universities and hospitals. Those results were then published in various scientific journals, as well as in periodicals that were exclusively devoted to topics of hypnology.

In Milan, Italy, in 1958, the A.M.I.S.I. (Italian Medical Association for the Study of Hypnosis) was established, exclusively reserved for medical professionals and, in Verona, in 1965, the 'H. Bernheim' was set up, in connection with it.

Later, when the Centre became an Institute, it also represented the Italian division of the Institute for Research on Hypnosis in New York.

The A.M.I.S.I. promoted, from 1960 to 1971, theoretical-practical teaching courses and some national congresses (the first in Rome in 1967, the second in Turin in 1969 and the third in Pavia in 1971).

From 1966 onwards, the 'Bernheim' Centre organised annual preparatory specialisation courses and many lectures for graduates in medicine and surgery, one of which was part of the 2nd national congress of the Italian Society of Psychosomatic Medicine in Verona in 1969.[92]

The scientific output from these associations was extensive. A significant amount of authors from these associations distinguished themselves particularly, with contributions of various kinds that were published by the magazines 'Rassegna di Ipnosi e Medicina Psicosomatica', an official entity of the A.M.I.S.I., and by 'Psychosomatic Medicine', an official entity of the Italian Society of Psychosomatic Medicine (S.I.M.P.).

University institutes (the Dental and Neuropsychiatric Clinic at the University of Pavia, the Institute of Psychology at the Catholic University of Rome, the Neuropsychiatric Clinic at the University of Modena), as well as many distinguished professors and hospital institutes (the Regional Hospital of Verona, the Provincial Hospital of Vercelli, where a Clinical and Experimental Hypnosis Centre was in operation) have also very actively expressed their interest in the study, teaching and use of hypnosis, in multiple ways, further endorsing them .

"It can therefore be said that hypnosis," writes Guantieri, "in the text that we summarise here – is now favourably regarded among the Italian medical profession. Even from a religious point of view," he adds, "there are no longer any qualms surrounding hypnosis and hypnology".

---

[92] There is an extensive account of the 'Bernheim' Centre-Institute in Chapter 2 of this text.

In fact, the Pope at the time – Pius XII – recognized hypnosis as an object of scientific research and as a medical practice with clinical purposes, reserved for serious scholars who respect the moral limits that are valid for any scientific activity.

Despite this reassuring recognition, especially compared to the situation a few decades earlier, the study of hypnosis was not yet officially or firmly included in Italian university programs.

The reasons for this are many: some that continued to hinder the path of hypnology in the past, and others due to a lack of Italian legislation in terms of hypnosis.

It should be noted that articles 613 and 728 of the Criminal Code (since updated and amended) have remained substantially unchanged.

They do not explicitly mention doctors or psychotherapists. In any case, today (as of 2024), they read as follows:

Art. 613 – Anyone who, by hypnotic suggestion or while awake, or by administering alcohol or narcotic substances, or by any other means, places a person, without their consent, in a state of incapacity to understand and express will, shall be punished by imprisonment for up to one year.

Art. 728 – Anyone who places someone, with their consent, in a state of narcosis or hypnotism, or performs a treatment on them that suppresses their conscience or will, shall be punished, if this results in danger for the person's safety, with a jail sentence from one to six months or with a fine of between €30 and €516.

We refer to Guantieri's comment on the matter, here: "Certainly it is implied that the use of hypnosis in medicine, as well as that of any other means, with negligence, inexperience, or imprudence always involves a professional fault, [...however] it is unthinkable that a doctor aware of the damage that they could do to their patient would consciously will it. In that case, they would simply be a criminal, aggravated by the specific position. Any medicine in the hands of a criminal can become dangerous and be an instrument of crime".

Noting the inadequacy of the legislation on hypnology, Guantieri concludes: "It seems [...] desirable to formulate a law which, also taking into account the contributions made by recent studies [... on] the nature of the hypnotic process and the possibility that it can allow, finally qualifies hypnosis as a scientific discipline, reserving its use and teaching exclusively to those who are truly competent".[93]

---

[93] Commenting, in the year 2022, on the sterile evolution that we tried to bring about with regards to the topic, we recall the Italian law, n. 4 of January 14, 2013. It *"understands the hypnologist as an intellectual freelancer and allows him to exercise the profession of hypnologist freely and legally, provided that the trance is used only as an induction and not as a therapy"*. According to this legislation, the hypnologist must be qualified and certified by recognized schools, and is a freelancer who carries out an activity related to personal improvement. He will thus be able to guide his client for an improvement of human and personal energy potential. Therapy is therefore reserved for those who carry out a health profession, but the hypnologist is not recognized as a therapist.

2. The phenomenology of hypnosis

Hypnosis as a state and as an interpersonal relationship

With the term hypnosis we can indicate a set of conditions, a psychophysical state and an interpersonal relationship simultaneously, though they are quite peculiar and intimately correlated with each other, following appropriate stimulations, through the succession of multiple phenomena, whether psychic or psychosomatic, which involve the person and their way of being, thus determining particular effects.

The state of hypnosis

The state of hypnosis can be conceived as the Fourth Organismic State; it differs from the other three states in which man, like animals, finds himself in: the waking state (1st state), that of non-REM sleep (2nd state), in which one sleeps but does not dream, the state of REM sleep (3rd state) in which oneiric activity is typical.

The hypnotic relationship

The hypnotic relationship is the mutual, interpersonal hypnologist-subject relationship that is established from the moment the hypnotic induction is initiated to the next step in which de-hypnotisation has come to an end.
Both the state and the hypnotic relationship are regressive in nature, as are, for example, sleep, disease and any doctor-patient relationship.
These conditions are characterised by simple, primitive modes of behavior, different from those of an adult who is, normally, in a waking state.

Correlations between state and hypnotic relationship

The state and the hypnotic relationship are inextricably linked: the relationship initiates the state and maintains it, the state in turn influences the relationship.
Variations of the subject in hypnosis imply experiences, attitudes, actions and the manner of the hypnologist, and vice versa.
For example, a permissive induction that causes agitation can convince those who propose it to change their behavior and propose additional, firmer and more directive stimuli.

The stages of depth in hypnosis

Many authors have distinguished various levels of hypnosis; there have been those who have described, in progression, the following phases: drowsiness, mild sleep or hypotxia, deep sleep or somnambulism; there are those who have listed three: lethargic, cataleptic, somnambular. These are hypothetical subdivisions that are not entirely well-founded, due to excessively analytical and organicistic mindsets. It is interesting, however, to think of the existence of different types of hypnosis, attainable in intensity ranging from minimal to maximal, and in short, medium or long periods of time, progressively realising more or less impressive phenomena such as vivid imagination, remarkable influences on visceral functions, resounding perceptual distortions, age regression and automatic writing.

Hypnotic phenomena

They can be divided into Expressions of Hypnosis (which do not appear in connection with verbal suggestions intentionally aimed at achieving them) and Hypnotic Effects (which instead manifest themselves as direct consequences of specific verbal stimuli).

Expressions of hypnosis

By expressions of hypnosis we mean spontaneous phenomena that do not appear in connection with verbal suggestions, intentionally aimed at achieving them.

Constant expressions of hypnosis

Attention is selectively polarised on the environment surrounding the hypnologist, and is unrelated to any other information coming from the outside, to which the subject does not respond, as a consequence. They become particularly sensitive, for example, to tactile and auditory stimuli, which therefore take on the significance of particularly valuable information.
The perception of oneself in external reality takes place for the subject in hypnosis through the voice of the hypnologist. It appears modified not only in respect to the surrounding environment, but also to one's own body and to time, which appears to the subject – once hypnosis has ended – usually considerably less than that actually elapsed; one's body or parts of it are perceived differently than in waking conditions.

Memory undergoes constant changes: it becomes absent or significantly reduced due to stimuli not related to the hypnologist.

Language is different from that used in waking conditions: the answers to the hypnologist's questions have a longer latency, are expressionless and refer to neutral topics in terms of content. Words are low in pitch and are fewer in individual sentences.

Emotional inhibitions and critical thinking gradually decrease spontaneously, while unconscious functions become prevalent. The state of vigilance of the ego, however, does not appear to be abolished, but on the contrary is well preserved (stimuli words that are not appropriate or are in contrast to certain principles of the subject determine a superficialisation of hypnosis and even an immediate cessation of it, even when it has become intense).

All these conditions constitute particularly suitable terrain for the production of particular images, definable as eidetic, that is to say of certain vividness, comparable to the real perception of an object, to the development of a particular learning process to produce certain responses, to the strengthening of the action of speech, which hypnosis itself shows to be a physiological and therapeutic factor of considerable value.

Variable expressions of hypnosis

Variable expressions of hypnosis are thus the intrinsic conditions present in each person, which determine other, purely individual phenomena.

The perception of the source of information (hypnologist) can be refined to the point that the ticking of a clock is heard as a deafening sound.

Phenomena of hyperesthesia can also be observed in various sensory organs.

The environment is not only perceived as alien, but it can be felt as infinite, without limits; one's body is perceived to be levitating, or feels heavy or even absent, in whole or in part.

The memory of intra-hypnotic experiences may be absent – once hypnosis has ended– for the whole situation experienced (total amnesia), for part of it (elective amnesia), for the origin and the way in which the experience occurred, but not for the content (amnesia of the source).

Imaginative and fantastical activity can be enhanced, producing figurative mental representations, experienced as real.

The subject's appearance is often similar to that of a person who is deeply immersed and immobile in physiological sleep, or of someone who is relaxed (passive hypnosis); sometimes there is a certain ability to move (active hypnosis).

At other times, there is an increase in muscle tone or the occurrence of contractions. Alongside the neuromuscular changes, neurovegetative phenomena can also be observed, such as changes in temperature, sweating, breathing, heart rate or blood pressure.

Once hypnosis is over, in very rare cases nausea, headache, vague malaise or numbness may be present.

Generally, however, after the cessation of hypnosis, especially when used for therapeutic purposes, improvement of the cenestesis, new hypnotic abilities, more profitable learning, favourable modifications of the interpersonal relationship and of the body are observed: all very important elements for therapeutic purposes.

The effects of hypnosis

Hypnotic effects, phenomena induced by specific verbal stimuli, can occur both during hypnosis (when the stimuli are given) and after its cessation.

Dynamics of hypnotic effects

The stimuli can determine psychic or somatic effects, directly or indirectly (ie. through the induction of images that represent a situation experienced by the subject, accompanied by the desired response).
Simple effects, such as "heaviness and immobility of a limb" can be reached with the mere suggestion that one's" limb will become heavy and immobile".
More complex effects, such as the loss of sensitivity to pain (analgesia), can instead be produced by intentionally eliciting, (once the subject has developed a certain training to produce hypnosis), mental images that depict situations in which pain sensitivity in a given body area has actually been reduced or abolished. For example, imagining an experience of pharmacological analgesia in hypnosis, such as that experienced before a tooth extraction, or a modification of sensitivity, such as when a surface of the body comes into contact with a cold medium, effectively translates into analgesia, which can be objectively confirmed (if one stimulates the affected area with a large needle, it does not cause any pain).
As in a dream, in hypnosis the imagination also comes to constitute a subjective experience, experienced as an interior reality so intense and exclusive that it completely replaces the external reality.
The more different the desired effects are, the more complex (especially in therapy) the modalities to follow become.
If the procedure is carried out correctly, most of the body's functions can be changed, as long as there is sufficient willingness on the part of the subject from both a neurophysiological and psychological aspect.

"Intra-hypnotic" effects

Attention and memory can be reduced, abolished or enhanced by any stimulus.
Significant material referring to childhood can be recalled more quickly in hypnosis. It is also possible that clear memories of past experiences are accompanied by the emotions felt during those experiences (regression).
In fact, emotionality can be significantly influenced in hypnosis.
Perception can be modified in different ways: it can be reduced, abolished or intensified by any stimulus, or even a single component of it; responses to non-existent stimuli in external reality (hallucinations), or erroneous perception of real stimuli (illusions) may be induced.[94]
The subject can thus develop visual, tactile, thermal, olfactory, gustatory and auditory sensations, even very intense ones, in the face of stimuli that would instead be barely felt, or even not perceived at all in a state of wakefulness; on the contrary, one can learn not to perceive very intense and lasting stimuli. For instance, it is possible to perceive a non-existent odor, light or noise, or perceive an unpleasant smell such as ammonia as pleasant, to hear a low-pitched sound as a high-pitched ringing, to see the colour green as red, or to develop insensitivity in every sensory organ.
Among the changes in perception we can include inducible variations in tactile, thermal, and above all pain sensitivity; just as it is possible to achieve sensations of pain, tingling, burning, numbness, itching, hot, humid, cold or others, so it becomes possible to develop an insensitivity to pain (analgesia).
Muscle tone and motility are modifiable: both can be reduced, abolished or even increased, with occasional consequent phenomena of hypotonia, paresis or paralysis, contractions and contractures that can last a long time.
Cardiovascular and respiratory functions can be affected: suggestions of cold and heat can lead to vasoconstriction and vasodilation, respectively.
In gastrointestinal function, a tendency towards an increased production of hydrochloric acid and pepsin was noted, inducing satisfaction, or to decreased secretion, instead arousing anger or fear.
Induced phenomena that involve the entire psychosomatic unit are the so-called age regression and induced emotions. By age regression we mean the patient's return to previous periods of his or her life, for which their psychophysical behavior, both healthy and pathological, can become identical to that of the determined previous period, to which they were brought back by the hypnologist's appropriate suggestions.

---

[94] Let it be clear that we are not dealing here with psychotic symptoms. In hypnosis, hallucinations or illusions are induced for experimental, clinical or didactic reasons but are absolutely reversible.

"Post-hypnotic" effects

Post-hypnotic effects are inducible in hypnosis with appropriate verbal stimuli and can appear, using certain procedures in hypnosis, post-cessation, after some time. The moment of onset and the duration of these phenomena, so called as they can be observed after de-hypnotisation, are strictly related to what has been suggested in hypnosis.

3. The nature of hypnosis and some hypnotic phenomena

Neurophysiological interpretations of hypnosis

From a neurophysiological point of view, hypnosis is explained in terms of conditioning, inhibition, arousal and learning.

Hypnosis and cortical inhibition

Ivan Pavlov (1849-1936) places hypnosis along a continuum at the extremes of which are sleep and wakefulness as an expression of a widespread inhibition of the cerebral cortex (a process by which nerve cells are not available for the passage of the stimulus), which accompanies concentrated arousal of one area.
The existence of widespread inhibition prevents any interference of signals unrelated to the hypnologist's instructions and therefore any influence on circuits unrelated to the hypnotic project; moreover, it contributes to the copious production of images, intimately correlated with the information coming from the hypnologist and with the experience of the subject.
The practitioner's speech therefore, thanks to the aforementioned inhibition, due to its physical qualities and above all its semantics, is able to turn on, through the "relationship zone", "guard points", that is, certain underlying internal realities, previously experienced as external. These realities are thus experienced intensely as real, even on a somatic level. The switching on, for example, of an experiential circuit of heat, cold and analgesia, effectively produces corresponding states in the subject.
The interpretation of hypnosis as a process of inhibition and Pavlov's own experiences with a dog's conditioned reflexes greatly enabled many studies on the relationship between hypnosis and sleep and between animal hypnosis and human hypnosis.

Hypnosis and sleep

Studies on the relationship between hypnosis and sleep are justified by the fact that the inhibition of the cortex also characterises sleep, be it total (widespread inhibition), partial (coexistence of areas of arousal), or dispersed (when there is coexistence in the same zone of both prevailing inhibition and excitation).
In the onset of inhibition, we would pass from the phase characterised by a diffused irradiation of excitation (wakefulness), in which the organism responds more to intense stimuli than to light ones, to an intermediate stage, in which weak stimuli have the same effect as intense ones; subsequently, the end point would be that of the phase characterised by complete loss of action by the excitatory stimuli.
Referring to inhibitory stimuli, Pavlov states: "The monotonous, repeated, but on the other hand indifferent stimulation of a certain area of the cortex is capable of causing inhibition, then drowsiness, then subsequently hypnosis, and finally deep sleep".

Hypnosis and other states

There is no relationship between hypnosis and psychopathological states. If, for example, hysteria, compulsive neurosis or schizophrenia recall some expressions of hypnosis, post-hypnotic behavior, imagination and catalepsy have nothing to do with the healthy and reversible dynamism of hypnotic altered states of consciousness.

Hypnosis and learning

The realisation of hypnotic images is generally much quicker, easier and more vivid with each induction, as is the rapid and total abolition of pain.
These effects, even if the training that originally allowed them has been interrupted for a long time, reappear easily and quickly after one or two inductions, in a more brief timeframe than had previously been necessary, so so that they satisfactorily produce the effects felt the first time. By associating, for example, with stimuli that induce hypnosis or are responsible for a certain hypnotic effect, such as analgesia, another stimulus of any nature, such as music or light, the latter acquires the power to evoke hypnosis or that particular hypnotic effect (transfer of training).
Similarly, any stimulus that has been associated with hypnosis, experienced as well-being, is able to independently be felt as well-being, at a later time, outside of hypnosis. Inversely, a sound stimulation associated in hypnosis with a sensation, is consequently capable of producing, in a waking state, a reaction of fear.
In similar ways, a truly impressive variety of new conditioned reflexes can be created.

Socio-psychological interpretations of hypnosis

Hypnosis and suggestion

Some scholars have considered hypnosis an expression of suggestibility, therefore inducible by psychological means. Others believe that it is possible to induce hypnotic phenomena in predisposed subjects, by means of suggestions given in waking conditions. Still others believe that hypnosis is "something different" to suggestibility. There is certainly correlation, but not absolute identity, between suggestibility and hypnotisability.[95]

Hypnosis and "attitudes"

The transitory state of the hypnotic condition — thus absolutely dynamic and reversible — was considered of psychogenic dissolution as a regression to archaic behaviours. Some mentioned a poorly defined hypnotic attitude, which would explain the behavior of the hypnotised subject as an effort intended to produce a certain behavior, that is, that which is suggested to them by the hypnologist. This interpretation, although unsatisfactory, can be accepted in the sense that the subject, thanks to adequate motivations, is actually pushed to act in the way indicated by the hypnologist. Others believe that so-called involvement skills may be at play.

Hypnosis and "role theory"

From a sociological point of view, hypnotic conduct can be considered as role play by the subject: that is, they would act as society (to which they belong) expects a hypnotised person to act.
Hypnotic conduct, therefore, that is inseparable from the opinion that the community has of hypnosis in a given era, thus attributing fundamental value to socio-cultural factors.
Six psychological variables involved in hypnotic role play have been described:

---

[95] The influence of a prompter on another person does not always produce convictions devoid of arguments and logical foundations, determining in these situations that suggestion understood in its worst meaning; sometimes a good idea from a wise person can illuminate the subject who receives the information as imaginative, creative, suggestive, promotional. However, this can happen without the two interlocutors establishing hypnotic changes of consciousness in themselves and between them. It is also observed that the admiration of 14th-century frescoes, Renaissance paintings, Hellenistic sculptures, Gothic cathedrals, or listening to music by the great authors of 19th-century Romanticism, or even the contemplation of splendid geographical locations, nature and so on, can be suggestive. These too are cases in which the percipient does not necessarily fall into an induced hypnotic state.

1. Validity of the subject's expectations;
2. Precision in the perception of the task;
3. Relevant interpretative skills;
4. Congruence between role and subject;
5. Sensitivity to the requests that are made;
6. Sensitivity to the reinforcement provided by spectators.

These variables should also be valued in the clinical field: expectations play an important role which becomes particularly effective where there is the capacity for the actions to be performed, the congruence between the characteristics of the person and the requirements of the task, and finally the sensitivity to the requests that the latter involves, together with adequate motivations.

While it is important to study factors preceding and concurrent with induction, it is not possible to share the opinion of the non-specificity of hypnotic conduct supported by the role theory.

In fact, post-hypnotic amnesia, age regression, the free expression of unconscious content and other phenomena (spontaneous and induced), whether neuromotor, neurovegetative or sensorial, surely argue against this theory.

Psychoanalytic interpretations of hypnosis

Hypnosis and transfert

Sigmund Freud (1856-1939) initially interprets hypnosis as an "unconscious fixation of the subject's libido on the figure of the hypnotist, through the masochistic components of sexual instinct; subsequently, as an unconscious replacement by the hypnotist of the subject's Superego".

This conception is connected to the whole Freudian theory of the repression of instincts and to their possible translation onto another person, who generally represents the one, or those, who played the role of model in the subject's childhood (usually the father) and have contributed, together with the Real Ego, (the conscious part of the personality, as opposed to the Id, which instead represents the unconscious, instinctive part), to form the Superego.

The hypnotist, by exalting the image of the father, determines at the same time a considerable weakening or a real paralysis of the other component of the Superego (the one inherent in the sense of reality, or criticism) and hence the main characteristics of hypnosis provoked by this libidinal fixation: [an]"unawareness of the process, affective attachment to the operator, uncritical realisation of the suggested ideas".

Hypnosis and "loss of ego boundaries"

Lawrence Kubie (1896-1973) and Sydney Margolin (1909-1985) finally also come to value sensory factors such as the progressive particular modification of perception (induced by monotonous and repeated stimulation), which goes hand in hand with sensory deprivation, that is with a notable decrease in the supply of information from the external environment.
Through these methods, partial sleep would be established and the boundaries of the ego canceled, which would result in a psychological fusion between hypnotist and subject.
The sensory relationship with the environment and with the hypnologist and the person's activity during hypnosis would be similar to those considered to be characteristic of being a child in the face of its environment and parents.
For the above authors, hypnosis can be induced by exclusively physical means: transference would therefore not be necessary for the hypnosis process; when it exists, it would be a consequence of the same.

Hypnosis and regression

Merton Gill (1914-1994) and Margaret Brenman (1940-1994), moving decidedly away from Freudian positions, also attribute value to sensory and motor factors: however, these factors are considered in close correlation with transference, which in this case is believed to be, unlike for Kubie and Margolin, an essential element of hypnosis.
More precisely, they would argue hypnosis was a "particular type of regression that can be initiated by sensory, motor and ideational deprivation and by the stimulation of an archaic relationship with the hypnotist".
The theories of Kubie, Margolin, Gill and Brenman finally envisage a possible mutual correlation and integration, between neurophysiology and psychoanalysis respectively; between neurophysiology, experimental psychology and psychoanalysis. This convergence of different disciplines, certainly also fruitful for therapeutic purposes, undoubtedly allows the interpretation of several aspects and the enhancement of several factors, both constant and variable, thus improving the knowledge of a process, the approach to which, involving the whole person, can only be multidimensional.
Therefore, one can conclude by proposing "hypnosis as a learning process to develop multiple, closely related neuropsychological and neurophysiological phenomena, a possible expression of a regression in the service of the ego, which is both a state and an interpersonal relationship".
Learning to produce hypnosis and certain hypnotic effects takes place in accordance with certain principles and thanks to adequate physical and

psychological stimulations, respectively inducing a sensory, motor, ideational deprivation and activating adequate motivations.

Regression in the service of the ego (which in neurophysiological terms could be explained by a partial cortical inhibition, accompanied by a concentration of arousal of certain areas) would take place, from the psychological point of view, by the organization of a subsystem equipped with peculiar functions. This subsystem would depend on the hypnologist, while the remaining conscious part would continue to maintain the critical orientation that characterises it in waking conditions.

Precisely from the activity of this subsystem (or from the aforementioned modifications of the nervous circuits), initiated and maintained in a wholly particular way by the hypnologist's voice, multiple effects of a psychic and psychosomatic nature would be derived, widely and variously usable for the purposes of experimental research, prophylaxis, diagnosis and therapy.

Dynamics of some hypnotic phenomena

Spontaneous changes in attention, perception and memory

We might regard the polarisation of attention on the hypnologist's voice, in the first moments of induction, as an expression of an active concentration due to an intentional act of the subject; subsequently, however, as the induction proceeds, we might speak of passive application, as it is the voice that is attracting the attention of the subject.

Changes in behavior and attention also allow us to understand the altered perception of time, as well as an increased memory, extraneous to the relationship with the hypnologist.

Spontaneous amnesia would be related to regression, the inhibition of the articulation of words, the way in which the hypnotist establishes relations with the world, to different thought processes, referable to the dissociation that is established. in hypnosis, with repressive processes that have arisen to protect oneself from anxiety.

Source amnesia is comparable to subjective processes that occur as a result of traumatic experiences, when these events have not been integrated into the temporal and spatial context of individual consciousness.

Induced changes in perception

The ease with which images are produced in hypnosis is due to various factors, including meditative concentration, the memory of past experiences, one's reasons for the hallucinatory experience, involving the transition from the state of active attention to the condition of passive perception. These images are predominantly mental rather than perceptual.

Regarding analgesia, in which pain impulses are effectively blocked and not detected by brain structures, the underlying mechanisms are those of an elevation of the pain threshold, the phenomena of amnesia and the absence of anxiety.

Regression and "post-hypnotic" conduct

The regression results in evident changes in self-image.

This is due to the use of primitive mechanisms of the perception of reality that prevail over logical and rational processes.

The impressionability of certain structures by past emotional events and the way in which these structures have been modified is relevant: the particular fixation, for example, to an earlier stage of development, may in part clarify why certain behaviours reappear.

4. The induction of hypnosis

Hypnotisability

Hypnotisability is the susceptibility to developing hypnosis.

It is a characteristic trait of personality. Latent or manifest, it is different in each individual and can emerge with varying degrees of intensity, depending on the circumstances in which factors related to the subject and to the hypnotist are at play and mutually influence each other.

Factors related to the subject

Factors related to the subject are: the susceptibility to hypnosis, the capacity for involvement (i.e. the complete participation of one's whole being in particular activities or experiences), to identify with one's parental figures as a result of early family life experiences, training, obedience, motivations and resistance.

Factors related to the hypnotist

Some factors identified through research are: the hypnologist's tendency to particularly identify with their role, the desire they have to understand and assume the role of an authoritative parental figure, their sensitivity in establishing an intimate and detached but, at the at the same time, responsible relationship with the subject.

Evaluation and the possibility of increasing hypnotisability

Hypnotisability can be quantitatively assessed using standardised scales.
Regarding the possibility of an increase thereof, research shows that this is difficult unless there is a good starting point.
We have observed this predisposition in hypnologists in training, at the end of courses in which scientific information was given on hypnosis and its related phenomena, and during which an adequate positive interpersonal relationship was established.

Means of hypnotic induction

The means of hypnotic induction are stimuli that initiate the psycho-neuro-physiological processes of hypnosis.
They are divided into means that induce sensory, motor and ideational deprivation and means that stimulate the development of a particular interpersonal relationship.

Means that induce sensory-motor and ideational deprivation

These are the stimuli that restrict the subject's field of perception. With these means, attention converges and progressively diverts itself from the remaining external reality.
They can be weak, continuous and violent, or sudden; depending on the stimulated area, they are visual, auditory, etc.
Among the violent and sudden stimuli are the "steps" (that is, the gestures performed, in various ways, by the hypnotist in front of the patient) or the compression of the carotid sinus, modalities that have fallen into disuse because they are neither indispensable nor appropriate.
Weak, continuous stimuli, on the other hand, are particularly useful also as they can allow a non-authoritarian, persuasive approach.
Among the visual stimuli are shiny objects on which the subject is invited to fix their gaze: the rotating mirror, the hypnotic ball.
Among the sound stimuli are the beat of a metronome, the tuning fork, the helmet and the vibrating chair.

Pharmacological stimuli have been used, but with discouraging results as they produce artificial sleep which does not allow the hypnotic relationship to be established.

Whatever the means used, they must cause a narrowing of the field of perception, with consequent sensory-motor and ideational deprivation. These instruments therefore assume particular importance, more than just for their nature, but for their frequency, intensity, and for the way in which they are used.

Means that stimulate the development of a particular interpersonal relationship

These consist of verbal and mimic attitudes and expressions, which tend to establish an interpersonal relationship, in which and through which certain needs of the subject are satisfied, certain abilities are activated and imitative behaviours are also carried out.

Suggestions of tiredness, heaviness, relaxation, numbness, drowsiness or sleep, if addressed with an adequate timbre, tone, volume of voice and frequency of words, to a subject motivated to rest, can actually induce hypnosis or sleep.

The same can be said for those suggestions oriented towards sensations and movements; for example the stagger test or the arm levitation technique.

Verbal suggestions are all the more effective the more they take into account needs and attitudes, both specific, i.e. individual, and common to each subject.

Modes of hypnotic inductions and de-hypnotisation

The ways in which the means of hypnotic induction can be used are various: therefore there are numerous methods that have been developed to initiate hypnosis.

Hypnotic induction techniques

The techniques of hypnotic induction can be distinguished, according to the type of relationship that is established between the hypnotist and the subject, into authoritarian or permissive.

authoritarian techniques, particularly used in the past, are based on the use of violent or sudden stimuli and lead the subject to consider the hypnotist's so-called values as fundamental and to consider themselves to be a mere object of the latter's action.

Permissive techniques, preferred today, are usually based on the use of weak and continuous stimuli, and instead enhance the natural ability to develop hypnosis inherent in the subject, consequently initiating, in accordance with the evolution of the times, an approach that can be defined as "democratic".

Ideomotor and ideoplastic effects

The technique of visualising scenes consists in inviting the subject to imagine circumstances that are pleasant for them, by focusing their attention more and more on themselves, and therefore formulating adequate suggestions.

Principles relating to the induction of hypnosis and hypnotic effects

Most of the modern techniques of hypnotic induction are based on relaxation suggestions, aimed at the subject lying in an armchair or on a bed, in different ways, after having had the scientific reality of hypnosis and its purposes explained to them.

Once psychosomatic relaxation is achieved, it is then suggested to carry out increasingly complex tasks, following certain rules.

The suggestions must be clear, simple, precise, detailed and gradual, also in relation to the effects that are gradually produced in the phase in which the subject finds themselves.

That is to say, it is appropriate for the suggestions to become progressively less and less rational. The suggestion, for example, of numbness of a limb is certainly effective when a very light hypnosis has appeared; however, this is not the case in which analgesia can be induced.

The concepts gradually suggested must refer to realities already experienced by the subject: they are in fact likely to be transformed into concrete effects, only if the real situations to which they refer have been previously experienced, that is, if the relative dynamic stereotypes have been structured.

Physical contact, for example placing the hands on the shoulders of the subject during the staggering test, creating an undulatory movement, can facilitate the appearance of the desired phenomena, making the interpersonal relationship more intimate; however, in other cases they can be counterproductive, when they are perceived as an imposition or intrusion by the hypnologist or as a succession to it.

Hypnosis as a means of experimental investigation

Hypnosis in the study of dreams

It is possible to access, with appropriate suggestions, dream activity, inducing it, even on specific themes, facilitating memory or causing the subject to awaken at the very moment the dream begins, or to speak while dreaming, or in other ways, in any case allowing one to better control the dream process.

Hypnosis in the study of subliminal perception

The study of subliminal perception, a process by which certain stimuli, even if not consciously perceived, are nevertheless registered and can act on unconscious levels, is made possible through hypnosis, as it can allow the memory of such stimuli, not consciously perceived. or not remembered, thus demonstrating an unconscious registering and any consequences thereof.
For example, some volunteers were engaged in an experimental process, whereby they were induced into a hypnotic state and invited to engage in a number of tasks:
1st) to maintain an ongoing conversation;
2nd) shortly afterwards, they were engaged in learning lists of simple words;
3rd) asking them to describe drawings shown to them.

Upon awakening, a total amnesia of the tasks performed was noted. An attempt to recover memory was subsequently made, through a new induction of hypnosis; the result was a recognition of the drawings but no memory of the conversation or the learning of words.

Hypnosis in the study of "attitudes"

It is possible to suggest obedience, cooperation, interest, rivalry, dependence, extroversion, introversion, the ability to command, submission, upon which a change in the subject's attitudes in noted.

Hypnosis in the study of emotionality

The study of emotion, of emotional conflicts and of the relative effects on the person and on the organism, of how and why these effects occur, is of significance in medicine, especially in disorders in which the alteration of emotionality plays an important role.

There is no doubt that hypnosis is particularly suitable as a means for such a study: thanks to its qualities and characteristics, it allows the emergence, through the use of suitable methods, of completely genuine, orientable emotions of various kinds, that are also measurable in the spontaneous effects produced, and which are not otherwise inducible.

Hypnosis as a means of clinical investigation

Hypnosis has diagnostic value as it offers an expression of the person's profound realities, important for clarifying the genesis and dynamics of symptoms. They themselves can also be dynamically activated by special inductions.

In psychodiagnostics, the emergence of the profound is essentially characterised by unconscious and subconscious content, the awareness of which can be useful for various reasons.

Hypnosis allows greater productivity in the use of psychological tests and spontaneous hypnotic phenomena of diagnostic significance.

The questions that the subject poses after the experience, the images to which they relate and the same modality with which they conclude their hypnotic experience, are very useful elements in understanding how the subject has learned to establish personal relationships in their life, how they understand them and, therefore, how they face or flee situations that are important to them, and again, to know what their feelings, attitudes, motivations, repressions and defences may be.

Hypnosis also proves valuable as a projective test for the hypnologist, who can better understand their own unconscious psychological reality and orient themselves more precisely on what is underlying in the interpersonal relationship.

Spontaneous hypnotic phenomena of diagnostic significance

The induction of hypnosis and hypnosis itself constitute a vital situation in which various phenomena spontaneously develop, which, if carefully examined, provide information on the personality of the experiential subject.

Hypnotically induced phenomena with diagnostic significance

In psychodiagnostics, the emergence of the profound is essentially characterised by unconscious and subconscious content, an awareness of which can be useful for various reasons.

For this purpose, mental associations and emotions can be induced with visualisations of scenes, evoking of the emotions felt at the time, age regression, automatic writing and drawing.
Of course, these methods must be placed within a psychodynamic project.

Hypnosis and psychological "tests"

The relationship between hypnosis and psychological tests is bidirectional: on the one hand, the former can allow a greater understanding of the subject's personality, on the other, the latter allow for further checks on what can be produced in hypnosis.
On this relationship, the T.A.T. (Thematic Apperception Test) and the Rorschach (countless cases are cited in the manual, Ed.) are interesting.

5. Hypnosis as a therapeutic means

Hypnotherapy for somatic disorders

Hypnotherapy can be directed towards physical or psychic symptoms, as a direct expression of the disease itself or a consequence of its physical manifestations.
Indeed, every somatogenic disease induces regression, which can lead to emotional disturbances.

Principles of hypnotherapy in somatic disorders

The most important criterion is to induce motivation to heal.
Somatic symptoms can be beneficially influenced by means of simple suggestions for the improvement, reduction, abolition or displacement of the symptoms themselves.
The second criterion, much simpler, more practical and productive, consists of the induction of hypnosis as sleep, without making any other specific suggestions.

Practical applications of hypnotherapy in somatic disorders

Favourable results are reported in scientific literature regarding the use of hypnotherapy in somatic disorders.
Hypnosis in these cases is intended as a means of parallel and integrative clinical use of – and certainly not a substitute for – traditional psychosomatic medical treatments.

The outcomes are achieved in different ways, depending on the symptoms and the etiopathogenesis.

Painful syndromes of various kinds, such as multiple sclerosis, epilepsy, neuritis, myositis and other modifications of skeletal muscles, cardiac and vascular disorders, vomiting during pregnancy, haemophilia, diabetes insipidus, Reynaud's disease and other afflictions have been treated through its use.

Beneficial effects on pain have been recorded, for example, by inducing hypnotic relaxation associated with suggestions directed toward initiating more positive attitudes in the face of pain, an acceptance of the pain, or to encourage new interests that distract the subject's concentration on a body in suffering.

In certain cases, suggestions of dissociation to isolate the areas affected by pain have proved useful.

In others, indications directly aimed at focusing patients on their recovery prospects have proved effective.

Pain hypnotherapy, an expression of neoplasm, has considered inductions aimed at reducing the need for pharmacological analgesics and at bringing people to an acceptance of illness.

Here are some examples of hypnotherapeutic applications to somatic disorders (among the many described in Guantieri's text):

In multiple sclerosis: by suggestions of muscle relaxation in certain areas, or by acquiring conditioning signals to be used when awake, for example, the idea that whenever the patient clenches their right hand in a fist, their muscles will relax;

In epilepsy: asking the subject to remember scenes they have lived through and to report their memories of them;

In cases of skeletal muscle disorders: through hypnosis aimed at achieving analgesic and relaxation effects;

Similarly, hypnosis has been considered a means of rehabilitation in muscular paralysis, helping the patient to reconsider their own body image and motivating them to resume their place in society;

In heart attacks: with the aim of modifying the way the subject considers their heart, helping them to develop a belief which, alongside increased kidney function, achieved progressive improvement in cardiovascular conditions;

In cases of vomiting in pregnancy: diversifying the interventions according to whether they are regurgitations or an expression of emotional conflicts, rather than abnormal outcomes of the new particular neurovegetative situation that characterises pregnancy;

in the case of myocardial infarction: where hypnotherapy can be used to reassure and reeducate; Similarly, with biliary stone colic and subsequent liver dysfunction: suggesting the idea of biliary secretions (actually found through instrumental monitoring), and imagining food ingestion.

Hypnotherapy in psychosomatic disorders

Psychosomatics is a holistic approach to the person, whether healthy or sick, that takes into account the living body, one's emotions and the environment in which one lives.

It is therefore a discipline that studies reactions and diseases that manifest themselves in the soma as an expression of disturbances in the psychic sphere.

Treating psychosomatic disorders with hypnosis usually means striving for therapeutic goals through a clinical means that can be used in various ways, vis-à-vis the underlying emotional alterations of the symptoms, such as anxiety, agitation, depression, aggression, or frustration.

Beyond the signal, then, using this approach, attention is focused on the dynamics of these anomalies, the symptoms being only a reflection of them.

However, there are still minimal cases in which the symptoms, as conditioned reflexes, can be directly treated as they have become abnormal habits, even if in such cases psychosomatic knowledge is indispensable, if only to arrive at differential diagnoses between the two types of disorders, in the first case due to conflicting situations, in the second as results of subordinate behaviour.

The principles of psychosomatic medicine Psychosomatic etiopathogenesis

Bronchial asthma, migraine, certain forms of vomiting and diarrhoea and other symptoms may be the expression of an emotional conflict, or, more simply, of abnormal conditioned reflexes.

An example relating to this case is that of a child who begins to display enuresis, originally as a clear expression of an emotional conflict, because they were — or felt — abandoned early on, due to the birth of a younger brother or sister. Where said conflict has been resolved, persistence of the symptom continues. At that point it can be considered that nocturnal incontinence has become a simple expression of a series of conditioned reflexes, or an abnormal habit.

The conditioned reflex consists of the response elicited by a stimulus which, although usually ordinarily inadequate, is presented together with another biologically adequate one, thus becoming an effective substitute for the latter.

For example, any food placed in a dog's mouth produces saliva; this process is a natural reflex. If a certain number of times, in identical circumstances, we precede the administration of food with the ringing of a bell or the switching on of a light, elements which in themselves have no effect on the salivary glands, after a certain amount of time these stimuli take on the meaning of a signal of the arrival of food, a signal capable of producing salivation in itself. This second case is a conditioned reflex.

Its dynamics were, for Ivan Pavlov (1849-1936), a coupling of the stimuli, establishing an excitatory conversion that can sometimes work in the presence of only one of the two stimuli.

The narrowing of the pupil is an innate involuntary act, for example, caused by a light beam, which is absolutely excitatory. However, if the verbal repetition of the phrase "my pupil will narrow" is associated with this a certain number of times, in perfect concomitance with this natural stimulus, it is subsequently able to cause the narrowing by itself. By perfecting this training, it is then sufficient to obtain the effect with only the mental repetition of the sentence; finally, the mere thought that the pupil will narrow is enough to bring about its contraction.

Vladimir Bechterew (1857-1927), conditioned muscle spasms in the hands and feet to electrical stimuli; other researchers were able, by means of verbal conditioning, not only to prevent the effects of pharmaceutical drugs, but also to obtain pharmacological effects by administering a simple saline solution.

One, with the simple command "get ready to work", induced increased lung ventilation; having induced this hyperventilation by having the subject breathe several times for eight hours in a closed environment, so that the carbon dioxide rate increased, then noticed the same respiratory modification in the same closed room even when the carbon dioxide content was equal to that of the external environment. He also observed that brachycardia induced by the compression of the eyeballs could also be caused by an acoustic stimulus, if this had previously been associated with the aforementioned compression.

Conditioning is inextricably linked to learning, which can affect both motor and visceral functions.

By associating stimuli-reinforcement, that is, rewards, to spontaneous variations of the heart rhythm, it can be seen that animals learn to produce these variations in order to obtain the reward.

Once established, the conditioned reflex is maintained stably if it is fostered: in the case of the aforementioned conditioned salivation, so that the sound or light does not lose its acquired meaning as a signal, it is necessary to offer a reinforcement, that is, to administer food from time to time after the stimulation, sound or light.

The extent of a conditioned response depends on the intensity of the stimulus, on non-interference in it by other agents, on the number of repetitions of the stimulus-response experience, on the characteristics of the species or of the individual animal, in which motivations must also be present for the effect of the stimulus. For example, it is much less easy to condition salivary secretion in a satiated animal than in a hungry one.

Psychosomatic diagnosis

Psychosomatic diagnostic investigation aims to shed light on the nature, onset and evolution of symptoms, on the patient's personality, on environmental conditions, etiology being as it is multi-factor, in which biological, psychological and relational factors are linked together.

Only from this perspective is it possible to engage in psychosomatic medicine and, more generally, to assume a psychosomatic clinical attitude: "a special way of seeing, concerning medicine, which certainly does not pay less attention to the body, but rather more consideration of the psyche".

Psychosomatic investigation is aimed at linking biological, psychological and social factors together with the greatest possible caution, in order to avoid diagnostic and consequently therapeutic errors. A functional syndrome can be present at the same time as a somatic disease; intestinal or cardiovascular syndromes can be observed in chronic infections; diabetes, nephropathy, multiple sclerosis, or a carcinoma can express themselves at the outset solely in functional conditions.

With psychosomatic investigation, which is based on an adequate interpersonal relationship, the aim is to first establish the presence or absence of pathological somatic findings; secondly, to record certain data that can testify to psychosomatic etiopathogenesis; thirdly, to fix elements that offer the possibility of framing the disorder according to the psychological source.

Psychosomatic investigation is carried out by means of the psychosomatic anamnesis, physical examination and clinical interview.

It consists of an accurate biological and psychological-social history, aimed at correlating the most varied factors inherent in past events.

Physical examination is focused on the body and psyche; it uses traditional means (radiological, laboratory, personality tests, etc.).

The clinical interview is conducted by creating a favourable emotional atmosphere, listening to the patient, without judging them, participating in their suffering, observing their mimic, phonetic and neurovegetative expressions, their gaze, posture, etc., carefully asking indirect and brief questions, aware of the inductive effects that words can have.

Thus the patient will be more readily willing to show their feelings, hopes, anxieties and fears.

By proceeding in this way it is possible to understand their deep and unsolved psychic problems — the true reasons for their psychosomatic suffering.

The doctor-patient relationship is productive not only for diagnostic purposes but also, simultaneously, for therapeutic purposes. It puts the suffering subject in a positive disposition, so they may feel considered more as a healing person, rather than an ailing neurophysiological unit.

A fourth means of psychosomatic investigation can now also be offered through hypnosis, if used following a psychodynamic approach.

Consider, for instance, the case of a child who, under certain circumstances of psychological and relational distress, presents with abdominal pain and diarrhoea. From an initial examination of the situation, even before asking whether these symptoms can be interpreted as specific organ language, a disturbance in the family atmosphere emerges, that could be frustrating for the subject. In a situation of this kind, the first measure to be taken, whenever possible, is to intervene in the environment. In this regard, it should be remembered that essential hypertension — at the basis of which would lie repressed hostilities, alongside constitutional factors — can improve or heal simply by changing the environmental conditions.

Hypertension in black communities, though rare in Africa, has become a very common disease in the United States.

Undoubtedly, there may be more than one explanation, but consider that the living conditions of African Americans require an extraordinary degree of self-control.[96]

Delving deeper into these issues, let us examine some fundamental differences that distinguish four different patients, all suffering from psychosomatic bronchial asthma.

Two patients suffered the onset of asthma after the death of their spouse; the third, where marriage was imminent; the fourth during childhood, coinciding with the birth of a younger brother.

In the first two patients the disease, due to grief, was typically depressive in one case; in the other, due to a conflict between a sense of liberation and a sense of guilt. In the former it is a matter of simply offering human help, in the second it is essential to act on the conflict.

In the third case, clinical work could highlight a conflict centred on an excessive dependence on the mother that finds the patient torn between a desire to indulge in the affections of a new bond and the sense of guilt for the "betrayal" towards the parent, (here, too, therapy must be directed towards conflict); in the fourth patient, asthma was an expression of acute jealousy in childhood, although this later was resolved. In this latter case, therapy is aimed at the after-effects of the conflict, that is to say, it involves acting on the abnormal residual conditioning, on the habit acquired by the patient of "having asthma", a habit which can often be seen as fuelled by self-suggestion.

Finally, consider the case of a woman who suffered from migraines before sexual intercourse. From the clinical investigation, taking into consideration the patient's personality type, the symptom was deemed a manifestation of repressed anger. Since this conflict is pre-eminent, it is on its dynamics that we mainly act, and not on the migraines themselves. This is to avoid the risk that a potential, difficult direct suppression of this may give rise to other, perhaps even more serious,

---

[96] How timely this consideration is! Today, in the 2020s, many seem to be losing this self-control.

symptoms (tachycardia, genital problems, hypertension, fear of heart attack, etc.), again in order to avoid sexual intercourse.

Naturally, absolute prudence is required in proposing profound psychotherapy, especially if the patient's ego is particularly weak: doing so could aggravate the illness, triggering psychotic episodes.

Psychosomatic therapy

Psychosomatic therapy should point in several directions, considering that the influences on man are endogenous, psychological, social, and exogenous (not least atmospheric and cosmic).

However, since of these influences some are unknown, some are not yet well known to science, and some are of secondary importance, we can distinguish two basic possibilities of psychosomatic therapy: 1st) psychological 2nd) pharmacological.

No therapy, however, can do without a doctor-patient relationship that is also therapeutic in itself.

It should also be noted that each preparation to which the subject attributes any action has a pure, psychological effect, regardless of its pharmaco-dynamic action.

Medication therapy may be of some use in moderating symptoms, however, the patient's dependence on the doctor should be avoided, not least because the persistence or aggravation of symptoms can occur, when in fact these symptoms can be a useful in gaining interest and affection, avoiding situations of inferiority, expressing willpower and satisfying one's competitive needs.

On this level, requests made to the therapist for unnecessary surgical interventions could occur, where the patient is not motivated or culturally geared towards psychotherapy.

Psychotherapy of psychosomatic disorders is now implemented following two fundamental directions: one with a psychodynamic approach, the other behavioural.

The former is scientifically structured and differs from suggestion, which is a process that is more or less involved in a large number of therapeutic treatments, including those of a certain clinical utility.

At the basis of psychoanalytic methods are the interpretation of symptoms, introspection (insight), awareness, emotional experiences induced by the doctor-patient relationship (which allows the patient to strengthen their ability to relate to the world).

It is important for the therapist to re-evaluate the significance of current situations in relation to the patient's childhood conflicts, while remaining neutral, or rather, a supporter of the patient's ego.

Behavioural-oriented psychotherapy addresses behavior and symptoms: it seeks to modify them by way of de-conditioning and de-sensitisation techniques.

In treatment, by using relaxation techniques, they can be repeated, with gradual intensity, so that over time they are better tolerated and resolved. In other cases, two joint stimuli can be associated with the pathological manifestations that are to be eliminated: an unwelcome stimulus and a welcome one, so as to produce mutual inhibitions of the effects of the different inputs, as it is impossible, for example, for fear and of well-being to coexist in the same moment.

Behavioural therapy sometimes makes use of reinforcement, aimed at a general improvement of the personality by overcoming incorrect behaviours that have produced abnormal habits.

The two approaches, psychodynamic and behavioural, can today be integrated, through the common denominator of learning: that is, if it sometimes appears appropriate to implement psychodynamic-oriented psychotherapy the suppression of the symptom is not to be disdained, when this appears to be supported exclusively from an abnormal conditioning, an expression more of a neurotic superstructure than of a true neurosis.

Nor should we underestimate the reduction of symptom intensity, obtained with a behaviourist-type methodology, to enhance and shorten psychodynamic psychotherapy.

Principles of hypnotherapy in psychosomatic disorders

Hypnosis can be efficiently applied to psychodynamic, behavioural or even analytical psychotherapy, to make these therapeutic modalities possible or facilitate, enhance, accelerate them.

The use of hypnosis is implemented when it appears useful or necessary, on the basis of elements (willingness of the patient, strength of the ego, dynamics of symptoms, therapies carried out without results, etc.) that the therapist's information, psychological training, clinical experience and intuition make it possible to detect. These factors also contribute to determining the choice of specific modalities to be adopted on a case-by-case basis and from time to time, as psychotherapy is a highly dynamic process, which can occasionally bring new elements, progressively changing the patient's behaviour.

A good interpersonal relationship, curative in itself (as it properly satisfies certain emotional needs), can in fact also allow the emergence of significant material from a diagnostic point of view. Awareness of a certain situation, by both the doctor and the patient, can improve the therapeutic aspect of the relationship, modifying conflict situations.

Psychotherapy is not a coldly objective one-sided procedure, but rather a combination of objectivity and subjectivity, both on the part of the patient and the therapist.

The psychotherapeutic situation is a learning process, primarily for the patient, secondly for the therapist and the hypnosis used is a process that facilitates the learning of new understandings.
Hypnotherapeutic techniques used in focused on the emotional causes underlying the symptoms.

Procedures targeting symptoms

Conditioning and desensitisation are proposed and have symptomatic therapeutic significance: that is, they aim to abolish, reduce, replace or displace symptoms, manipulating them directly together with the anxiety that feeds them.
This can be sought in various ways: for example, having obtained intense hypnotic relaxation, anxiogenic situations are induced for the patient under waking conditions, of gradually increasing intensity from session to session; the patient is then gradually brought closer to them, or to some of their aspects. In this way, on the basis of the principle that one cannot be relaxed and tense at the same time, the anxious responses to increasingly anxious situations gradually decrease in hypnosis (and then outside of it), from session to session; that is, a kind of "vaccination" takes place.

Procedures targeting emotional causes

These hypnoanalytic procedures, instead of the underlying symptoms or anxiety, are focused on the emotional causes involved and can be used in the course of a psychoanalytic therapy proper, or independently of this.
For instance, the use of hypnosis in the course of psychoanalytic treatment may be advised in the following situations: when the patient loses motivation for therapy, or refuses to start treatment if they do not feel rapid symptomatic relief, or do not develop a productive interpersonal relationship; when they are unable to verbalise sufficiently, to produce free associations, to remember dreams, or are blocked in the production of further meaningful material, or have repressed traumatic memories, the clarification of which can aid the therapeutic process; when, in the end, they have difficulty ceasing therapy.
The ultimate goal of hypnoanalytic techniques is not necessarily always that of becoming aware of profound situations which, in fact, even if they occur, are not always accompanied by an improvement in symptoms, at times they may not be possible or even contraindicated, but rather that of integrating conscious functions with unconscious functions.
These psychoanalytic techniques are also numerous: visualisation of scenes, the "emotional bridge", hypnodrama, the induction of dreams, etc.

The "affect bridge" is a procedure that uses common elements, ie. acts as a "bridge" between present and past emotional experiences. Particularly used when psychoanalysis has led to an intellectual but not an emotional insight, it facilitates the associative process, helping the patient to move from current experiences that are rooted in the past, to their origins. It consists of bringing the subject back to a recent situation, such as a source of conflict, and of making them relive this situation emotionally, focusing all attention on it. The patient is then regressed to a phase of their life in which an identical emotion was experienced for the first time, inviting them to verbalise, referring to the place, time and events that are taking place at that moment. We therefore also try to positively influence the emotional state with suitable suggestions, possibly inviting them to regress even further.

Hypnodrama is nothing other than psychodrama performed under conditions of hypnosis; that is, it consists of improvising, on a given theme, in the presence of an audience, a dramatic performance in which the leader of the group is also involved; conflicts thus come to be externalised in expressions and attitudes. This is advisable when patients cannot express their deep inner content through other techniques.

Sensory hypnoanalysis consists of using sensory responses, in the context of analytical work, particularly in subjects who have difficulty verbalising, that spontaneously arise in hypnosis.

Dream induction, on the other hand, is where dreams have been induced depicting the patient's problems, associating suggestions aimed at achieving, very gradually, a greater clarity of one's dream, a desensitisation of the subject from the emotions that accompany the dream activity and convey as much as possible their psychic energies in the interpersonal relationship with the therapist.

Practical applications of hypnotherapy in psychosomatic medicine[97]

Cardiovascular Disorders

Cardiovascular disorders in particular have been taken into consideration and treated hypnotherapeutically, as well as tachycardia, extrasystoles, headaches and migraines.

All this also in the light of the knowledge on the various relationships existing between myocardial excitability, pressure variations, modification of basal caliber and emotional states such as anxieties, fears and repressed aggression, caused by a wide range of varied factors.

---

[97] The summary relating to this series of disorders is almost always limited simply to a listing of them. It should be noted that in Guantieri's text, summarised here, there are many applied examples of hypnotherapy used in these categories of suffering.

Observations were made on subjects with modest essential hypertension undergoing hypnotherapy. Results demonstrated a spontaneous reduction in blood pressure by 20 millimetres Hg, already shown at the end of initial inductions.

Respiratory disorders

Among the various respiratory disorders, particular attention was paid to bronchial asthma, in the etiopathogenesis of which, in fact, it is possible to detect often suggestively striking evidence of psychic factors that act, according to the case in question, as predisposing, favouring or even determining.
Satisfactory results were also achieved with hypnotherapy in pollen allergies.

Gastrointestinal disorders

Among gastrointestinal disorders, duodenal ulcers, gastritis, colitis, vomiting and other dysfunctions are treated with hypnosis, appropriately distinguishing cases due to abnormal conditioned reflexes from dysfunctions due to somatic affections.

Urinary disorders

Of the urinary disorders treated favourably with hypnotherapy, nocturnal enuresis, particularly frequent in children takes the foreground.

Sexual disorders

In this field, sexual disorders such as vaginismus, frigidity, impotence and premature ejaculation have been treated.
These disorders often express unconscious rejections of sexual intercourse, repressed aggressive impulses, feelings of guilt and the consequent need for punishment.

Skin disorders

Eczema, neuro-dermatitis, hives, herpes, warts, anal and vulvar itching, alopecia and psoriasis are just a few disorders that affect the skin.
The psyche exerts a great influence on such a sensitive organ that reveals emotions, conditions of stress, tension, anguish and other emotional restlessness.

Neuromuscular disorders

Tics, stuttering, paralysis and psychosomatic contractures associated with joint dysfunctions, such as stiff neck, low back pain and sciatica, not sustained by objective injuries, are disorders that have been widely treated by hypnotherapy.

Endocrine and nutrition disorders

With regard to obesity, hypnological literature shows that the results obtained with hypnotic treatment are significantly more satisfactory than those that can be achieved with traditional therapies.
Even anorexia, if it is not an expression of psychosis, can be treated with a view to achieving a better psychosomatic balance.
Hypnotherapy, in the case of diabetic patients, can promote not only an acceptance of the disorder, but also a reduction in the amount of insulin required for treatment.
Thyroid diseases can also obtain considerable benefit through hypnosis.

Hypnotherapy for mental disorders

Indications and methods of use

Certain psychoneuroses such as hysteria and generic depression have shown significant susceptibility to the influence of hypnotherapy.
Positive results have also been recorded in cases of sexual perversions, drug addictions and psychopathic personalities.
The problem was also addressed, with the necessary prudence and gradualness, in the use of hypnosis in selected cases of schizophrenia and paranoia.

Practical applications

In Guantieri's text there are many accounts of hypnotherapeutic interventions: cases of insomnia, phobias, even very serious neuroses, depression associated with headaches, hysterical conversions, drug addiction, alcohol addiction and smoking.
Cases of the use of hypnosis with schizoid subjects are also reported.
There is no shortage of contraindications: in relation to delusional schizophrenias, overt paranoia, oligophrenic or demented subjects, partly because, with these

patients, the possibility of establishing a good interpersonal relationship, so important in hypnotic therapy, can be difficult to achieve.

6. Other practical applications of hypnosis in medicine

The use of hypnosis in obstetrics

Hypnosis can be used in obstetrics:

1) To treat disorders such as insomnia, anorexia, nausea, vomiting, fatigue, back pain and cramps, which often accompany pregnancy;
2) To induce calm, serenity and trust;
3) To facilitate the puerperium by positively influencing milk supply, when low or excessive;
4) To reduce or abolish pain in childbirth.

Combined psychoprophylactic and hypnotic instruction, with childbirth under hypnosis or in the waking state, is carried out with methods that are all based on the following principles:

1) Starting from the sixth or seventh month of pregnancy, the pregnant woman is progressively de-conditioned by those psychological orientations and attitudes that have led her, over the years, to consider pregnancy almost synonymous with illness;
2) In parallel, inducing psychosomatic relaxation by means of hypnosis;
3) Subsequently teaching her in hypnosis to contract the abdominal muscles and to relax the perineal muscles;
4) Eventually developing analgesia.

This latter effect can be achieved by employing procedures similar to those used to induce anaesthesia during surgery. One can, for example, first induce analgesia of one hand and, having made this effect as intense and extensive as possible, it is made to persist after the cessation of hypnosis, so that it can be objectively ascertained by the pregnant woman. The analgesia is then transferred, through appropriate suggestions, to the abdominal region and to others.

The pregnant woman is subsequently trained to reproduce the insensitivity to pain in hypnosis or self-hypnosis, by means of a conditioned stimulus, after being suggested in hypnosis and associated with analgesia in conjunction with the onset of this (for example by suggesting to the pregnant woman that the gradual contraction in the first of one hand, carried out at the onset of each contraction, will facilitate the contraction, depriving it of pain).

The use of hypnosis in surgery

Hypnosis can be used in surgery:

1) To reduce or eliminate pre-operative anxiety and its consequences, in combination with drugs or in place of them;
2) To induce analgesia or anaesthesia in combination with chemicals (balanced anaesthesia), or without them;
3) To facilitate the post-operative journey and thus accelerate healing, since hypnosis can positively affect complications such as vomiting, cough, pain, paresis of the alvus, insomnia, and anorexia;
4) To simultaneously strengthen motivations to heal.

When hypnosis is to be employed as the sole anaesthetic means, the procedure becomes more complex than in balanced anaesthesia: once analgesia is achieved, it is extended and intensified as much as possible; it is then transferred to the area where the surgery will take place and to other areas of the body. The patient is also trained to produce anaesthesia on their own in any part of the body, using stimuli that, previously associated in hypnosis with the onset of this insensitivity, in perfect conjunction with this, have become so conditioned. Finally, the various phases of the operation are explained and "post-hypnotic" suggestions are formulated, designed to act both during the intervention and after it.

The use of hypnosis in dentistry

The use of hypnosis in dentistry is advisable in order to facilitate certain results, or to enable them when traditional means are insufficient, in order to make treatment more effective.

The main indications are the following:

1) Easing anxiety, which accompanies or precedes the first visit, (sometimes even preventing it) and / or subsequent procedures;
2) Eliminating gag reflex;
3) Reducing salivary secretion;
4) Immobilising the tongue and cheeks;
5) Facilitating the production of mouth molds;
6) Performing radiographs and fitting prostheses;
7) Reducing or eliminating post-operative complications.

These outcomes are pursued through relaxation, visualisations, and "post-hypnotic" suggestions.

Not only can the "fear of the dentist" be prevented and overcome, but also vomiting, sialorrhea, incorrect habits such as interposition of the tongue between the teeth, and bruxism, as long as there are no serious emotional conflicts at the base of the manifestations. In this case, in fact, as well as in others of a psychosomatic nature that affect the oral cavity, the use of hypnosis implies notions and experiences that transcend the competence of the dentist.

In fact, in these cases, it is essential to get to know the patient's personality and the dynamics of the symptoms and to establish hypnosis with them, in addition to psychotherapy.

The dentist, as well as other specialists (for example, the dermatologist, the orthopedist or the ophthalmologist), must be adequately prepared from a psychological and psychotherapeutic point of view in order to proceed with caution in the use of hypnosis, otherwise, not only would they not achieve their goals, but they would risk serious negative consequences for their clients.

Appendix – Animal Hypnosis

The possibility of developing hypnosis in animals among the most diverse species (fish, amphibians and reptiles, birds or mammals) has been discovered and affirmed by several scholars.

In fact, various vertebrates and invertebrates spontaneously produce a cataleptic state that some authors – questionably – define as the biological antecedent of human hypnosis.

Man too can induce this state in animals by natural means; an example of this is the result that snake charmers obtain through intense gaze fixation.

Many studies have been carried out and research continues in this field.

The detectable characteristics regarding the effects that this hypnosis produces relate to the postures assumed, the frequency of breathing, heart rate, electroencephalographic changes and the conditioning they bring about.

Both biological and evolutionary factors are at play.

The nature of animal hypnosis today is still fundamentally considered in terms of cortical inhibition and fear paralysis.

There are various theories that offer explanations and interpretations of animal hypnosis; we believe that, to date, an identification between human and animal hypnosis is not possible, nor that there is sufficient correlation between them.

Supplement

Holistic conception of the person in neonatology, psychomotricity and neuroscience

1. Introduction

In chapter three, entitled "Epistemological foundations of Guantierian Hypnology", we pointed out that one of the main pillars of Gualtiero Guantieri's scientific paradigm was his humanistic conception of the person. In fact, we asked ourselves what was his vision of man, noting how he always considered him in his complexity, from an essentially holistic perspective therefore, as an entity that is body and psyche well rooted in a contextual environment that defines to a large extent its very identity.

This supplement to our text, then, intends to account for how that way of considering man, since Guantieri's time, has been improving, and we account for this by considering examples from neonatology, psychomotricity and neuroscience. The holistic consideration of the person, understood as a single and inseparable organism, considers man – in body and mind – an integral unity, inserted in a specific context of life.

Therefore, the body is man, its vitality is simultaneously psyche, that cannot disregard its own somatic dimension, but also that of relationship and communication; indeed, it is the first instrument of message transmission in that it precedes language, and then continually integrates it. Man talks to himself, being at the same time a communicator and interlocutor, his own internal notes (for example hunger, thirst, cold, physical pain, bodily desires that express their requests), while expressing externally, towards the other, experiences that mask them, supporting intentions, sometimes truth, replacing or integrating words in need of support and integration of their insufficiency.

The body is not pure physical matter, it is alive, and it is a constitutive part of the person, it manifests will and emotions, it recounts its own history, culture and identity.

It represents meanings; for example, if a body moves back and forth, here and there aimlessly, it reveals indecision and emptiness, if it is clumsy it signals internal confusion, if it walks in a tired tired and shaky way, it indicates disinterest, if it tries to hide from the gaze of others, it denounces shame or similar feelings: every bodily expression is always non-verbal communication.

The body records in itself every instant of the passage of time.

An immobile body that is relaxed in an armchair, is a body that has the experience of a lived and present time.[98] However, it also summarises all the experiences of the past that remain embodied and current stresses – as James Hilmann (1926-2011) argues – "as if to reproduce an 'imprinting' effect which is a

---

[98] Malesani P.G., *Tempo concitato e tempo rilassato*, ReS magazine, Verona, year IX, n. 2, 2003.

distinctive mark of origin and individuality and which reproduces and repeats ourselves and it becomes a coded relational system".[99]

The author also affirms a point of view that turns common thinking on its head, and writes that it is not the spirit that inhabits the body but it is the latter "who strolls in that garden which is the soul".[100]

Otto Kernberg (1928-2006) emphasises how the biological aspects of the person constitute the matrix within which the psychological aspects develop. He also claims that "the body, love, death ... are one [...;] they are time".[101]

The body expresses pragmatic and relational communication that is aimed at the world in order to significantly influence it, to promote or determine its behaviours, evaluating them, esteeming them, judging them, appreciating them, sometimes even rebuking them.

The semiology of non-verbal language, the study of the signs produced by this type of communication, of course has to do with the body, with its tone, its postural attitudes, movement, mimicry, gesture, paralinguistic productions and the weather.

Paola Loreto (b. 1964) wrote 'The Awakening', a song about the body, which says: "No one needs to tell me what happens. The body speaks its special phrases of when it wakes up in spring and looks around in amazement. The body knows that life wants life, it calls for it, demands it. I have to say yes. I must go (and then, if anything, stay)".[102]

The body wants to live and survival instinct is strong.

The body cannot bear to turn to ashes in a crematorium.

Piero Iotti (1926-2016), recounts the first night he spent, interned by the Nazis during the Second World War, in a barrack in the Mauthausen concentration camp, when he witnessed the hanging of a man and did not sleep a wink, but he claims that if he had seen the same scene after three months in captivity, he would have remained indifferent and would not even have turned his head towards the crime.[103]

In the body, reason and inhibitions, impulses and chills, desires and fears, dreams and reality are mixed in a melting pot of body-time, body-space and body-soul.

The body, in relation to time, can fear it to the point of being frightened. For example, when, as the mind becomes blind and does not understand, the body stiffens into military postures: harsh, inflexible and intolerant.

If it is time for light, the body says so and it is brilliant, remembering mistakes never to be repeated, and it learns, and listens, and relates and compares, and

---

[99] Hilmann J., *La forza del carattere (The force of character)*, Adelphi, Milan, 2000.
[100] Idem, c.s.
[101] Kernberg O., *Relazioni d'amore*, Raffaello Cortina, Milan, 1995.
[102] Loreto P., *La memoria del corpo*, Crocetti Editions, Milan, 2007.
[103] Iotti P., Masoni T., *Sono dov'è il mio corpo. Memoria di un ex deportato a Mauthausen (I am where my body is: Memory of an ex-deportee to Mauthausen)*, Giuntina, Florence, 1995.

gives weight and meaning to life.

With the time of light the body expresses, with its language, its warnings, hopes, attitudes of transcendence and sanctification.
And the body knows about the past and present and remembers what the mind can forget.[104]
The body of omens may tremble or become excited, the body of the spirit reverberates from a transcendent time and becomes sick if it is not in harmony with the spirit.[105]
Simona Vinci (b. 1970) meditates on the immature bodies of those who are not yet "grown up", and writes: "In adolescence the body begins to make noise, from identity problems to the assumption of one's gender, from somatic manipulations to self-harm, from risky behaviours to suicide attempts... The body feels everything and allows us to express ourselves beyond silence and words".[106]
The Milanese writer, in another passage, tells of a woman who says: "I'm sitting here. The naked eyes, the abandoned hands, the body offered to the light, to the movements of the day. It seems that the body, while it vibrates, knows and speaks its own language...". [107]

2. Neonatology

Neonatology deals with primordial intelligence.
The prenatal condition consists, according to the studies carried out by this discipline, of a fusion of ego-love-loathing which is one with the mother-matter that surrounds it.
Man is a being made up of a whole, which is motherhood, generativity and creation. There is an epistemology of neonatology that considers the unborn child an omnipotent embryo-node, destined to encounter pain, to a bang of being, which will necessarily experience the time of labor, already at birth, when there will be the forced renunciation of the maternal Eden and the wandering pilgrimage to a motherland that will restore identity, and relief will begin.

---

[104] This is the case, for example, of a 30-year-old woman who, in a hypnotherapeutic session, relived the experience of a previously forgotten surgery, which she underwent at the age of four.
[105] It is a transcendent body that is recounted by Anne Cameron (b. 1938), a Canadian Indian woman of the Nootka tribe. The writer describes cyclical times, the time of the earth, and the time of the female body and its flows in a temporal order that refers to the quality of the body and its humoral, liquid physiology. And she writes of young women who, during their menstrual cycle, celebrated in sacred places, isolated, and far from their villages. There, they sat on the earth that was soaked in their blood, in a ritual that represented a sort of restitution of energy, being the blood, the menstrual cycle and the earth, strongly linked together in a primordial intertwining called *Time of the Moon*, (Cameron A., *The Daughters of the Copper Woman*, Edizioni Terra di Mezzo, Milan, 2003).
[106] Vinci S., *In tutti i sensi come l'amore*, Einaudi, Turin, 1999.
[107] Vinci S., Idem, c.s.

According to this thought, this would essentially give rise to a regret for the lost paradise that universal man cannot avoid.

The expectant mother, experiencing desires, suffering and fear, involves the newborn child, on a psychic and bodily level, with relational, bodily, somatic, tonic, prenatal and pre-mental effects that form a vital imprinting as early as gestation and lasting forever.

These contributions suggest to us how prenatal experience, movement and sensoriality are knowledge that precede the shaping of cognitive intelligence, while at the same time preparing its foundations.

Before conscious knowledge, an enteroceptive and exteroceptive, visceral and sensorial intelligence would operate, which is already 'being in the world'.

In the nascent, the senses, the muscles, the axial tone, the neuromuscular system and the respiratory, cardiovascular and immune systems, etc., are always all involved, totally, inextricably in the body and with the body that exists, in its unity and complexity that it gradually acquires.

The foetus listens to the world and learns.

The intelligence of the tone − of all and each of the organs participating in vital experiences − from the very beginning, acts by determining memory and therefore biological, somatic, emotional , albeit unconscious, knowledge, but which is essential for the purposes of overall evolution.

The nervous system and the brain specialise their characteristics, qualities and functions, not before, nor after, nor alone, but simultaneously and in parallel with the overall evolution of the whole being that is incessantly involved and shaped by infinite, organic interactions that are psychic, natural and cultural.

Joseph Le Doux (b. 1949) argues that "in the early stages of human development, experiences are not cognitive but essentially emotional and based on interactive exchanges. They leave bodily traces, not necessarily written only in terms of brain engrams". [108]

John Bowlby (1907-1970), for his part, states that "already in the first hours of neonatal life, prolonged mother-infant contact identifies the senses as an essential driver of attachment behavior. The very essence of tonic dialogue is given by bodies in contact that speak".[109]

The mother represents, for the child, a pre-verbal opportunity for knowledge strongly emotionally connoted. She is the child's first emotional and psychic mirror. For the child, perceiving means following and controlling the environment and what happens to them, but the newborn has neurophysiological mechanisms and primordial psychological devices at their disposal, depending on the evolutionary stage reached.

---

[108] Le Doux J., *Il cervello emotivo. Alle origini delle emozioni,* Baldini Castoldi Dalai Edizioni, Milan, 2003.
[109] Bowlby J., *Attaccamento e perdita,* Bollati Boringhieri, Turin, 1972.

The being exists already, it is at the beginning of its time and interacts and operates with an intelligence that is very intuitive and as time passes, it also integrates this with rational intelligence.
Even before there is cognition, precursors are built, which is corporeality that acts intelligently and records memory.
Stanley Greenspan (1941-2010) states that at the very foundation of the development of intelligence there are precisely those emotional interactions that are experienced from birth with the people around us. If you grow up in an environment that is lacking in feelings, you also risk deficiencies from an intellectual point of view".[110]

3. Psychomotricity

The body is not simply inert somatic nature, and in its own right, but a vibrant and constitutive part of the person.
It is directly from the body that the individual, physical and psychic needs of each emerge and they are preparatory to the organization of life itself, on a motory and cognitive, emotional, behavioural and relational level.
The body is therefore a cognitive entity, it constitutes the foundation for the development of affectivity, thought, intelligence, communication and interpersonal relationships. At the same time, it serves these personality traits and expresses all the conscious and hidden realities of the person.
The body is a mnestic parchment on which all the events, wounds and kindnesses, pleasures and dramas, anxieties and torments, joys and enthusiasms experienced in individual history are inscribed and annotated. And therefore it is the mind, a metaphor of the same, a visible photograph of the history of each one.
The body is a psychic place and also a psyche tout court.
Its posture and tone are an expression, a function of the emotional state. Emotions change the body.
Tone highlights the sensory condition of the moment and communicates it in a way that can be observed and touched, seen and felt, so that the other receives affective information with respect to which they experience emotions and feelings.
There is an innate tonic system: it automatically registers pleasant and unpleasant sensations; primitive discomforts dissolve with appropriate parental interventions that attribute physiological and psychological meanings to what manifests itself in the body, progressively differentiating physical sensations from correlated mental activities.

---

[110] Greespan S.I., *L'intelligenza del cuore,* Mondadori, Milan, 1997.

In bodies, the psychological and emotional systems and the organic, tonic and motor organizations are not only connected to each other, but intertwine in an inextricable, unitary whole.

Henri Wallon (1879-1962) considers emotions as a "formation of postural origin that has muscle tone as its fabric", while Julian de Ajuriaguerra (1911-1986), states that "the role of the tonic state is extremely important in organising personality".

They are joined by Jean Piaget (1896-1980) who suggests that emotion is proof of the existence of the relationship, indicating its property of "tying together different systems: affection, facial expressions, posture, hormonal modifications".[111]

Tone and feelings are mediated by sensations, with the result that the Self organises its relational, communicational, social, significant and semiotic motor activity of the emotional system.

Tone simultaneously has an intra-psychic function and a relationship with the outside world, so as to demarcate one's own psychological spaces and the individual affective space.

The psychic sphere inhabited by the subject necessarily and simultaneously places them in relationship with their own internal and external dimension, thus constituting delimitations of individual body and psychic areas, preluding, constituting, strengthening the Self, the Ego and one's own personality which, again, are expressed, represented and communicated to the world by the body, in primordial form.

Here, then, is how tonic dialogue starts to take place.

Here hypertonia is a protection, a defensive armour and a conflict between desire and repression. This is how the psychic holding arranged by the mother affects the tonic and therefore emotional condition of the child.

Relational situations of bodies that move are grafted onto it and in which one carries the other, puts him or her to bed, offers them food, thus creating a sentimental relationship, which is sometimes very satisfying and gratifying or in some cases frustrating and sad. And it is psychomotricity. And it is the manifestation of sensory conditions and experiences: tactile, visual, olfactory, gustatory, auditory, minimal and delicate or decisive, sometimes opposing, such as tremors, vibrations, prehensile reactions, affectionate or reproachful looks, perfumed or stinking smells[112], tastes that are delicious or disgusting, musical or

---

[111] This paragraph is mainly inspired by the writings of Franco Boscaini (b. 1948). In particular: Boscaini F., Boscaini F., *Corpo ed emozione. Primo spazio di comunicazione e rappresentazione,* ReS magazine, Year VI, n. 3 and year VII n. 1, Verona, 1998-1999, which cites, among others, Wallon, Ajuriaguerra and Piaget.
[112] In this regard, the story by Patrick Süskind (b.1949) about a protagonist who, deeply conditioned by bad smells when he was a child, abandoned on a pile of garbage, later became a world-famous perfumer when he grew up, (Süskind P., *Il Profumo,* Longanesi, Milan, 1985). Even more shocking is the direct testimony of Ennio Mancini (b.1938) - survivor of the inhumane Nazi-massacre of Sant'Anna di Stazzema (Lucca) in August 1944 - who tells of that acrid smell which so affected him then, and which he still remembers, to the point he can't bear to cook meat on the grill, (Minoli G., (Edited by), *Una mattina d'agosto,* from the series *La storia siamo noi,* www.raiplay.it/video/2013).

loud sounds. And it is non-verbal communication, once again a meaningful and intense relational modality.

In this way, the needs and impulses of movement in which the subject situates themselves and lives are expressed.

Through these paths, the body schema and self-image are built, the first being the neuropsychological support of the second, which includes feelings, affective sensations and libidinal experiences aroused by the body.

Psychomotricity knows how to fit into these communication contexts, read their contents, give them meaning, interpret these psychophysical, psychosomatic states, therefore, grasp and measure these degrees of tonic tension, use this information and requests that pulsating bodies address to those who can, or should, understand them.

Psychomotricity skills are therefore able to grasp psychomotor indicators that denounce normality or psychic disorders, psychosomatic functioning, levels of psychomotor skills relating to balance, walking, running, jumping, identifying difficulties in which to intervene.

It is therefore interested in physiological behaviours, manipulations, the use of objects, as functional, affective and cognitive realities and as signals of the state of health and well-being of the subject being cared for.

Psychomotricity studies praxis, such as dressing or washing oneself, building games, graphism (for example doodling while drawing), body language, i.e. non-verbal and speech, the use of hands, the laterality of one's writing, reading, as well as psychophysiological, behavioural, language and communication mechanisms.

This procedure makes it possible to diagnose, from a psychomotor point of view, such disorders as disharmonies and delays, imbalances in the mind-body relationship, disturbances between the individual and the environment, irregularities in physiological functions, disorders of tone and motor skills, incorrect use of objects, inhibitions, instability, stuttering, tics, language delays and disorders, learning difficulties, or relationship problems.

On these bases, it is possible to establish prevention, management and psychomotory care.

It is a systemic approach considering that, in the case of children, parents, family members, educators and teachers are directly or indirectly involved.

They, by working introspectively on themselves, can help improve the child's psychomotor organization and personality.

4. Neuroscience

Antonio Damasio (b. 1944) asserts that neuroscience considers intelligence as a "complex interacting and structured set of second-level body-brain-mind, as an integration of simpler basic constitutive systems".[113] He offers a spectacular metaphor for this complexity and writes: "All emotions use the body as [a] theatre".[114]

Candace Pert (1946-2013) describes neuroscience as follows: "It considers the body broadly in connection with the mind. Not only the belly, but all the organs of the body [...] are in connection with the mind, as if there were a 'moving brain'".[115]

She has identified psychic molecules present in every cell of the body and writes that, since the body and mind together constitute the seat of memory, we also find a possible trauma inscribed, engraved, marked, sculpted in the quivering body which therefore also constitutes a place where to seek repressed truths.

Many painful stories are stored in different places in the body.

"The whole body is alive, intelligent and conscious," says Candace Pert. "Each cell feels pleasure or pain and develops metabolic strategies for the collective well-being of the organism".[116]

Psycho-Neuro-Endocrine-Immuology (P.N.E.I.) accounts for the close relationships between the psyche and nervous, endocrine and immune systems, highlighting how the mediators of information and emotions are active proteins: neuropeptides. They are present in all individual cells: in the blood, in the immune system, in the intestine and in the nervous system.

From these findings, it can be deduced that all states of mind are faithfully reflected in the physiological states of the various organismic systems: immune, digestive, circulatory, nervous etc. The conclusion is the following: the whole body is the psyche!

Each cell, each organ and system, the individual parts of the body and the entire organic whole think, feel, feel emotions, process their own psychophysical information and disseminate them within the living complex through a very dense structure of intertwining and totalising connections.

The models and paradigms of Damasio and Pert do not neglect the cultural context in which the person lives, simultaneously influenced in the mind and soul and, directly, in the body.

The effect of the cultural context is evident: for instance, can a European ever become a true Hindu? Truthfully, it would be very complicated!

Gian Marco Carenzi (b. 1961), a neuroscience expert, states: "The cells of the body, from conception onwards, inform each other as they grow, so that the

---

[113] Damasio A., *L'errore di Cartesio. Emozione, ragione e cervello umano*, Adelphi, Milan, 1995.
[114] Idem, c.s.
[115] Pert C., *La chimica delle emozioni*, in www.ceepsib.org/PNEI
[116] Pert C., *Molecole di Emozioni*, Tea Libri, Milan, 2005.

feelings, emotions and sensations of the birth scenario remain imprinted on them [...,] there to forever influence what we become, what we do and how we relate".[117]

Vincenzo Di Spazio (b. 1962) hypothesised a spinal clock, capable of recording the traumatic experiences lived throughout the course of life, through tangible physical traces. It would be found in the "spinal Plates", there, to record the "time of our lives", like tree rings. [118]

He quotes Giuseppe Calligaris (1876-1944) who maintains that: "Our body is a faithful mirror of our spirit, and this of that".[119]

Everything that is experienced, including situations of great suffering, are therefore stored, not only in the brain and the spino-medullary area, but also in the chest, jaw, shoulders, abdomen, pelvis, etc. All our memories are invisibly tattooed on the brain and throughout the nervous system, but also in the flesh, in the bowels of the body and on the skin, there to document the history and identity of each of us.

Maurice Merleau-Ponty (1908-1961) succeeds well in intuiting and anticipating this knowledge, stating that: "The body is the only means you have to go to the heart of things",[120] after all, where we could go, and how we could live without a body?

5. Conclusions

Neuroscience, neonatology, modern paediatrics and psychomotricity suggest that the child is a full-bodied intelligent.

Of course, when they grow up, the child continues to live in the adult.

Their rational and cerebral intelligence do not take into account the total experience of man.

This betrays their abstraction from the real world, it is disembodied, it makes them an automaton, which disengages itself with great speed and ease in solving calculation problems, but transferred into existence, it provides partial and often disappointing results, because even the body knows, it has its own intelligence, with other connotations than logic and mathematics.

The attempt to translate life, the concrete reality of the body, into intellectual structures reduced at the neurological level is impractical.

Each content or experience is born in the body and its environment and with its own language, outside of which it does not exist.

---

[117] Carenzi G. M., *Il respiro che guarisce,* Tecniche Nuove Editore, Milan, 2000.
[118] Di Spazio V., *Il meridiano del tempo,* Giannone, Milan, 2002.
[119] Di Spazio V., *Il corpo-specchio secondo Calligaris,* in www.vega2000.it/art_dispazio.html, 2008._
[120] Merleau-Ponty M., *Il corpo vissuto, l'ambiguità dell'esistenza, la riscoperta della vita percettiva, la carne del mondo. Dalle prime opere a L'occhio e lo spirito,* (Anthology by Fergnani F.), Il Saggiatore, Milan, 1979.

After all, the experience is always unrepeatable, it carries with it an immediate emotional charge, which cannot be expressed in terms of logical-rational knowledge.

An idea: if the wisest science gives us back the body, a more sensitive concomitant humanism will allow other returns, such as: myth, history, autobiographical testimonies, the modest and fragmentary reality of everyday life. And there will be room for Olympus and its divinities who continue to live and be there.

Alda Merini (1931-2009) is a poet who made intuitive contributions to the science of intelligence. Her verses are useful, as long as the scientist is sometimes able to leave the laboratory, to stop for a while and close their eyes.

Here is one of her poems: "Your memory is a petal / that rests on the heart and upsets it / Goodbye, like every evening / beyond the fractures there is an erect corpse of speech / it looks like a fragment of euthanasia / but you kill me as always / love, and reopen my eternal deposits / The sepulchres of Foscolo, the farewells / of certain hands that are not buried / and emerge futile from nowhere / to ask for justice of words / your memory is a petal".

There is a gap between the power of the intuitive intelligence of poetry and the stumbling block of a certain science that is relentless in producing artificial languages and forgets the words of the body.

Life is not, reductively, miserably, a neuronal fact, if memory upsets hearts, causes the wounds of abandonment to bleed continuously, arouses feelings of death, moves the hands, cries out the protest of incomprehension and fuels the pretence to speak again.

General Bibliography

- AA.VV., Proceedings of the Conference: *Ipnologia Guantieriana e i suoi sviluppi nel tempo*. San Martino B.A (Verona), 15 novembre 2008, in *Acta Ipnologica* magazine, Year XII n. 3, 2008 e Year XIII, n. 1, 2009.
- AA.VV., *Il training autogeno applicato*, Proceedings of the I Congresso Internazionale di Campione d'Italia, Publisher CISSPAT, Padua, 1976.
- AA.VV., *L'esperienza dell'ipnosi*, Publisher Astrolabio, Rome, 1990.
- AA. VV., Proceedings of the XX Congresso S.I.M.P. Dedicato a Gualtiero Guantieri, *L'ansia nella clinica e nella società attuale*, Editions S.I.M.P., Verona, 20-23 October 2005.
- AA. VV., *Verità del corpo. Una domanda sul nostro essere*, Editions Pro Santitate, Rome, 2008. See the contributions of: Natoli G., *l'uomo nella sua dimensione psicosomatica secondo la programmazione neuro-linguistica (P.N.L.)*; Caltagirone C., *"Avere" ed "Essere" corpo. Il contributo neuroscientifico di Antonio R. Damasio*.
- Abbozzi P., *La forza delle parole*, Publisher Airone, Rome, 1996.
- Abbozzi P., *Tecniche di autoipnosi pratica*, Publisher Airone, Rome, 2003.
- Abstract Book of XX Congresso S.I.M.P. Dedicato a Gualtiero Guantieri, *L'ansia nella clinica e nella società attuale*, Publisher S.I.M.P., Verona, 20-23 October 2005.
- Airaudi O., *Corso di ipnosi in 13 lezioni*, Publisher Med, Padua, 1988.
- Albisetti V., *Il training autogeno per la quiete psicosomatica*, Publisher Paoline, Milan, 1994.
- Araoz D.L., *Ipnosi e terapia sessuale*, Publisher Astrolabio, Rome, 1984.
- Arena M., *Il linguaggio ipnotico nella comunicazione terapeutica*, in *Acta Ipnologica* magazine, Year I, n. 3, 1997.
- Argyle M., *Il corpo e il suo linguaggio*, Publisher Zanichelli, Bologna, 1978.
- Auriol B., *Tutti i metodi di rilassamento*, Publisher Red, Como, 1989.
- Balaskas J., *Manuale del parto attivo: gli esercizi per arrivare al parto con la sicurezza e le energie necessarie*, Publisher Red, Como, 1983.
- Bányai É.I., *The Interactive Nature of Hypnosis: Research Evidence for a Social Psychobiological Model*, in *Contemporary Hypnosis* magazine, 1985.
- Bányai É.I., *On the Adaptive Value of Hypnosis: A Social Psychobiological Model*, Invited address presented at the 12th International Congress of Hypnosis, Jerusalem, Israel, 25-31 July 1992.
- Bányai É.I., *The Interactive Nature of Hypnosis: Research Evidence for a Social Psychobiological Model*, in *Contemporary Hypnosis* magazine, 1998.
- Bányai É.I., *Toward a Social-Psychobiological Model of Hypnosis*, in Lynn SJ, Rhue JW, *Theorie of Hypnosis. Current Models and Perspectives*, New York, London: The Guilford Press.
- Bányai É.I., Mészáros I. e Csókay L., *Interaction between Hypnotist and Subject: A social Psychophysiological Approach, (Preliminary report)*, in Waxman D., Misra P.C.,

- Gibson M., Basker M.A., *Modern Trends in Hypnosis,* New York, London: Plenum Press, 1985.
- Beggiora S., (edited by), *Il cosmo sciamanico. Ontologie indigene fra Asia e Americhe,* Series S.T.R.A.D.E.: Spiritualità e Tradizioni Religiose. Approcci, Discipline, Etnografie, Publisher Franco Angeli, Milan,1919.
- Bernheim H., *De la suggestion hypnotique dans l'état hypnotique et dans l'état de veille,* Publisher Doin, Paris, 1884.
- Bernheim H., *De la suggestion et de ses applications à la thérapeutique,* Publisher L'Hartmattan, Paris, 2005.
- Bernt H., *Manuale di training autogeno,* Publisher Astrolabio, Rome, 1980.
- Bertoldi P., *Meditazione. Riscoprire la gioia,* Publisher Demetra, Colognola ai Colli (Verona), 1999.
- Biermann G., *Il training autogeno in età pediatrica,* Editions CISSPAT, Padua, 1989.
- Bizzotto M., *Il grido di Giobbe. L'uomo, la malattia, il dolore nella cultura contemporanea,* San Paolo Editions, Cinisello Balsamo (Milan), 2001.
- Boccali G., *Forse lo sciamano ha qualcosa da dirci,* Sunday supplement, *Il Sole 24 Ore,* Milan, 21 March 2021.
- Boscaini F., *Il rilassamento psicomotorio e psicosomatico secondo G.B. Soubiran,* dossier by CISERPP, Verona, 1990.
- Boscaini F., *Corpo ed emozione. Primo spazio di comunicazione e rappresentazione,* ReS magazine, Year VI, n. 3 and Year VII, n. 1, Verona, 1998-1999.
- Boscaini F., *Storia della psicomotricità,* Publisher AIF, Verona, 2001.
- Bowlby J., Attaccamento e perdita, Publisher Bollati Boringhieri, Turin, 1972.
- Brenner H., *Rilassamento progressivo e desensibilizzazione sistematica dell'ansia,* Publisher Paoline, Milan, 1992.
- Brugnoli A., *Possibilità terapeutiche nel dolore psicosomatico,* in *Anoressia e obesità,* (edited by Antonelli F. and Guantieri G.), Vol. II, n. 15, Publisher Società Editrice Universo (S.E.U.), Rome, 1969.
- Brugnoli A., *Etica del dolore e della sofferenza alle soglie del terzo millennio,* in *Acta Ipnologica* magazine, Verona, Year III, n. 1, 1999.
- Brugnoli A., *Stati di coscienza modificati,* Editions Istituto Italiano Studi di Ipnosi Clinica e Psicoterapia 'H. Bernheim', Scuola di Ricerca e Formazione, San Martino B.A. (Verona), 2000.
- Caldironi B., Widmann C., *Visualizzazioni guidate in psicoterapia,* Publisher Piovan, Abano Terme (Padua), 1980.
- Cameron A., *Le Figlie della Donna di Rame,* Publisher Terra di Mezzo, Milan, 2003.
- Carletti C., Piazza C., *Ipnosi e poesia. Un uso del ritmo e della metafora in una esperienza di gruppo. Hypnosis and Poetry. A use of rhythm and metaphor in a group training experiences,* in *Acta Ipnologica* magazine, Year X, n. 2-3, May-September 2006.
- Carenzi G.M., *Il respiro che guarisce,* Publisher Tecniche Nuove, Milan, 2000.

- Carnevali R., *Il training autogeno*, Publisher Universitarie Massi, Milan, 1982.
- Casiglia E., *Trattato di ipnosi e altre modificazioni di coscienza*, Publisher Cleup, Padua, 2015.
- Castaneda C., *A scuola dallo stregone*, Publisher Astrolabio, Rome, 1970.
- Castellani P., *La luce di Ippocrate*, Publisher Cisalpino, Milan-Varese, 1962.
- Crock R., *Rilassamento per bambini*, Publisher Red, Como, 1995.
- Crosa G., *Il training autogeno di Schultz nel trattamento delle caratteropatie*, in *Rivista di psichiatria*, Publisher Il Pensiero Scientifico Editore, Rome, 1968.
- Damasio A., *L'errore di Cartesio. Emozione, ragione e cervello umano*, Publisher Adelphi, Milan, 1995.
- D'Avila T., *Il Castello interiore*, Publisher Paoline, Turin, 2011.
- De Benedittis G., *In Memoriam del Prof. Gualtiero Guantieri*, in *International Journal of Clinical and Experimental Hypnosis*, Publisher Taylor & Francis Inc., Philadelphia, U.S.A., 1995.
- De Bussingen D.R., *Distensione e training autogeno*, Publisher Edizioni Mediterranee, Rome, 1980.
- De Chirico G., *Training autogeno*, Publisher Red, Como, 1984.
- De Fontaine B., (Bernardo di Chiaravalle), *Sermones super Cantica Canticorum*, Editiones Cistercienses, Rome, 1957.
- Dei Benedetti J., (*Iacopone da Todi), Amor de caritate*, Publisher Laterza, Bari, 2006.
- Desoille L.R., *Sogno da sveglio guidato*, Publisher Astrolabio, Rome, 1974.
- De Yepes Álvarez J., (Giovanni della Croce), Notte oscura, Publisher Città Nuova, Rome, 2006.
- Dietmar O., *Rilassamento muscolare progressivo*, Publisher Red, Como, 1996.
- Di Spazio V., *Il meridiano del tempo*, Publisher Giannone, Milan, 2002.
- Dogs W., *Rilassamento del training autogeno*, Publisher Hermes, Rome, 1987.
- Duran De Busingen R., *I metodi di rilassamento*, Publisher Paoline, Rome, 1996.
- Eberlein G., *Sani con il training autogeno*, Publisher Feltrinelli, Milan, 1975.
- Eberlein G., *Training autogeno per progrediti, esercizi di grado superiore*, Publisher Feltrinelli, Milan, 1977.
- Èdelstein G.M., *Trauma, trance, trasformazione. Guida clinica all'ipnoterapia*, Publisher Astrolabio, Rome, 1982.
- Emmerick A.K., *La dolorosa Passione del Nostro Signore Gesù Cristo*, Publisher Shalom, Camerata Picena (Ancona), 2015.
- Erickson M.H., *La mia voce ti accompagnerà*, Publisher Astrolabio, Rome, 1978/a.
- Erickson M.H., *Le nuove vie dell'ipnosi*, Publisher Astrolabio, Rome, 1978/b.
- Erickson M.H., *Opere: la natura della suggestione*, Publisher Astrolabio, Rome, 1978/c.
- Erickson M.H., *La comunicazione mente-corpo in ipnosi*, Publisher Astrolabio, Rome, 1978/d.

- Erickson M.H., *A scuola di ipnosi*, Publisher Boringhieri, Turin, 1983.
- Erickson M.H., Rossi E.L., *L'esperienza dell'ipnosi*, Publisher Astrolabio, Rome, 1985.
- Erickson M.H., Rossi E.L., *Tecniche di suggestione ipnotica*, Publisher Astrolabio, Rome, 1989.
- Erickson M.H., Rossi E.L., *Ipnoterapia*, Publisher Astrolabio, Rome, 1990.
- Faretta E., Parietti P., *Ben Essere e Sviluppo delle Risorse Personali. Tecniche dal Mal Essere al Ben Essere Consapevole*, Publisher Alpes Italia, Rome, 2012.
- Farné M., Calderaro G., Pozzi U., T.A. *Il Training Autogeno di J.H. Schultz*, Publisher Giunti e Barbera, Florence, 1980.
- Fieschi Adorno C., (Caterina da Genova), *Trattato del purgatorio e altri scritti*, Publisher Gribaudi, Milan, 2010.
- Filiputti A., *Ipnosi*, Publisher Horus, Turin, 1991.
- Filiputti A., *Ipnosi a mappe cerebrali*, Publisher Demetra, Colognola ai Colli (Verona), 1994.
- Filiputti A., *Ipnosi, dilatare la mente per conoscere e trasformare la realtà*, Publisher Demetra, Colognola ai Colli (Verona), 1999.
- Gastaldo G., Ottobre M., *Il training autogeno in quattro stadi*, Publisher Armando, Rome, 1994.
- Gatto S., *L'ipnosi*, Publisher Selenia, Milan, 1993.
- Geussman De Bussingen A., Il *rilassamento progressivo di E. Giacobson*, Publisher Paoline, Milan, 1977.
- Giorda G., Benizzi M., *Il training autogeno. Teoria e pratica*, Publisher Città Nuova, Rome, 1979.
- Gocci G., *Gruppi di individuazione, (l'officina dell'immaginario)*, in *Acta Ipnologica* magazine, Year IX, n. 1-2, January-May 2005/a.
- Gocci G., *Psicologia del femminile*, in *Acta Ipnologica* magazine, Year IX, n. 1-2, January-May 2005/b.
- Gocci G., *L'anima perduta*, in *Acta Ipnologica* magazine, Year IX, n. 1-2, January-May 2005/c.
- Gocci G., *Buddismo, cristianesimo ed individuazione*, in *Acta Ipnologica* magazine, Year IX, n. 1-2, January-May 2005/d.
- Gocci G., *Un vomito che non voleva cessare*, in *Acta Ipnologica* magazine, Year IX, n. 1-2, January-May 2005/e.
- Gocci G., Piazza C., *Corpo, sogno e immagine in ipnosi senza trançe. Body, Dream and Image in Hypnosis whidout Trance*, in *Acta Ipnologica* magazine, Year III, n. 1, January 1999.
- Gocci G., Piazza C., *Ipnosi moderna e comunicazione. Modern Hypnosis and Comunications*, in *Acta Ipnologica* magazine, Year VI, n. 1, January 2000.
- Goldwurm G.F., Sacchi B., Scarlatto A., *Le tecniche di rilassamento nella terapia comportamentale*, Publisher Angeli, Milan, 1986.
- Granone F., *Trattato di ipnosi*, Publisher Boringhieri, Turin, 1979.

- Green J.P., Lynn S.J., *Hypnotic responsiveness: Expectancy, attitudes, fantasy proneness, absorption, and gender*, in International Journal of Clinical and Experimental Hypnosis, 2011.
- Greespan S.I., *L'intelligenza del cuore*, Publisher Mondadori, Milan, 1997.
- Groddeck G., *Il libro dell'Es*, Publisher Adelphi, Milan, 1966.
- Guantieri G., *Le insuline*, in *Il Fracastoro*, Bulletin of Hospital Institutes of Verona, Verona, 1953.
- Guantieri G., *Il trattamento dell'ipertensione arteriosa con i diidroalcaloidi della segale cornuta*, in *La riforma medica* magazine, 1954.
- Guantieri G., *La terapia del diabete pancreatico*, in *Il Fracastoro*, Bulletin of Istituti Ospitalieri di Verona, Verona, 1954.
- Guantieri G., *L'emozione in medicina: considerazioni su di un caso di interesse psicosomatico*, in *Medicina psicosomatica* magazine, n. 8, Società Editrice Universo (S.E.U.), Rome, 1963.
- Guantieri G., *Contributo allo studio della eziopatogenesi del diabete giovanile: indagine psicosomatica sulla insorgenza e sul decorso di un caso*, in *Annali di Neuropsichiatria e Psicoanalisi* magazine, Year X, n. 4, 1963.
- Guantieri G., *Contributo allo studio della eziopatogenesi e terapia della enuresi essenziale: indagine psicosomatica su di un caso portato a guarigione con l'ipnosi*, in Rivista di Psicologia Normale e Patologica, Publisher Zanichelli, Bologna, n. 1-2, 1963.
- Guantieri G., *Origine e sviluppo della medicina psicosomatica e suo valore nell'epoca attuale*, rivista *Il Policlinico – Sezione Pratica*, Publisher *Biblioteca Nazionale Centrale*, Rome, n. 120, 1963.
- Guantieri G., Proceedings of the 16th Congresso dell'Associazione Otorinolaringologi Ospedalieri Italiani (A.O.O.I.), Verona, May 1963, *Contributo allo studio della eziopatogenesi e terapia della balbuzie, indagine psicologica su di un caso*, in *Annali di Laringologia* magazine, Year LXII, n. 4, 1963.
- Guantieri G., *Contributo allo studio della eziopatogenesi e terapia della enuresi essenziale: indagine psicosomatica su di un caso portato a guarigione con ipnosi*, in *Revista de Psycologia Normal y Patologica*, Pontifícia Universidade Católica de São Paulo (Brasil), n. 1-2, 1963.
- Guantieri G., *Contribution to the Study of Psychosomatic Disorders in Children and their Treatment: General Considerations and Report of a Case*, Proceedings of VI Congresso Internazionale di Psicoterapia, London, August 1964.
- Guantieri G., *L'ipnosi e le sue applicazioni in medicina*, in *Panorama Medico* magazine, Publisher Arnaldo Mondadori, Milan, December 1965.
- Guantieri G., *L'ambiente familiare come fattore patogeno: indagine psicosomatica su di un caso gravissimo di malattia dei tics*, in *Minerva Medica* magazine, n. 56, 1965.
- Guantieri G., *Indagine psicosomatica su di un caso di gastroduodenite*, in *Medicina Psicosomatica* magazine, Year I, n.10, 1965.
- Guantieri G., P*sicodinamica ed ipnosi*, Proceedings of the III Convegno Centro Bernheim, Lazise (Verona), June 1967.

- Guantieri G., *Uber die induktion der hypnose: beitrag zur verwirklichung einer induktionsmethode, besonders geeignet fuer didaktische zweche*, Proceedings of the Congresso Internazionale di Medicina Psicosomatica e Ipnosi di Kyoto, Japan, Juli 1967.
- Guantieri G., *Sull'ipnoterapia dei disordini psicosomatici*, in Antonelli F., Ancona L., (edited by) Proceedings of the VII Conferenza Europea sulla Ricerca Psicosomatica, Rome, September 1967.
- Guantieri G., *Principi per una didassi dell'ipnosi*, Proceedings of the I Congresso dell'Associazione Medica Italiana per lo Studio della Ipnosi (A.M.I.S.I.), Rome, September 1967.
- Guantieri G., *L'ipnosi come mezzo di psicoprofilassi ostetrica*, Proceedings of the Symposium della Società Italiana di Psicoprofilassi Ostetrica, Rome, 1967.
- Guantieri G., *Sull'ipnoterapia dei disordini psicosomatici*, in Antonelli F., Ancona L., (edited by), Proceedings of the VII European Conference on Psychosomatic Research, Rome, Publisher S.I.M.P., 1967.
- Guantieri G., *Sull'induzione di ipnosi: contributo alla realizzazione di un metodo valido sotto il profilo didattico*, in *Rassegna di Ipnosi e Medicina Psicosomatica* magazine, Publisher University "La Sapienza", n. 59, Rome, 1968.
- Guantieri G., *Ipnosi medica. Introduzione allo studio e alla pratica dell'ipnosi in medicina*, in *Opera medica* magazine, Publisher A. Wassermann S.p.A., Milan, Year LVI, April-September, n. 130, 1968.
- Guantieri G., *L'ipnosi: caratteristiche e possibilità di impiego* in *Medicina, Miscellanea*, magazine, Year I, n. 179, 1968.
- Guantieri G., *L'induzione di ipnosi*, in Antonelli F., Businco L. (edited by), *Aggiornamenti in Psicosomatica*, in *Quaderni di Psicosomatica*, Publisher Società Editrice Universo (S.E.U.), Rome, 1969.
- Guantieri G., *Modalità di approccio e di terapia del paziente psicosomatico mediante ipnosi*, in Antonelli F., Guantieri G., (edited by), *Anoressia e Obesità*, in *Quaderni di Psicosomatica* magazine, Società Editrice Universo (S.E.U.), Rome, 1970.
- Guantieri G., *Fondamenti e prospettive dell'ipnologia medica*, in AA.VV., *Lezioni di apertura del Corso di Aggiornamento in Ipnologia medica, Verona, 7-9 maggio 1971*, dossier by Istituto Italiano Studi di Ipnosi Clinica e Psicoterapia 'H. Bernheim', Scuola di Ricerca e Formazione, Verona, 1971.
- Guantieri G., *Lezioni di Psicosomatica*, in Antonelli F., Lapiccirella V., (edited by), *Allucinogeni e Psicosomatosi*, Publisher Società Editrice Universo (S.E.U.), Rome, 1972.
- Guantieri G., *La formazione psicologica del medico*, *Medicina Psicosomatica* magazine, Società Editrice Universo (S.E.U.), Rome, n. 18, 1973.
- Guantieri G., *L'ipnosi, come oggetto di studio e mezzo di impiego in medicina*, Publisher Rizzoli, Milan, 1973.
- Guantieri G., *Fenomenologia dell'ipnosi*, in *Rassegna di Ipnosi Medicina Psicosomatica* magazine, Società Editrice Universo (S.E.U.), Rome, n. 24, 1974.

- Guantieri G., *Ipnosi e psicosomatica: correlazioni sperimentali e cliniche,* in *Rassegna di ipnosi e Medicina Psicosomatica,* in *Minerva Medica* magazine, Turin, n. 25, 1974.
- Guantieri G., *L'ipnosi medica: problemi antichi, fondamenti e prospettive attuali,* in *Rassegna di Ipnosi e Medicina Psicosomatica,* in *Minerva Medica* magazine, Turin, n. 25, 1974.
- Guantieri G., *Formazione psicosomatistica del medico e training ipnotico,* in *Rassegna di Ipnosi Medicina Psicosomatica,* in *Minerva Medica* magazine, Turin, n. 25, 1974.
- Guantieri G., *Posizione e ruolo della ipnosi in psicosomatica,* in *Rassegna di Ipnosi e Medicina Psicosomatica,* rivista *Medicina Psicosomatica,* in *Minerva Medica* magazine, Turin, n. 20, 1975.
- Guantieri G., *Ipnosi e Medicina Psicosomatica come oggetto di studio e di insegnamento universitario,* in *Rassegna di Ipnosi e Medicina Psicosomatica,* in *Minerva Medica* Magazine, Turin, n. 31, 1976.
- Guantieri G., *Training Ipnotico e Training Autogeno,* Proceedings of the International Congress CISSPAT, Campione d'Italia (Como), 1976.
- Guantieri G., *Hypnosis and Psychodinamics,* in Antonelli F., (edited by), Proceedings of the III Congresso Internazionale di Medicina Psicosomatica, Florence, Publisher Pozzi, Brescia, 1977.
- Guantieri G., *Possibilità terapeutiche della ipnosi in alcune disfunzioni sessuali,* in Salvati A., (Edited by), *I 500 perché della donna, Minerva Medica* magazine, Rome, 1978.
- Guantieri G., *L'ipnosi quale modalità di terapia psicosomatica,* Proceedings of the I European Congress of Hypnosis in Psychotherapy and Psychosomatic Medicine of Malmö, Sweden, 1978.
- Guantieri G., *Ipnosi e terapia psicosomatica,* Proceedings of Convegno di Psicoterapia e Psicosomatica, in *Collana di Medicina Psicosomatica,* Publisher Maccari, Parma, 1979.
- Guantieri G., *L'ipnosi quale modalità psicoterapeutica,* Proceedings of the V Convegno Nazionale Medicina, *Studi sulla ipnosi clinica,* A.M.I.S.I., Milan, 1979.
- Guantieri G., *Ipnosi e Sessuologia,* in *Rivista di Sessuologia Clinica* magazine, Publisher Franco Angeli, Milan, n. 4, 1980.
- Guantieri G., *L'ipnosi in terapia,* in Colli F., Quattrocchi S., (Edited by), *Il fenomeno ipnosi,* Publisher Nuova Spada, Rome, 1980.
- Guantieri G., *The Value of Placebos in Chronic Pain Therapy,* Proceedings of the *International Practical Refresher Course on Pain Therapy,* Vicenza, 1982.
- Guantieri G., *L'induzione di ipnosi in medicina psicosomatica,* Proceedings of the IX International Congress of Hypnosis and Psychosomatic Medicine of Glasgow, *Rivista Italiana di Ipnosi Clinica Sperimentale,* Publisher Franco Angeli, Milan, n. 2, 1982.
- Guantieri G., *Rilassamento, ipnosi, formazione psicosomatista,* Proceedings of the II Convegno Sezione Toscana della S.I.M.P., Florence, in *La formazione*

psicosomatica, Collana di Igiene Mentale, Publisher Università of Messina, n. 1, 1984.

- Guantieri G., *Hypnosis in Psychotherapy and Psychosomatic Medicine*, Proceeding of the 3rd European Congress on *Hypnosis in Psychotherapy and Psychosomatic Medicine*, Abano Terme (Padua), 22-27 May 1984, Publisher Il Segno, Negrar (Verona), 1985.
- Guantieri G., *Opening address*, Proceedings of the III European Congress on *Hypnosis in Psychotherapy and Psychosomatic Medicine*, Abano Terme (Padova), 22-27 May 1984, Publisher Il Segno, Negrar (Verona), 1985.
- Guantieri G., *How and why Hypnosis in Psychosomatic Medicine*, Proceedings of the III European Congress on *Hypnosis in Psychotherapy and Psychosomatic Medicine*, Abano Terme (Padua), 22-27 May 1984, Publisher Il Segno, Negrar (Verona), 1985.
- Guantieri G., *Farewell address, Hypnosis in Psychosomatics*, Proceedings of the III European Congress on *Hypnosis in Psychotherapy and Psychosomatic Medicine*, Abano Terme (Padua), 22-27 May 1984, Publisher Il Segno, Negrar (Verona), 1985.
- Guantieri G., in AA.VV. (edited by Guantieri G.), *Hypnosis in Psychotherapy and Psychosomatic Medicine, Il linguaggio del corpo in ipnosi*, Publisher Il Segno, Negrar (Verona), 1985.
- Guantieri G., *Il setting ipnotico in prospettiva psicodinamica, Il linguaggio del corpo in ipnosi*, (edited by Guantieri G.), Proceedings of the Symposium X Congresso Nazionale *Società Italiana di Medicina Psicosomatica* (S.I.M.P.), Publisher Il Segno, Negrar (Verona), 1985.
- Guantieri G., *Il linguaggio del corpo in ipnosi*, (edited by Guantieri G.), Proceedings of the Symposium X Congresso Nazionale *Società Italiana di Medicina Psicosomatica* (S.I.M.P.), Publisher Il Segno, Negrar (Verona), 1985.
- Guantieri G., *Greeting by Authorities, Messaggio di benvenuto e di apertura del congresso*, in Guantieri G., Ischia S., (edited by), *L'ipnosi nelle istituzioni. Ruolo e contributo,* Proceedings of the I Congresso Nazionale di Ipnosi di Verona, 21-22 December 1985, Edition Istituto Italiano Studi di Ipnosi Clinica e Psicoterapia 'H. Bernheim', Scuola di Ricerca e Formazione, Verona, 1987.
- Guantieri G., *L'ipnosi oggi*, in Guantieri G., Ischia S., (edited by), *L'ipnosi nelle istituzioni. Ruolo e contributo*, Proceedings of the I Congresso Nazionale di Ipnosi di Verona, 21-22 December 1985, Editions Istituto Italiano Studi di Ipnosi Clinica e Psicoterapia 'H. Bernheim', Scuola di Ricerca e Formazione, Verona, 1987.
- Guantieri G., *Tavola rotonda*, in Guantieri G., Ischia S., (edited by), *L'ipnosi nelle istituzioni. Ruolo e contributo,* Proceedings of the I Congresso Nazionale di Ipnosi di Verona, 21-22 December 1985, Editions Istituto Italiano Studi di Ipnosi Clinica e Psicoterapia 'H. Bernheim', Scuola di Ricerca e Formazione, Verona, 1987.

- Guantieri G., *Ipnosi e terapia del dolore*, Newsletter magazine, Vol. II, n. 2, October 1989.
- Guantieri G., *Ipnosi e terapia del dolore*, in Newsletter magazine, Volume II, n. 2, October 1989.
- Guantieri G., *L'emozione in prospettiva psicosomatica*, in Newsletter magazine, Volume IV, n. 1, April 1991.
- Guantieri G., *Fondamenti e prospettive dell'Ipnologia – 1967*, in Acta Ipnologica magazine, Year II, n. 2-3, May-September 1998/a.
- Guantieri G., *Schema di tecnica induttiva ipnotica*, in Acta Ipnologica magazine, Year II, n. 2-3, May-September 1998/b.
- Guantieri G., *Fondamenti e prospettive dell'Ipnologia*, in Acta Ipnologica magazine, Year II, n. 2-3, 1998/c.
- Guantieri G., Abrescia N., *L'ipnosi nella preparazione della gestante*, Convegno della Società di Medicina e Chirurgia Veronese, Verona, September 1961.
- Guantieri G., Angelozzi A., *Un fondamento e una prospettiva. Il Centro 'H.Bernheim' e l'evoluzione concettuale dell'ipnosi*, Editions Istituto Italiano Studi di Ipnosi Clinica e Psicoterapia 'H. Bernheim', Scuola di Ricerca e Formazione, Verona, 1985.
- Guantieri G., Angelozzi A., *Hypnosis: a Base a Way Forward*, Editions The 'H. Bernheim' Institute for Research in Clinical Hypnosis and Psychotherapy, School for Research and Training, Verona, 1988.
- Guantieri G., Bartoloni A., Seminara B., Ischia S., *Tecniche di sedazione psicologica in anestesia loco-regionale*, Acta Anaesthesiologica Italica & Anaesthesia and Intensive Care, Editions La Garangola, Padua, 1978.
- Guantieri G., Bartoloni A., Seminari B., Ischia S., Pasetto A., *On a case of Cholecistectomy under Hypnosis*, in Pajntar M., Roskar E., Lavric M., (edited by), Hypnosis in Psychotherapy and Psychosomatic Medicine, Proceedings of the 2nd European Congress of Hypnosis held in Dubrovnik, Croatia, University Press, Lubiana, Slovenia, 1980.
- Guantieri G., Benatti G., *Il lavoro medico italiano nel campo dell'ipnosi nel XX secolo*, in Rassegna di Ipnosi e Medicina Psicosomatica magazine, n. 31, 1976.
- Guantieri G., Bottoli A., Azzini V., *Su un caso di ritenzione urinaria trattato con ipnosi*, Proceedings of the IX International Congress of Hypnosis and Psychosomatic Medicine of Glasgow, in Rivista Italiana di Ipnosi Clinica Sperimentale magazine, n. 2, 1982.
- Guantieri G., Caliari P., Mosconi G.P., *Bibliografia italiana sulla ipnosi 1973-1983*, in Rivista Italiana di Ipnosi Clinica Sperimentale magazine, n. 2, 1983.
- Guantieri G., Forghieri P.L., *Trattamento ipnotico di turbe del sonno di pazienti neuropsichiatrici ricoverati in ambiente specialistico*, Proceedings of the IX International Congress of Hypnosis and Psychosomatic Medicine of Glasgow, in Rivista Italiana di Ipnosi Clinica Sperimentale magazine, n. 2, 1982.
- Guantieri G., Forghieri P.L., *Teaching Self Hypnosis as a Valid Instrument to Improve Therapeutical Results in Neuropsychiatric Ward Patients*, in Guantieri G.

- (edited by), *Hypnosis in Psychotherapy and Psychosomatic Medicine*, Proceedings of the 3rd European Congress of Hypnosis, held in Abano Terme (Padua), 22-27 May 1984, Publisher Il Segno, Negrar (Verona), 1985.
- Guantieri G., Gambacciani A., *L'ipnosi nel trattamento riabilitativo di un caso di malattia di Guillain-Barrè*, Proceedings of the IX International Congress of Hypnosis and Psychosomatic Medicine of Glasgow, in *Rivista Italiana di Ipnosi Clinica Sperimentale* magazine, n. 2, 1982.
- Guantieri G., Gasparini D., Lafisca S., *Possibilità di applicazioni forensi dell'ipnosi alla luce del nuovo Codice di Procedura Penale*, in *Newsletter* magazine, Volume II, n. 2, October 1989.
- Guantieri G., Guerra G., *Contributo alla conoscenza e all'impiego del rilassamento in varie situazioni esistenziali*, in *Giornale di Medicina Militare* magazine, n. 6, 1981.
- Guantieri G., Guerra G., Simonelli F., Sarao G., Tagliaro F., Luisetto G., *Livelli plasmatici di beta-endorfine e analgesia ipnotica*, in Proceedings of the IX International Congress of *Hypnosis and Psychosomatic Medicine* of Glasgow, in *Rivista Italiana di Ipnosi Clinica Sperimentale*, n. 2, 1982.
- Guantieri G., Bottoli A., Azzini V., *On a Case of Urinary Retention Treated by Means of Hypnosis*, in D. Waxman et al., *Modern Trends in Hypnosis*, Plenum Press, New York, 1985.
- Guantieri G., Ischia S., (edited by), *L'ipnosi nelle istituzioni. Ruolo e contributo*, Proceedings of the I Congresso Nazionale di Ipnosi di Verona, 21-22 December 1985, Edited Istituto Italiano Studi di Ipnosi Clinica e Psicoterapia 'H. Bernheim', Scuola di Ricerca e Formazione, Verona, 1987.
- Guantieri G., Parietti P, *La preparazione del medico ipnologo*, in Antonelli F. (edited by), Proceedings of the III International Congress of *Hypnosis and Psychosomatic Medicine,* Publisher Pozzi, Brescia, 1977.
- Guantieri G., Parietti P., *Psicoterapia e ipnosi*, in *Rassegna di Ipnosi e Medicina Psicosomatica* magazine, n. 13, 1977.
- Guantieri G., Parietti P., *Problems and Perspectives of Solution in the Teaching of Hypnosis*, in Pajntar M., Roskar E., Lavric M. (edited by), *Hypnosis in Psychotherapy and Psychosomatic Medicine,* Proceedings of the 2nd European Congress of Hypnosis, Dubrovnik, Croatia, University Press, Lubiana, Slovenia, 1980.
- Guantieri G., Pasetti C., *L'ipnosi come mezzo di ausilio nella riabilitazione funzionale delle paralisi spastiche* in *Rassegna di Igiene Mentale* magazine, Year I, n. 4, 1979.
- Guantieri G., Roncaroli P., *Livelli di interazione nel rapporto interpersonale ipnotico*, in *Rassegna di Igiene Mentale* magazine, Year I, n. 4, 1979.
- Guantieri G., Roncaroli P., *Hypnosis as a Method of Multidimensional Analysis in Psychotherapy*, in Pajntar M., Roskar E., Lavric M., (edited by), *Hypnosis in Psychotherapy and Psychosomatic Medicine,* Proceedings of the 2nd European Congress of Hypnosis, held in Dubrovnik, Croatia, University Press, Lubiana, Slovenia, 1980.

- Guantieri G., Roncaroli P., *Ipnosi e curva erotica femminile*, in *Rivista di Sessuologia Clinica*, n. 5, 1980.
- Guantieri G., Seminara G., Ischia S., Bartoloni A., Pasetto A., *On a Case of Cholecistectomy under Hypnosis*, in Pajntar M., Roskar E., Lavric M., (edited by), *Hypnosis in Psychotherapy and Psychosomatic Medicine*, Proceedings of the 2nd European Congress of Hypnosis, held in Dubrovnik, Croatia, University Press, Lubiana, Slovenia, 1980.
- Guerra G., *Ipnosi e sofferenza umana*, in *Acta Ipnologica* magazine, Year I, n. 1, 1997.
- Gullotta G., *Techniques of hypnotic influence upon the subject: argumentative and mystifying aspects*, in Proceedings of the 3rd European Congress on *Hypnosis in Psychotherapy and Psychosomatic Medicine*, Abano Terme (Padua), 22-27 May 1984, Publisher Il Segno, Negrar (Verona), 1985.
- Gullotta G., *Ipnosi e psicologia: rimuginandoci*, in *Rassegna di Ipnosi e Medicina Psicosomatica*, Turin, 1973.
- Gullotta G., *Ipnosi sperimentale*, in AA.VV. in Guantieri G., Ischia S., (edited by), Proceedings of 1rd Congresso Nazionale, *L'ipnosi nelle istituzioni, ruolo e contributo*, Verona, 21-22 December 1985.
- Gullotta G., *Commemorazione di Rolando Weilbache*, Conference, Verona, 21.10.2016.
- Gulotta G., *Techniques of hypnotic influence upon the subject: argumentative and mystifying aspects*, in AA.VV. (edited by Guantieri G.), *Hypnosis in Psychotherapy and Psychosomatic Medicine*, Proceedings of the 3rd European Congress on *Hypnosis in Psychotherapy and Psychosomatic Medicine*, Abano Terme (Padua), 22-27 May 1984, Publisher Il Segno, Negrar, (Verona), 1985.
- Haley J., (Tr. It. da Loriedo C.), *Terapie non comuni. Tecniche ipnotiche e terapia della famiglia* (*Uncommon Therapy: The Psychiatric Techniques of Milton H. Erickson*, Paperback), Publisher Astrolabio, Rome, 1978.
- Hartland J., *Ipnosi in medicina e odontoiatria*, Publisher Monduzzi, Bologna, 1977.
- Heap M., *Does Clinical Hypnosis Have Anything to Do with Experimental Hypnosis?* in *The Journal of Mind Body Regulation*, 2011.
- Hilgard E.R., *Psicologia. Corso introduttivo*, Publisher Giunti, Florence, 1971.
- Hillman J., *La forza del carattere*, Publisher Adelphi, Milan, 2000.
- Hoffman B.H., *Manuale di training autogeno*, Publisher Astrolabio, Rome, 1996.
- Imbasciati A., Manfredi P., *Il feto ci ascolta... e impara. Genitorialità, transgenerazionalità e ricerca sperimentale*, Publisher Borla, Rome, 2004.
- Iotti P., Masoni T., *Sono dov'è il mio corpo. Memoria di un ex deportato a Mauthausen*, Publisher Giuntina, Florence, 1995.
- Jacobson E., *L'arte del rilassamento. Come si affronta la tensione della vita moderna*, Publisher Casini, Rome, 1952.

- James W., *Principi di Psicologia*, Publisher Società Editrice Libraria, Milan, 1901.
- Jung C.G., *Ricordi, sogni, riflessioni*, Publisher Il Saggiatore, Milan, 1965.
- Kernberg O.F., *Relazioni d'amore*, Publisher Raffaello Cortina, Milan, 1995.
- Kirsch I., Lynn S.J., *Dissociation theories of hypnosis*, in *Psychological Bulletin*, 1998.
- Kline M.V., *The roots of modern Hypnosis*, self-published, New York, 1961.
- Kuhn T.S., *La struttura delle rivoluzioni scientifiche*, Publisher Piccola Biblioteca Einaudi, Turin, 1962.
- Lamaze F., Accouchement sans douleur avec la méthode psychoprophylactique, in Encyclopédie médicale chirurgicale française, 1956.
- Lankton S.R, *Training in Therapy-Induction Without Scripts*, in *The American journal of clinical*, 2017.
- Le Doux J., *Il cervello emotivo. Alle origini delle emozioni*, Publisher Baldini Castoldi Dalai, Milan, 2003.
- Lemaire G., *Il rilassamento. Rilassamento e rieducazione psico tonica*, Edition Celuc Libri, Padua, 1977.
- Lipton B., *La biologia delle credenze*, Publisher Macro Edizioni, Diegaro di Cesena, Forlì-Cesena, 2006.
- Lodetti M.P., *Mio padre medico studioso mistico. Romolo Lodetti. La scienza a servizio della pace*, Publisher Editrice Veneta, Vicenza, 2019.
- Lombardi Vallauri L., *Meditare in Occidente. Corso di mistica laica*, Publisher Le Lettere, Florence, 2015.
- Loreto P., *La memoria del corpo*, Publisher Crocetti, Milan, 2007.
- Loriedo C., *The Use of Metaphor in Indirect Hypnotherapy*, Proceedings of the 3rd European Congress on *Hypnosis in Psychotherapy and Psychosomatic Medicine*, Abano Terme (Padua), Publisher Il Segno, Negrar (Verona), 1985.
- Loriedo C., Gulotta G., *Hypnosis in Italy*, in Hawkins P., Heap M., *Hypnosis in Europe*, Whurr Publishers Ltd., London, 1998.
- Malesani P.G., *Self-hypnosis and abreaction: exposition and a case discussion*, in AA.VV. (edited by Guantieri G.), *Hypnosis in Psychotherapy and Psychosomatic Medicine*, Proceedings of the 3rd European Congress on *Hypnosis in Psychotherapy and Psychosomatic Medicine*, Abano Terme (Padua), 22-27 May 1984, Publisher Il Segno, Negrar (Verona), 1985.
- Malesani P.G., *L'ipnosi*, in ReS magazine, Year VII, n. 3, 1999 e Year VIII n. 1, 2000.
- Malesani P.G., *L'emergenza della memoria attraverso il Rilassamento*, in ReS magazine, Year XI, n. 1, 2003.
- Malesani P.G., *Tempo concitato e tempo rilassato*, in ReS magazine, Verona, Year XI, n. 2, 2003.
- Malesani P.G., *Psicosomatica dell'apprendimento*, in ReS magazine, Year IX, n. 3, 2003.
- Malesani P.G., *Il Rilassamento è gioco?* In ReS magazine, Year XII, n. 1, 2004.

- Malesani P.G., *Quiete e tempeste dell'essere*, Publisher ReS-C.I.S.E.R.P.P., Verona, 2004.
- Malesani P.G., *Guantieri: Uno sciamano benefico?* In Proceedings of the XX Congresso *L'ansia nella clinica e nella società attuale*, della Società Italiana di Medicina Psicosomatica, Verona, 2005.
- Malesani P.G., *Dissimmetrie nelle esperienze di rilassamento*, in ReS magazine, Year XIII, n. 3, 2005.
- Malesani P.G., *L'emozione corporea negli stati di rilassamento e nell'ipnosi*, in ReS magazine, Year XIV, n. 1, 2006.
- Malesani P.G., *Conosci il corpo, esplora il mondo*, in ReS magazine, Year XV, n. 1, 2007.
- Malesani P.G., *Il Maestro ipnologo*, in Acta Ipnologica magazine, Year XII, n. 3, September 2008 e Year XIII, n. 1, January 2009.
- Malesani P.G., *Réflexion sur des liens entre la psychomotricité et l'hypnose*, in Évolutions Psychomotrices magazine, Paris, Volume 22, n. 90, 2010.
- Malesani P.G., *Ipnosi sciamanica tra bene e male. Terapia e manipolazione*, in Acta Ipnologica magazine, Year XV, n. 1, May 2011/a.
- Malesani P.G., *Corpo, natura, mente: interazioni sistemiche tra pulsioni e logiche culturali*, in ReS magazine, Editions C.I.S.E.R.P.P., Verona, Year XIX, n. 1, 2011/b.
- Malesani P.G., *Spazi ampi ed angusti dell'inconscio*, in ReS magazine, Year XX, n. 1, 2012/a.
- Malesani P.G., *L'inconscio nelle parole, le parole dell'inconscio*, in ReS magazine, Year XX, n. 2, 2012/b.
- Malesani P.G., Malesani M., *Autoipnosi. La gioia dentro*, Publisher Vita Nuova, Verona, 2005.
- Marchi L., *Teoria e pratica del training autogeno*, Publisher Edizioni La Casa Verde, Sommacampagna (Verona), 1988.
- Markhman U., *La visualizzazione*, Publisher Edizioni Selenia, Milan, 1993.
- Meneghini A.M., *Meditazione e broaden-and-build theory*, in ReS, magazine, Verona, Year XXI, n. 1, 2013.
- Merini A., *Un'anima indocile*, Publisher Edizioni La vita Felice, Milano, 1996.
- Merleau-Ponty M., *Il corpo vissuto, l'ambiguità dell'esistenza, la riscoperta della vita percettiva, la carne del mondo. Dalle prime opere a L'occhio e lo spirito*, (Anthology by Fergnani F.), Publisher Il Saggiatore, Milan, 1979.
- Modenese M., *Sogno e ipnosi*, in Acta Ipnologica magazine, Verona, Year anno III, n. 2-3, 1999.
- Modenese M., *Ipnosi immaginativa in psicoterapia: tra mentale e corporeo. Imaginative hypnosis in psychotherapy: between mind and body*, in Acta Ipnologica magazine, Year X, n. 2-3, May-September 2006.
- Mosconi G., *L'ipnosi per partorire*, Publisher Piccin, Padua, 1974.

- Muzi P., Angelozzi A., *Costruire la trançe. Mezzi linguistici e modelli esplicativi. Building the trance. Linguistic Means and Illustrative Models*, in *Acta Ipnologica* magazine, Year I, n. 2, May 1997.
- Nardone G., Loriedo C., Zeig J., Watzlavick P., *Ipnosi e terapie ipnotiche. Misteri svelati e miti sfatati*, Publisher Salemi, Milan, 2012.
- Odini G., (edited by) *Hippolyte Bernheim, Della suggestione nello stato ipnotico e nello stato di veglia*, Publisher Sometti Editoriale, Mantova, 2017.
- Ohm D., *Rilassamento muscolare progressivo*, Publisher Red, Como, 1984.
- Pardell S.S., *Psychology of the hypnotist*, in *The Psychiatric quarterly* magazine, 1950.
- Peresson L., *Trattato di psicoterapia autogena*, Publisher Piovan, Padua, 1985.
- Peresson L., (edited by), *Il training autogeno nelle sue applicazioni non cliniche, educazione, sport, lavoro, applicazioni speciali*, Editions CISSPAT, Padua, 1988.
- Pert C.B., *Molecole di Emozioni*, Publisher Edizioni Tea Libri, Milan, 2005.
- Piazza C., *L'ipnosi come strumento di formazione per l'operatore socio-sanitario; un'esperienza con operatori psichiatrici. Hypnosis as a Training Instrument for the Socio-sanitary Operator; an experience with Psychiatric Operators*, in *Acta Ipnologica* magazine, Year II, n. 1, January 1998.
- Piazza C., *Esperienze di ipnosi senza trançe in gruppo. Group Hypnotic Experiences whithout Trance*, in *Acta Ipnologica* magazine, Year III, n. 2-3, May-September 1999/a.
- Piazza C., *Aspetti di rilievo nella formazione del personale impiegato nel trattamento di soggetti con problemi psichiatrici: la relazione ipnotica come strumento. Relevant Aspects of Training Psychiatric Operators*, in *Acta Ipnologica* magazine, Year III, n. 2-3, May-September 1999/b.
- Piazza C., *Dalla frammentazione specialistica alla comunicazione unificante; l'ipnosi nell'ottica psicosomatica. From the Fragmentation of the Specialisation to the Unifying Communication; Hypnosis from a Psychosomatic Poin of View*, in *Acta Ipnologica* magazine, Year IV, n. 1, January 2000.
- Piazza C., *Ipnosi e psicosomatica. Hypnosis and Psychosomatics*, in *Acta Ipnologica* magazine, Year VI, n. 2-3, May-September 2002/a.
- Piazza C., *Ipnosi e psicosomatica. Hypnosis and Psychosomatics*, in *Acta Ipnologica* magazine, Year VI, n. 2-3, May-September 2002/b.
- Piazza C., *Consapevolezza e guarigione. Awareness and Recovery*, in *Acta Ipnologica* magazine, Year VII, n. 2-3, May-September 2003.
- Piazza C., *Le depressioni. Esperienze cliniche e di vita. Depressions. Clinical and Life Experiences*, in *Acta Ipnologica* magazine, Year VIII, n. 3, September 2004.
- Piazza C., *Incoscio e approccio olistico*, in *Acta Ipnologica* magazine, Year XI, n. 1-2, January-May 2007/a.
- Piazza C., *Disturbo psichiatrico e comunicazione alterata*, in *Acta Ipnologica* magazine, Year XI, n. 1-2, January-May 2007/b.
- Piazza C., *Psicoterapia immaginativa nell'ansia prestazionale*, in *Acta Ipnologica* magazine, Year XI, n. 1-2, January-May 2007/c.

- Piazza C., *L'ansia normaloide*, in *Acta Ipnologica* magazine, Year XI, n. 1-2, January-May 2007/d.
- Piazza C., *Per una semeiotica dell'inconscio*, in *Acta Ipnologica* magazine, Year XI, n. 1-2, January-May 2007/e.
- Piazza C., *Il dolore esistenziale, terra di confine tra corpo, mente e spirito; tecniche immaginative e di rilassamento in gruppo per l'approccio al dolore e alla malattia*, in *Acta Ipnologica* magazine, Year XIII, n. 2, May 2009.
- Piazza C., *Il dolore esistenziale, terra di confine tra corpo, mente e spirito; tecniche immaginative di rilassamento in gruppo per l'approccio al dolore e alla malattia*, in *Acta Ipnologica* magazine, Year XIII, n. 2, May 2010.
- Piazza C., Carletti C., *Un'esperienza integrata tra analisi immaginativa Junghiana e psicoterapia ipnotica Ericksoniana, (An integration experience between Junghian imaginative analysis and Ericksonian hypnotic psychotherapy)*, in *Acta Ipnologica*, magazine, Year X, n. 2-3, May-September 2006.
- Piazza C., Modenese M., *Esperienze di Trance ipnotica in attività di gruppo a mediazione corporea. Experiences of Hypnotic Trance in Bodily Mediated Group*, in *Acta Ipnologica* magazine, Year VI, n. 1, January 2002.
- Piscicelli U., *Training autogeno respiratorio e psicoprofilassi ostetrica*, Publisher Piccin, Padua, 1982.
- Popper K.R., Eccles J.C., *The self and its brain*, Publisher Springer-Verlag Berlin and Heidelberg GmbH & Co. K, 1977.
- Rolla E., Manca M., *Il rilassamento muscolare*, Publisher Omega, Turin, 1986.
- Rosa K.R., *Cos'è il training autogeno*, Publisher Sugar, Milan, 1975.
- Sapir M., and Oders, *Il rilassamento*, Publisher Astrolabio, Rome, 1980.
- Sbriglio V.S., *Psicoprofilassi autogena della maternità. Guida sinottica per le gestanti dei corsi di preparazione al parto con il "training autogeno" di J.H. Shultz*, Publisher Cortina, Turin, 1980.
- Schultz J.H., *Il training autogeno: esercizi inferiori*, volume I, Publisher Feltrinelli, Milan, 1968.
- Schultz J.H., *Il training autogeno: esercizi superiori*, volume II, Publisher Feltrinelli, Milan, 1971.
- Shon R., *La tecnica dell'autoipnosi*, Publisher Astrolabio, Rome 1982.
- Sonato R., *Terapie tecniche naturali per combattere ansia, stress, insonnia*, Publisher Demetra, Colognola ai Colli (Verona), 1993.
- Soskis D., *Insegnare l'autoipnosi*, Publisher Astrolabio, Rome 1987.
- Sugarman L.I., Schafer P.M., Alter D.S., Reid D.B., *Learning Clinical Hypnosis Wide Awake: Can We Teach Hypnosis Hypnotically?* In *The American journal of clinical hypnosis*, 2018.
- Süskind P., *Il profumo*, Publisher Longanesi, Milan, 1985.
- Thomas K., *Autoipnosi e training autogeno*, Publisher Edizioni Mediterranee, Rome, 1976.
- Varga K., *Possible Mechanisms of Hypnosis from an Interactional Perspective*, in *Brain Sciences* magazine, 2021.

- Vinci S., *In tutti i sensi come l'amore,* Publisher Einaudi, Turin, 1999.
- Viziale E., *Tecniche di rilassamento,* Publisher SIAD, Milan, 1985.
- Waxman D., *Hartland's Medical and Dental Hypnosis,* Baillière Tindall Publisher, London, 1988.
- Widmann C., *Manuale di training autogeno,* Publisher Piovan, Padua, 1980.
- Zin L., *L'arte della respirazione,* Publisher Red, Como, 1998.

Bibliography of the studies of the 'Bernheim' institute in the period 1988-1993

Taken from *Newsletter* magazine, Editions of the Italian Institute of Clinical Hypnosis and Psychotherapy 'H. Bernheim', School of Research and Training, Verona.

Original works

- Angelozzi A., *Ipnosi e psicosi endogene (parte prima). Considerazioni generali,* in *Rivista Italiana di Ipnosi Clinica e Sperimentale* magazine, n. 2, 1983.
- Angelozzi A., *Therapeutic Applications of Hypnosis on Psychotic and Borderline Patients,* in Guantieri G. (edited by), *Hypnosis in Psychotherapy and Psychosomatic Medicine,* Proceedings of the 3rd European Congress of Hypnosis, Abano Terme (Padua). Publisher Il Segno, Negrar (Verona), 1985.
- Angelozzi A., *Ipnosi e psicosi endogene (parte prima). Considerazioni generali,* in *Rivista Italiana di Ipnosi Clinica e Sperimentale* magazine, n. 2, 1985.
- Angelozzi A., Guantieri G., *L'ipnosi: un fondamento ed una prospettiva,* Editions 'Bernheim', Verona, 1985.
- Angelozzi A., Guantieri G., *Hypnosis: a base and a way forward,* Editions 'Bernheim', Verona, 1985.
- Angelozzi A., *La comunicazione non verbale in Milton H. Erickson,* in Guantieri G., (edited by), *Il linguaggio del corpo in ipnosi,* Proceedings of the X Congresso della Società Italiana di Medicina Psicosomatica (S.I.M.P.), Publisher Il Segno, Negrar (Verona), 1985.
- Angelozzi A., *L'approccio Ericksoniano fra terapia sistemica e psicodinamica,* in Loriedo C., Angiolari C., Martini L. (edited by), Proceedings of the Congresso Internazionale *Ipnosi e Terapia della Famiglia,* Roma, 1985, Publisher L'Antologia, Napoli, 1987.
- Angelozzi A., Guantieri G., *Notes on the Birth and Development of the 'H. Bernheim' Centre for Research in Clinical Hypnosis and Psychotherapy,* X International Congress of Hypnosis and Psychosomatic Medicine, Toronto, Canada, 1985.
- Angelozzi A., Guantieri, G., *L'ipnosi nelle Istituzioni,* Corso di Ipnosi del C.I.I.C.S., Turin, 1986.
- Angelozzi A., *Ipnosi, relazione e transizione di stato,* in Guantieri G., Ischia S., (edited by), *L'ipnosi nelle istituzioni. Ruolo e contributo,* Proceedings of the I Congresso Nazionale, Verona, 1985, Editions Istituto 'Bernheim', Verona, 1987.
- Angelozzi A., *L'aggressività in ipnosi: dalla interpretazione alla costruzione relazionale,* XI Congresso Nazionale della Società Italiana di Medicina Psicosomatica

- (S.I.M.P.), Messina, 1987, in *Rassegna di Igiene Mentale* magazine, Year XI, 1989.
- Angelozzi A., *Hypnotherapeutic Approach in Psychotherapeutic Relationship,* Proceedings of the IV European Congress of Hypnosis in Psychotherapy and Psychosomatic Medicine, Oxford, England, 1987.
- Angelozzi A., *Relation and Transition of State of Consciousness in Hypnosis,* Proceedings of the IV European Congress of Hypnosis in Psychotherapy and Psychosomatic Medicine, Oxford, England, 1987.
- Angelozzi A., *Immagini corporee e immagini del mondo,* Proceedings of the II Convegno Internazionale *Mente-Corpo,* Milan, 1987.
- Angelozzi A., Muzi P.G., *How to Do Trance with Words,* Proceedings of the XI International Congress of Hypnosis and Psychosomatic Medicine, Leiden, Holland, 1988.
- Angelozzi A., Roncaroli P., *Hypnotic Regression and Childish Structures of Thinking,* Proceedings of the XI International Congress of Hypnosis and Psychosomatic Medicine, Leiden, Holland, 1988.
- Angelozzi A., Muzi P.G., *Che ci fa il mio cervello nel laboratorio di neurofisiologia?* Proceedings of the XII Congresso Nazionale Società Italiana di Medicina Psicosomatica (S.I.M.P.), Milan, 1989.
- Angelozzi A., Guantieri G., *Note sull'origine e l'evoluzione del Centro Studi 'H.Bernheim'* in *Newsletter* magazine, Editions 'Bernheim' Year II, n. 1, 1989.
- Angelozzi A., *L'ipnosi in Psicoterapia,* in Santonastaso P., (edited by), *Manuale di Psicoterapia,* Publisher Masson, Milan, 1993.
- Arrigucci E., Gocci G., *L'ipnosi come processo psicodinamico (euipnosi),* in *Rivista Italiana di Ipnosi Clinica e Sperimentale* magazine, n. 2, 1982.
- Bado F., *Il rapporto psiche-soma nell'anoressia mentale,* Proceedings of the XIII Congresso Nazionale Società Italiana di Medicina Psicosomatica (S.I.M.P.), Bologna, 1991.
- Bado F., *Training autogeno e visualizzazioni: dal soma alla psiche,* Proceedings of the II Convegno Internazionale *Mente-Corpo,* Milan, 1987.
- Bartoloni A., Pasetto, A., Passerelli M., Ischia S., *Tecniche di sedazione psicologica in anestesia locoregionale,* in *Acta Anaesthesiol Italica* magazine, n. 29, 1978.
- Bartoloni A., Pasetto A., Guantieri G., Seminara B., Ischia S., *On a case of Cholecistectomy under Hypnosis,* in Pajntar M., Roskar E., Lavric M., (edited by), *Hypnosis in Psychoterapy and Psychosomatic Medicine,* Proceedings of the II European Congress of Hypnosis, Dubrovnik, Croatia, Editions University Press, Lubiana, Slovenia, 1980.
- Bartoloni A., Pasetto A., Luzzani A., Passerelli M., Remondini P., Rigotti L., Antonello L., *Responsività ipnotica e valutazione del dolore,* in Guantieri G., Ischia S., (edited by), *L'ipnosi nelle istituzioni. Ruolo e contributo,* Proceedings of the I Congresso Nazionale, Verona, 1985, Editions Istituto 'Bernheim', Verona, 1987.

- Benassai I. and others, *Transfert e ipnosi*, Proceedings of the XII Congresso Nazionale Società Italiana di Medicina Psicosomatica (S.I.M.P.), Milan, 1989.
- Benatti G., *Considerazioni pratiche e psicoterapia dell'obesità*, in *Medicina Psicosomatica* magazine, n. 14, 1969.
- Benatti G., *La diuresi nella psicodinamica indotta in un caso di edema polmonare acuto*, in *Rassegna di Medicina Psicosomatica* magazine, n. 15, 1970.
- Benatti G., *Aspetti psicosomatici del megacolon in due casi osservati*, in *Rassegna di Medicina Psicosomatica* magazine, n. 13, 1970.
- Benatti G., *Frigidità e note anatomo-fisio-psicologiche*, in *Rassegna di Medicina Psicosomatica* magazine, n. 16, 1971.
- Benatti G., *Stato comportamentale delle mani e psicoterapia con ipnosi*, in *Rassegna Medicina Psicosomatica* magazine, n. 18, 1972.
- Benatti G., Minella E., *Una manovra antalgica sulla partoriente condizionata in ipnosi*, in *Rassegna Medicina Psicosomatica* magazine, n. 18, 1972.
- Benatti G., *Ipnosi e disordini somatici*, in *Rassegna Medicina Psicosomatica* magazine, n. 24, 1974.
- Benatti G., *Ipnosi e disordini somatopsichici*, in *Rassegna Medicina Psicosomatica* magazine, n. 24, 1974.
- Benatti G., *Igiene mentale e igiene della famiglia. Considerazioni su un caso di mutacismo risolto mediante ipnosi*, Proceedings of the IV Congresso Nazionale Società Italiana di Medicina Psicosomatica (S.I.M.P.), Publisher S.E.U., Rome, 1974.
- Benatti G., *Il travaglio di parto condotto in ipnosi con audio a circuito chiuso*, Proceedings of the IV Congresso Società Italiana di Psicoprofilassi Ostetrica, in *Aggiornamenti Ostetricia Ginecologia* magazine, n. 7, 1974.
- Benatti G., Guantieri G., *Il lavoro medico italiano nel campo dell'ipnosi nel XX secolo*, in *Rassegna di Medicina Psicosomatica* magazine, n. 31, 1976.
- Benatti G., *L'ipnosi nella diagnostica. La tecnica della doppia anamnesi in medicina psicosomatica*, in *Rassegna di Medicina Psicosomatica* magazine, n. 34, 1977.
- Benatti, G., *L'anamnesi e la diagnosi nelle colonpatie psicosomatiche*, in *Rassegna di Medicina Psicosomatica* magazine, n. 35, 1978.
- Benatti G., *Misura e effetti diagnostici della comunicazione prima e dopo il rilassamento psicosomatico indotto*, Proceedings of the V Convegno Nazionale A.M.I.S.I., Milan, 1979.
- Benatti G., *Le tensioni psicosomatiche nella storia dell'iperteso*, Proceedings of the VII Congresso Società Italiana di Medicina Psicosomatica (S.I.M.P.), Ancona, 1980.
- Benatti G., *La diagnosi pediatrica di asma bronchiale, quale? E la terapia più opportuna, come?* Proceedings of the VIII Congresso Nazionale Società Italiana di Medicina Psicosomatica (S.I.M.P.), Venezia (edited by Cerotti R., Bruno S.), in *Riza Psicosomatica* magazine, Milan, 1981.

- Benatti G., *Parto cesareo e ginecologia psicosomatica*, Proceedings of the VIII Congresso Nazionale Società Italiana di Medicina Psicosomatica (S.I.M.P.), Venice (edited by Cerotti R., Bruno S.), in *Riza Psicosomatica* magazine, Milan, 1981.
- Benatti G., *La diagnosi psicosomatica è già terapia?* Proceedings of the Congresso Internazionale Ipnosi e T.A., Editions C.I.S.S.P.A.T., Padua, 1981.
- Benatti G., *Grandi messaggi nelle piccole reazioni psicosomatiche mimiche o segmentali*, in Guantieri G. (edited by), *Il linguaggio del corpo in ipnosi*, Proceedings of the X Congresso Nazionale Società Italiana di Medicina Psicosomatica (S.I.M.P.), Publisher Il Segno, Negrar (Verona), 1985.
- Benatti G., *Motivazione e creatività nella psicoterapia della riabilitazione*, Proceedings of the IX Congresso Nazionale Società Italiana di Medicina Psicosomatica (S.I.M.P.), Turin, 1983, Editions Università degli Studi, Turin, 1985.
- Benatti G., *Il linguaggio del corpo in ipnosi e sua importanza diagnostica: un contributo clinico di depressione mascherata*, Proceedings of the 36th Congresso Nazionale della Società Italiana di Psichiatria, Milan, 1985, Editions UNICOPLI, Milan, 1987.
- Benatti G., *L'aggressività nel simbolismo dell'oggetto transizionale per la clinica dell'ipnosi in medicina psicosomatica*, XI Congresso Nazionale Società Italiana di Medicina Psicosomatica (S.I.M.P.), Messina, 1987, in *Rassegna di Igiene Mentale* magazine, Year XI, 1989.
- Benatti G., *La lettura del vissuto attraverso il corpo parlato quale oggetto transizionale*, Proceedings of the II Convegno Internazionale *Mente-Corpo*, Milan, 1987.
- Benatti G., *Ipnosi e neuroendocrinologia*, Proceedings of the XII Congresso Nazionale Società Italiana di Medicina Psicosomatica (S.I.M.P.), Milan, 1989.
- Benatti G., *L'ipnosi per la tempestività dello scatto individuale nell'agonismo di gruppo*, Proceedings of the VIII Congresso A.I.P.S., 1990.
- Benatti G., *L'induzione ipnotica "mirata" nelle urgenze da panico*, Proceedings of the IX Congresso Nazionale di Ipnosi Clinica e Sperimentale A.M.I.S.I., Monastier (Treviso), 1991.
- Benatti G., *L'ipnosi nella crisi degli affetti mancati e qualità della vita*, Proceedings of the XIII Congresso Nazionale Società Italiana di Medicina Psicosomatica (S.I.M.P.), Bologna, 1991.
- Bottoli A., Azzini V., Guantieri G., *Su un caso di ritenzione urinaria trattato con ipnosi*, IX Congresso Internazionale Ipnosi e Medicina Psicosomatica, Glasgow, England, in *Rivista Italiana di Ipnosi Clinica Sperimentale* magazine, n. 2, 1982.
- Brugnoli A., *Possibilità terapeutiche nel dolore psicosomatico*, in Antonelli F., Guantieri G., (edited by), *Anoressia e obesità*, Vol. II, Publisher S.E.U., Rome, 1969.

- Brugnoli A., *Tecniche di terapia ipnotica del dolore*, in *Rassegna Medicina Psicosomatica* magazine, n. 24, 1974.
- Brugnoli A., *Ipnoterapia del dolore*, in *Rassegna Medicina Psicosomatica* magazine, n. 25, 1974.
- Brugnoli A., Galeazzi L., *Uso differenziato del rinforzo dell'Io in ipnosi*, in *Rassegna Medicina Psicosomatica* magazine, n. 31, 1976.
- Bulgarini G., *L'ipnosi*, in Bulgarini G., *Psicologia, Malattia e Salute*, Publisher La Scuola, Brescia, 1983.
- Bulgarini G., *Dal linguaggio verbale al linguaggio non verbale in ipnosi*, in Guantieri G. (edited by), *Il linguaggio del corpo in ipnosi*, Proceedings of the X Congresso Nazionale Società Italiana di Medicina Psicosomatica (S.I.M.P.), Publisher Il Segno, Negrar (Verona), 1985.
- Bulgarini G., *L'ipnosi nella terapia del paziente psichiatrico ricoverato. Report di un'esperienza presso i Servizi Psichiatrici di Brescia*, in Guantieri G., Ischia S. (edited by), *L'ipnosi nelle istituzioni. Ruolo e contributo*, Proceedings of the I Congresso Nazionale, Verona, 1985, Editions Istituto 'Bernheim', Verona, 1987.
- Bulgarini G., *Brief Psychotherapy Using Hypnosis as Preparation for Surgical Operations*, Proceedings of the V European Congress of Hypnosis in Psychotherapy and Psychosomatic Medicine, Costanza, Germany, 1990.
- Caldironi B., *Contributo all'esplorazione del profondo mediante ipnosi*, in *Rassegna Medicina Psicosomatica* magazine, n. 10, 1969.
- Caldironi B., *Regressione in ipnosi ad uno stato determinato da L.S.D.*, Proceedings of the V Congresso Internazionale di Ipnosi e Medicina Psicosomatica, Mainz, Germany, Publisher Springer, Berlin-HeidelbergNew York, 1973.
- Caldironi B., *Modalità ipnoterapeutiche e psiconevrosi*, in *Rassegna Medicina Psicosomatica* magazine, n. 24, 1974.
- Caldironi B., Widmann C., *Visualizzazioni guidate in psicoterapia*, Publisher Piovan, Abano Terme (Padua), 1980.
- Caldironi B., Lisanti S., *Imprinting and Hypnosis in Psychotherapy*, in Guantieri G. (edited by), *Hypnosis in Psychotherapy and Psychosomatic Medicine*, Proceedings of the 3rd European Congress of Hypnosis, Abano Terme (Padua), Publisher Il Segno, Negrar (Verona), 1985.
- Caliari P., Guantieri G., Mosconi G.P., *Bibliografia italiana sull'ipnosi 1973-1983*, in *Rivista Italiana di Ipnosi Clinica Sperimentale*, n. 2, 1983.
- Campanella G., *Neuropsicologia ed ipnosi*, in *Newsletter* magazine, Year III, n. 1, 1990.
- Campanella G., *La relazione medico-paziente nel malato di cancro. L'impiego dell'ipnosi*, in Romoli M., Bausi C. (edited by), *Il dolore e la sofferenza nel malato di cancro*, Publisher La Mandragola, Siena, 1990.
- Campanella G., *Hypnosis and Cancer Pain*, Proceedings of the 5th European Congress of Hypnosis in Psychotherapy and Psychosomatic Medicine, Costanza, Germany, 1990.

- Campanella G., Roncaroli P., *Psico-oncologia e relazione terapeutica*, Proceedings of the XIII Congresso Nazionale Società Italiana di Medicina Psicosomatica (S.I.M.P.), Bologna, 1991.
- Campanella G., *Ipnosi e dolore oncologico*, in *Algos* magazine, 1991.
- Castagna G., *Ipnoterapia della componente psicosomatica dell'asma bronchiale*, in *Medicina Psicosomatica* magazine, n. 15, 1970.
- Castagna G., *Trattamento dei postumi funzionali articolari con ipnosi*, in *Rassegna Medicina Psicosomatica* magazine, n. 13, 1970.
- Castagna G., Vannoni S., *Rieducazione funzionale psicosomatica in ortopedia*, in Antonelli F., Lapiccirella V. (edited by), in *Allucinogeni e Psicosomatosi*, Vol. III, Publisher S.E.U., Rome, 1972.
- Castelli P., Modenese M., *Rilassamento e visualizzazioni in un gruppo di allievi ISEF*, Proceedings of the VIII Congresso Nazionale Associazione Italiana di Psicologia dello Sport, Senigallia (Ancona), 1990.
- Castelli P., Modenese M., *Ipnosi e psicoterapia*, Proceedings of the Associazione Psicologi Veronesi, Verona, 1991.
- De Benedetti L., *Hypnosis as a Relationship with the Self and the Other*, in Guantieri G. (edited by), *Hypnosis in Psychotherapy and Psychosomatic Medicine*, Proceedings of the 3rd European Congress of Hypnosis, Abano Terme (Padua), Publisher Il Segno, Negrar (Verona), 1985.
- De Benedetti L., *Possibilità di riabilitazione e di apprendimento ideomotorio per mezzo dell'ipnosi*, in Guantieri G., Ischia S. (edited by), *L'ipnosi nelle istituzioni. Ruolo e contributo*, Proceedings of the I Congresso Nazionale, Verona, 1985, Editions Istituto 'Bernheim', Verona, 1987.
- De Benedetti L., *Motivazioni all'apprendimento dell'ipnosi*, Proceedings of the IX Congresso Nazionale di Ipnosi Clinica e Sperimentale A.M.I.S.l., Monastier (Treviso), 1991.
- De Benedetti L., Guantieri G., *Learning of Hypnosis: Correlations and Personalities*, Proceedings of the 5th European Congress of Hypnosis in Psychotherapy and Psychosomatic Medicine, Costanza, Germany, 1990.
- De Benedetti L., Gambacciani A., *Handicaps e qualità della vita*, Proceedings of the XIII Congresso Nazionale Società Italiana di Medicina Psicosomatica (S.I.M.P.), Bologna, 1991.
- De' Lutti P., *Un approccio psicosomatico nella terapia riabilitativa dell'etilista cronico*, Proceedings of the II Convegno Internazionale *Mente-Corpo*, Milan, 1987.
- De' Lutti P., *Il femminile ed i suoi simboli*, Proceedings of the II Giornata di Medicina Psicosomatica Rivana, Riva del Garda (Trento), 1989.
- De' Lutti P., *Il cervello ed i suoi simboli*, Proceedings of the III Giornata di Medicina Psicosomatica Rivana, Riva del Garda (Trento), 1990.
- De' Lutti P., *Il sonno ed i suoi sogni*, Proceedings of the IV Giornata di Medicina Psicosomatica Rivana, Riva del Garda (Trento), 1991.

- De' Lutti P., *Per un approccio psicosomatico nella riabilitazione del paziente etilista,* Proceedings of the XIII Congresso Nazionale Società Italiana di Medicina Psicosomatica (S.I.M.P.), Bologna, 1991.
- De Stavola W., *Ipnoterapia in due casi di tics,* in Antonelli F., Ancona L. (edited by), Proceedings of the della Settimana Psicosomatica Internazionale, Editions S.I.M.P., Rome, 1967.
- De Stavola W., *Terapia con ipnosi in alcuni casi di nevrosi ansiosa,* in Antonelli F., Ancona L. (edited by), Proceedings of the Settimana Psicosomatica Internazionale, Editions S.I.M.P., Rome, 1967.
- De Stavola W., *Considerazioni neurofisiologiche in tema di traversate a nuoto su lunghe distanze,* in Antonelli F. (edited by), Proceedings of the Simposio Internazionale Medicina Psicosomatica Sportiva, Editions S.I.M.P.), Rome, 1967.
- De Stavola W., *La parola come fattore fisiologico e terapeutico (parte prima). Rassegna sintetica dell'opera omonima di Platonov,* in *Medicina Psicosomatica* magazine, Year 13, 1968.
- De Stavola W., *La parola come fattore fisiologico e terapeutico (parte seconda),* in *Rassegna sintetica dell'opera omonima di Platonov, Medicina Psicosomatica* magazine, Year 14, 1969.
- De Stavola W., *La parola come fattore fisiologico e terapeutico (parte terza),* in *Rassegna sintetica dell'opera omonima di Platonov, Medicina Psicosomatica* magazine, Year 14, 1969.
- De Stavola W., *Basi neurodinamiche dell'ipnosi,* in *Rassegna di Ipnosi e Medicina Psicosomatica* magazine, n. 11, 1969.
- De Stavola W., *L'ipnologo di fronte alle terminologie psicoanalitiche e reflessologiche,* in *Rassegna di Ipnosi e Medicina Psicosomatica* magazine, n. 13, 1970.
- De Stavola W., *L'ipnologo di fronte alle psicoterapie brevi,* in *Rassegna di Ipnosi e Medicina Psicosomatica* magazine, n. 15, 1970.
- De Stavola W., *Principi di reflessologia condizionata,* in Antonelli F., Lapiccirella V. (edited by), *Allucinogeni e Psicosomatosi,* Publisher S.E.U., Rome, 1972.
- De Stavola W., *L'ipnosi come risposta condizionata,* in *Rassegna di Ipnosi e Medicina Psicosomatica* magazine, n. 24, 1974.
- De Stavola W., *Ipotesi e considerazioni sulla neurofisiologa dell'ipnosi condizionata,* in *Rassegna di Ipnosi e Medicina Psicosomatica* magazine, n. 65, 1974.
- Di Donato R., *Ipertensione: problema psicosomatico,* in *Medicina Psicosomatica* magazine, Year 16, 1971.
- Di Donato R., *La sindrome psicovegetativa,* in *Medicina Psicosomatica* magazine, Year 18, 1973.
- Di Donato R., Ligabue A., *Risposta cortisolemica e trattamento farmacologico e ipnotico dell'asma bronchiale,* in *Medicina Psicosomatica* magazine, Year 18, 1973.
- Di Donato R., *Ipnosi e ipertensione,* in *Rassegna di Ipnosi e Medicina Psicosomatica* magazine, n. 12, 1976.

- Di Donato R., Agresta F., Barone M., Nattarella C., *Between Hypnosis and Psychoanalysis: the Relaxation. Its use for Therapy of Psychosomatosis,* in Guantieri G. (edited by), *Hypnosis in Psychotherapy and Psychosomatic Medicine,* Proceedings of the 3rd European Congress of Hypnosis, Abano Terme (Padua), Publisher Il Segno, Negrar (Verona), 1985.
- Di Donato R., *Il rilassamento ad ispirazione analitica,* Proceedings of the XII Congresso Nazionale Società Italiana di Medicina Psicosomatica (S.I.M.P.), Milan, 1989.
- Fayenz S., *Possibilità dell'applicazione dell'ipnosi in endoscopia digestiva,* in *Newsletter* magazine, Year V, n.1, 1992.
- Fayenz S., *L'Ipnosi in endoscopia digestiva,* Proceedings of the Convegno Internazionale *Mente-Corpo: la relazione terapeutica in Medicina Psicosomatica,* Milan, 1987.
- Ferioli W., *Training autogeno ed ipnosi: rileggendo Schultz,* Proceedings of the XII Congresso Nazionale Società Italiana di Medicina Psicosomatica (S.I.M.P.), Milan, 1989.
- Ferioli W., *Modalità di ipnoterapia in due casi di vomito psicogeno,* in Antonelli F., Ancona L. (edited by), Proceedings of the Settimana Psicosomatica Internazionale, Editions S.I.M.P., Rome, 1967.
- Ferioli W., *Orientamenti metodologici dell'ipnoterapia dei disordini psicosomatici dell'età scolare,* in *Medicina Psicosomatica* magazine, Year 15, 1970.
- Ferioli W., *Ipnoterapia e disordini psicosomatici,* in *Rassegna di Ipnosi e Medicina Psicosomatica* magazine, n. 24, 1974.
- Ferrari F., *Costruttivismo, ipnosi e psicoterapia,* in *Newsletter* magazine, Year IV, n. 2-3, 1991.
- Fiori A., *Stati di coscienza e stati alterati: la fenomenologia dello stato ipnotico,* in *Newsletter* magazine, Year IV, n. 1, 1991.
- Fiori A., *L'immagine in psicoterapia. Valore e funzione delle immagini in psicoterapia,* in *Newsletter* magazine, Year II, n. 3, 1989.
- Forghieri P.L., Guantieri G., *Trattamento ipnotico di turbe del sonno in pazienti neuropsichiatrici ricoverati in ambiente specialistico,* Proceedings of the IX Congresso Internazionale di Ipnosi e Medicina Psicosomatica, Glasgow, Scotland, in *Rivista Italiana di Ipnosi Clinica e Sperimentale* magazine, n. 2, 1982.
- Forghieri P.L., Guantieri G., *Teaching Self Hypnosis as a Valid Instrument to improve Therapeutical Results in Neuropsychiatric Ward Patients,* in Guantieri G. (edited by), *Hypnosis in Psychotherapy and Psychosomatic Medicine,* Proceedings of the 3rd European Congress of Hypnosis, Abano Terme (Padua), Publisher Il Segno, Negrar (Verona), 1985.
- Forghieri P.L., *Ipnosi ed anoressia mentale,* Proceedings of the IX Congresso Nazionale di Ipnosi Clinica e Sperimentale A.M.I.S.I., Monastier (Treviso), 1991.

- Forghieri P.L., *Hypnosis: Possible Institutional Therapy?* Proceedings of the 5th European Congress of Hypnosis in Psychotherapy and Psychosomatic Medicine, Costanza, Germany, 1990.
- Forghieri P.L., *Anorexia and Hypnosis*, Proceedings of the 5th European Congress of Hypnosis in Psychotherapy and Psychosomatic Medicine, Costanza, Germany, 1990.
- Forghieri P.L., *Impiego dell'ipnosi in Casa di Cura Neuropsichiatrica: realtà e prospettive*, in Guantieri G., Ischia S. (edited by), *L'ipnosi nelle istituzioni, Ruolo e contributo*, Proceedings of the I Congresso Nazionale, Verona, 1985, Editions Istituto 'Bernheim', Verona, 1987.
- Galardi L., *L'immagine in psicoterapia. Il R.E.D. di Desoille e l'ipnoterapia non direttiva: spunti critici e riflessioni*, in *Newsletter* magazine, Year II, n. 3, 1989.
- Galardi L., *Stati di coscienza e stati alterati: la fenomenologia dello stato ipnotico (Parte prima)*, in *Newsletter* magazine, Year IV, n. 1, 1991.
- Galvano O.M., Perego P., *Utilizzo delle tecniche ipnotiche nell'ambito psichiatrico pubblico*, Proceedings of the 5th European Congress of Hypnosis in Psychotherapy and Psychosomatic Medicine, Costanza, Germany, 1990.
- Galvano O.M., *La resistenza all'uso dell'ipnosi*, Proceedings of the IX Congresso Nazionale di Ipnosi Clinica e Sperimentale A.M.I.S.I., Monastier (Treviso), 1991.
- Gambacciani A., *Hypnosis in Treatment of Multiple Sclerosis: Observation on a Case*, in Pajntar M., Roskar E., Lavric M. (edited by), *Hypnosis in Psychotherapy and Psychosomatic Medicine*, Proceedings of the 2nd European Congress of Hypnosis, Dubrovnik, Croatia, University Press, Lubiana, Slovenia, 1980.
- Gambacciani A., *Dolore e Ipnosi*, Proceedings of the I Corso Nazionale Aggiornamento *La terapia del dolore*, S.I.M.F.E.R., Milan, 1981.
- Gambacciani A., *L'ipnosi nel trattamento riabilitativo di un caso di malattia di Guillain-Barrè*, IX Congresso Internazionale Ipnosi e Medicina Psicosomatica, Glasgow, Scotland, in *Rivista Italiana di Ipnosi Clinica e Sperimentale* magazine, n. 2, 1982.
- Gambacciani A., *Rehabilitation and Hypnosis*, in Guantieri G., *Hypnosis in Psychotherapy and Psychosomatic Medicine*, Proceedings of the 3rd European Congress of Hypnosis, Abano Terme (Padua), Publisher Il Segno, Negrar (Verona), 1985.
- Gambacciani A., *Possibilità dell'approccio ipnotico in fisiatria*, in Guantieri G., Ischia S. (edited by), *L'ipnosi nelle istituzioni, Ruolo e contributo*, Proceedings of the I Congresso Nazionale, Verona, 1985, Editions Istituto 'Bernheim', Verona, 1987.
- Gambacciani A., *Ipnosi e psicoprofilassi ostetrica*, in Proceedings of the Convegno *Il parto e il dolore*, Editions CLEUP, Padua, 1986.
- Gambacciani A., *Esperienze ipnotiche in soggetti neurolesi*, Proceedings of the II Convegno Internazionale *Mente-Corpo*, Milan, 1987.

- Gambacciani A., Rupil S., *Ipnosi e riabilitazione*, Proceedings of the IX Congresso Nazionale di Ipnosi Clinica e Sperimentale A.M.I.S.I., Monastier (Treviso), 1991.
- Gambacciani A., De Benedetti L., *Handicaps e qualità della vita*, Proceedings of the XIII Congresso Nazionale S.I.M.P., Bologna, 1991.
- Gambacciani A., *Hypnosis and Rehabilitation*, Proceedings of the 5th European Congress of Hypnosis in Psychotherapy and Psychosomatic Medicine, Costanza, Germany, 1990.
- Genovese A., Mercurio A., *Il malato psicosomatico tra specialista e medico di base*, in *Newsletter* magazine, Year IV, n. 2-3, 1991.
- Gocci G., Arrigucci E., *L'ipnosi come processo psicodinamico (euipnosi)*, in *Rivista Italiana di Ipnosi Clinica e Sperimentale* magazine, n. 2, 1982.
- Gocci G., *Induzione ipnotica collettiva e tecniche meditative in un gruppo di universitari di Magistero*, in Guantieri G., Ischia S. (edited by), *L'ipnosi nelle istituzioni, Ruolo e contributo*, Proceedings of the I Congresso Nazionale, Verona, 1985, Editions Istituto 'Bernheim', Verona, 1987.
- Gocci G., *I gruppi di individuazione*, Proceedings of the II Convegno Internazionale *Mente-Corpo*, Milan, 1987.
- Gocci G., *Il corpo si immagina: immaginare per comunicare*, XI Congresso Nazionale S.I.M.P., Messina 1987, in *Rassegna di Igiene Mentale* magazine, Year XI, 1989.
- Gocci G., *Mente e corpo in ipnosi senza trance*, Proceedings of the XII Congresso Nazionale S.I.M.P., Milan, 1989.
- Gocci G., *Le basi psicodinamiche dell'ipnosi*, Proceedings of the Convegno C.E.I.S., Arezzo, 1991.
- Gocci G., *Incontro con la fiaba: i racconti che curano*, Proceedings of the Convegno, Marcon (Venezia), 1991.
- Gocci G., *Ipnosi e attività onirica*, Proceedings of the IX Congresso Nazionale di Ipnosi Clinica e Sperimentale A.M.I.S.I., Monastier (Treviso), 1991.
- Gramaccioni G.F., Lanari A., *Ipnosi e Visualizzazioni guidate nel calciatore*, Proceedings of the VI Congresso A.I.P.S., in *Movimento* magazine (Organo ufficiale dell'Associazione Italiana Psicologia dello Sport), n. 3, 1986.
- Gramaccioni G.F., Lanari A., *Allenarsi con l'ipnosi*, in *Riza Psicosomatica* magazine, n. 78, 1987.
- Gramaccioni G.F., *Visualizzazioni guidate nello sport*, Proceedings of the Congresso Nazionale *Ricerca e intervento in psicologia dello sport*, Verona, 1988.
- Gramaccioni G.F., Lanari A., *Ipnosi e visualizzazioni nello sport*, Proceedings of the XII Congresso Nazionale S.I.M.P., Milan, 1989.
- Gramaccioni G.F., *Settori operativi della psicologia dello sport. L'impiego dell'ipnosi nello sport*, Proceedings of the Tavola Rotonda *Ipnosi in ambito sportivo*, Verona, 1989.

- Gramaccioni G.F., *L'ipnosi nella preparazione mentale dell'atleta*, Proceedings of the VIII Congresso Nazionale dell'Associazione Italiana di Psicologia dello Sport, Senigallia (Ancona), 1990.
- Gramaccioni G.F., Lanari A., *Hypnosis and Ideomotor Training*, Proceedings of the 5th European Congress of Hypnosis in Psychotherapy and Psychosomatic Medicine, Costanza, Germany, 1990.
- Gramaccioni G.F., Lanari A., *Hypnosis and Mental Training for Sports Competitions*, Proceedings of the 5th European Congress of Hypnosis in Psychotherapy and Psychosomatic Medicine, Costanza, Germany, 1990.
- Gramaccioni G.F., *La performance atletica: aspetti psicologici e metodologie di intervento*, Proceedings of the V Meeting Nazionale di Medicina dello Sport, Porto S. Giorgio (Venezia), 1990.
- Gramaccioni G.F., *L'ipnosi e la formazione psicologica del medico di base*, Proceedings of the XIII Congresso Nazionale S.I.M.P., Bologna, 1991.
- Gramaccioni G.F., *Le basi psicologiche della performance dell'atleta ed il ruolo dell'ipnosi*, Proceedings of the IX Congresso Nazionale di Ipnosi Clinica e Sperimentale A.M.I.S.I., Monastier (Treviso), 1991.
- Grecchi V., *Verso una concezione integrata della psicologia scientifica: l'approccio psicobiologico e l'ipnosi terapeutica*, in *Newsletter* magazine, Anno V, n. 1, 1992.
- Guantieri G., *Origine e sviluppo della medicina psicosomatica e suo valore nell'epoca attuale*, in *Il Policlinico* magazine, Sez. Pratica, Vol. CXX, n. 34, 1963.
- Guantieri G., *L'emozione in medicina: considerazioni su di un caso di interesse psicosomatico*, in *Medicina Psicosomatica* magazine, n. 8, 1963.
- Guantieri G., *Contributo allo studio della eziopatogenesi del diabete giovanile: indagine psicosomatica sull' insorgenza e sul decorso di un caso*, in *Annali di Neuropsichiatria e Psicoanalisi* magazine, Year X, n. 4, 1963.
- Guantieri G., *Contributo all'eziopatogenesi e terapia della enuresi essenziale: indagine psicosomatica su di un caso portato a guarigione con ipnosi*, in *Revista de Psycologia normal y patologica* magazine, Year IX, n. 1-2, 1963.
- Guantieri G., *Contributo allo studio della eziopatogenesi e terapia della balbuzie: indagine psicologica su di un caso*, in *Annali di Laringologia* magazine, Year XII, n. 4, 1963.
- Guantieri G., *L'ipnosi e le sue applicazioni in Medicina*, in *Panorama Medico* magazine, n. 2, 1965.
- Guantieri G., *L'ambiente familiare come fattore patogeno: indagine psicosomatica su di un caso gravissimo di malattia dei tics*, in *Minerva Medica* magazine, n. 56, 1965.
- Guantieri G., *Indagine psicosomatica su di un caso di gastroduodenite*, in *Medicina Psicosomatica* magazine, n. 1, 1965.
- Guantieri G., *L'ipnosi come mezzo di psicoprofilassi ostetrica*, Proceedings of the Symposium Società Italiana di Psicoprofilassi Ostetrica, Rome, 1967.
- Guantieri G., *Sull'ipnoterapia dei disordini psicosomatici*, in Antonelli F., Ancona L. (edited by), Proceedings of the VII European Conference on Psychosomatic Research, Editions S.I.M.P., Rome, 1967.

- Guantieri G., *Principi per una didattica dell'ipnosi*, Proceedings of the I Convegno Nazionale Studi sulla Ipnosi Clinica A.M.I.S.I., Rome, 1967.
- Guantieri G., *Sull'induzione di ipnosi: contributo alla realizzazione di un metodo valido sotto il profilo didattico*, in *Rassegna di Ipnosi e Medicina Psicosomatica* magazine, n. 59, 1968.
- Guantieri G., *Ipnosi Medica: introduzione allo studio e alla pratica dell'ipnosi in Medicina*, in *Opera Medica* magazine, n. 130, Editions Wassermann, Milan, 1968.
- Guantieri G., *L'induzione di ipnosi*, in Antonelli F., Businco L. (edited by), in *Quaderni di Psicosomatica*, Vol. I, Publisher S.E.U, Rome, 1969.
- Guantieri G., *L'ipnosi: caratteristiche e possibilità di impiego in Medicina*, in *Miscellanea* magazine, n. 179, 1968.
- Guantieri G., *Ipnosi e Medicina*, in *Il Polso* magazine, Anno II, n. 4, 1969.
- Guantieri G., *Modalità di approccio e di terapia del paziente psicosomatico mediante ipnosi*, in Antonelli F., Guantieri G. (edited by), *Anoressia e Obesità*, in *Quaderni di Psicosomatica* magazine, Vol. II, Publisher S.E.U., Rome, 1970.
- Guantieri G., Antonelli F. (edited by), *Anoressia e Obesità*, in *Quaderni di Psicosomatica* magazine, Vol. II, Publisher S.E.U., Rome, 1970.
- Guantieri G., *Possibilità terapeutiche in medicina psicosomatica*, in *Lezioni di Psicosomatica*, appendice a Antonelli F., Lapiccirella V. (edited by), *Allucinogeni e Psicosomatosi*, Vol. III, Publisher S.E.U., Rome, 1972.
- Guantieri G., *La formazione psicologica del medico*, in *Medicina Psicosomatica* magazine, n. 18, 1973.
- Guantieri G., *L'ipnosi come oggetto di studio e mezzo di impiego in medicina*, Publisher Rizzoli, Milan, 1973.
- Guantieri G., *Fenomenologia dell'ipnosi*, in *Rassegna di Ipnosi e Medicina Psicosomatica* magazine, n. 24, 1974.
- Guantieri G., *L'ipnosi medica: problemi antichi, fondamenti e prospettive attuali*, in *Rassegna di Ipnosi e Medicina Psicosomatica* magazine, n. 25, 1974.
- Guantieri G., *Ipnosi Psicosomatica: aspetti clinici e sperimentali*, in *Rassegna di Ipnosi e Medicina Psicosomatica* magazine, n. 25, 1974.
- Guantieri G., *Formazione psicosomatica del medico e training ipnotico*, in *Rassegna di Ipnosi e Medicina Psicosomatica* magazine, n. 25, 1974.
- Guantieri G., *Posizione e ruolo della ipnosi in psicosomatica*, in *Medicina Psicosomatica* magazine, n. 20, 1975.
- Guantieri G., *Ipnosi e Medicina Psicosomatica come oggetto di studio e insegnamento universitario*, in *Rassegna di Ipnosi e Medicina Psicosomatica* magazine, n. 31, 1976.
- Guantieri G., Benatti G., *Il lavoro medico italiano nel campo dell'ipnosi nel XX secolo*, in *Rassegna di Ipnosi e Medicina Psicosomatica* magazine, n. 31, 1976.
- Guantieri G., *L'ipnosi da Mesmer ad oggi*, Proceedings of the Convegno E.S.P., 18 June 1976.
- Guantieri G., *Training ipnotico e training autogeno*, Proceedings of the Congresso Internazionale C.I.S.S.P.A.T., Campione d'Italia (Como), 1976.

- Guantieri G., *Hypnosis and Psychodinamics,* in Antonelli, F. (edited by), Proceedings of the III Congresso Internazionale Medicina Psicosomatica, Publisher Pozzi, Brescia, 1977.
- Guantieri G., Parietti P., *La preparazione del medico ipnologo,* in Antonelli F. (edited by), Proceedings of the III Congresso Internazionale Medicina Psicosomatica, Publisher Pozzi, Brescia, 1977.
- Guantieri G., Parietti, P., *Psicoterapia e Ipnosi,* in *Rassegna di Ipnosi Medica e Psicosomatica* magazine, n. 13, 1977.
- Guantieri G., *Possibilità terapeutiche dell'ipnosi in alcune disfunzioni sessuali,* in Salvati A. (edited by), *I 500 perché della donna,* Publisher Minerva Medica, Rome, 1978.
- Guantieri, G. *L'ipnosi quale modalità di terapia psicosomatica,* Proceedings of the I Congresso Europeo di Ipnosi in Psicoterapia e Medicina Psicosomatica, Malmö, Sweden, 1978.
- Guantieri G., *Ipnosi e terapia psicosomatica,* Proceedings of the Convegno Psicoterapia e Psicosomatica, Marostica (Vicenza), 1977, Vol. I, *Collana Medicina Psicosomatica,* Maccari (Parma), 1979.
- Guantieri G., *L'ipnosi quale modalità psicoterapeutica,* Proceedings of the V Convegno Nazionale Studi sull'ipnosi clinica A.M.I.S.I., Milan, 1979.
- Guantieri G., Roncaroli P., *Livelli di interazione nel rapporto interpersonale ipnotico,* Proceedings of the I Congresso Europeo di Ipnosi in Psicoterapia e Medicina Psicosomatica, Malmö, Sweden, in *Rassegna di Igiene Mentale* magazine, Year I, n. 4, 1979.
- Guantieri G., Pasetti C., *L'ipnosi come mezzo di ausilio nella riabilitazione funzionale delle paralisi spastiche,* I Congresso Europeo di Ipnosi in Psicoterapia e Medicina Psicosomatica, Malmö, Sweden, in *Rassegna di Igiene Mentale* magazine, Year I, n. 4, 1979.
- Guantieri G., *Ipnosi e Sessuologia,* in *Rivista di Sessuologia Clinica* magazine, n. 4, 1980.
- Guantieri G., Roncaroli P., *Ipnosi e curva erotica femminile,* in *Rivista di Sessuologia Clinica* magazine, n. 5, 1980.
- Guantieri G., *L'ipnosi in terapia,* in Colli F., Quattrocchi S. (edited by), *Il fenomeno ipnosi,* Publisher Nuova Spada, Rome, 1980.
- Guantieri G., Parietti P., *Problems and Perspectives of Solution Teaching of Hypnosis,* in Pajntar M., Roskar E., Lavric M. (edited by), *Hypnosis in Psychotherapy and Psychosomatic Medicine,* Proceedings of the 2nd European Congress of Hypnosis, Dubrovnik, Croatia, University Press, Lubiana, Slovenia, 1980.
- Guantieri G., Seminara B., Ischia S., Bartoloni A., Pasetto A., *On a Case of Cholecistectomy under Hypnosis,* in Pajntar M., Roskar E., Lavric M. (edited by), *Hypnosis in Psychotherapy and Psychosomatic Medicine,* Proceedings of the 2nd European Congress of Hypnosis, Dubrovnik, Croatia, University Press, Lubiana, Slovenia, 1980.

- Guantieri G., Roncaroli P., *Hypnosis as a Method of Multidimensional Analysis* in *Psychotherapy,* in Pajntar M., Roskar E., Lavric M. (edited by), *Hypnosis in Psychotherapy and Psychosomatic Medicine,* Proceedings of the 2nd European Congress of Hypnosis, Dubrovnik, Croatia, University Press, Lubiana, Slovenia, 1980.
- Guantieri G., Guerra G., *Contributo alla conoscenza e all'impiego del rilassamento in varie situazioni esistenziali,* in *Giornale di Medicina Militare* magazine, n. 6, 1981.
- Guantieri G., *The Value of Placebos in Chronic Pain Therapy,* Proceedings of the II Corso Pratico Internazionale di Aggiornamento sulla terapia del dolore, Vicenza, 1982.
- Guantieri G., *L'induzione di ipnosi in medicina psicosomatica,* IX Congresso Internazionale di Ipnosi e Medicina Psicosomatica, Glasgow, Scotland, in *Rivista Italiana di Ipnosi Clinica e Sperimentale* magazine, n. 2, 1982.
- Guantieri G., Guerra G., Simonelli F., Sarao G., Tagliaro F., Luisetto G., *Livelli plasmatici di betaendorfina e analgesia ipnotica,* IX Congresso Internazionale di Ipnosi e Medicina Psicosomatica, Glasgow, Scotland, in *Rivista Italiana di Ipnosi Clinica e Sperimentale* magazine, n. 2, 1982.
- Guantieri G., Bottoli A., Azzini V., *Su un caso di ritenzione urinaria trattato con ipnosi,* IX Congresso Internazionale di Ipnosi e Medicina Psicosomatica, Glasgow, Scotland, in *Rivista Italiana di Ipnosi Clinica e Sperimentale* magazine, n. 2, 1982.
- Guantieri G., Forghieri P.L., *Trattamento ipnotico di turbe del sonno di pazienti neuropsichiatrici ricoverati in ambiente specialistico,* IX Congresso Internazionale di Ipnosi e Medicina Psicosomatica, Glasgow, Scotland, in *Rivista Italiana di Ipnosi Clinica e Sperimentale* magazine, n. 2, 1982.
- Guantieri G., Caliari P., Mosconi G.P., *Bibliografia italiana sull'ipnosi 1973-1983,* in *Rivista Italiana di Ipnosi Clinica e Sperimentale* magazine, n. 2, 1983.
- Guantieri G., *Rilassamento, ipnosi, formazione psicosomatica,* II Convegno Sezione Toscana S.I.M.P., Florence, *La formazione psicosomatica, Collana di Igiene Mentale,* n. 1, Messina, 1984.
- Guantieri G., *How and why Hypnosis in Psychosomatic Medicine,* in Guantieri G. (edited by), *Hypnosis in Psychotherapy and Psychosomatic Medicine,* Proceedings of the 3rd European Congress of Hypnosis, Abano Terme (Padua), Publisher Il Segno, Negrar (Verona), 1985.
- Guantieri G., Angelozzi A., *L'ipnosi: un fondamento ed una prospettiva,* Editions Istituto 'Bernheim', Verona, 1985.
- Guantieri G., Angelozzi A., *Hypnosis: a base and a way forward,* Editions Istituto 'Bernheim', Verona, 1985.
- Guantieri G., Forghieri P.L., *Teaching Self Hypnosis as a Valid Instrument to Improve Therapeutical Results in Neuropsychiatric Ward Patients,* in Guantieri G. (edited by), *Hypnosis in Psychotherapy and Psychosomatic Medicine,* Proceedings of

- the 3rd European Congress of Hypnosis, Abano Terme (Padua), Publisher Il Segno, Negrar (Verona), 1985.
- Guantieri G., *Hypnosis in Psychotherapy and Psychosomatic Medicine,* Proceedings of the 3rd European Congress of Hypnosis, Abano Terme (Padua), Publisher Il Segno, Negrar (Verona), 1985.
- Guantieri G., *Il setting ipnotico in prospettiva psicodinamica,* in Guantieri G. (edited by), *Il linguaggio del corpo in ipnosi,* Proceedings of the X Congresso Nazionale S.I.M.P., Publisher Il Segno, Negrar (Verona), 1985.
- Guantieri G. (edited by), *Il linguaggio del corpo in ipnosi,* Proceedings of the X Congresso Nazionale S.I.M.P., Publisher Il Segno, Negrar (Verona), 1985.
- Guantieri G., Angelozzi A., *L'ipnosi nelle Istituzioni,* Corso C.I.I.C.S., Turin, 1986.
- Guantieri G., *L'ipnosi in psicoterapia,* in *Prospettive in Psicologia* magazine, n. 2, 1986.
- Guantieri G., *L'ipnosi oggi,* in Guantieri G., Ischia S. (edited by), *L'ipnosi nelle istituzioni. Ruolo e contributo,* Proceedings of the I Congresso Nazionale, Verona, 1985, Editions Istituto "Bernheim", Verona, 1987.
- Guantieri G., *L'ipnosi in prospettiva psicosomatica,* Proceedings of the *Rencontres Internationales* Federazione Internazionale Gruppi Balint, Ascona, Swiss, 1987.
- Guantieri G., *L'induzione di ipnosi quale comunicazione terapeutica,* XI Congresso Nazionale S.I.M.P., Messina, 1987, in *Rassegna di Igiene Mentale* magazine, Anno XI, 1989.
- Guantieri G., *Psychotherapy and Hypnotic Context,* Proceedings of the 4th European Congress of Hypnosis in Psychotherapy and Psychosomatic Medicine, Oxford, Scotland, 1987.
- Guantieri G., *Il vissuto del corpo in ipnosi,* Proceedings of the II Convegno Internazionale *Mente-Corpo,* Milan, 1987.
- Guantieri G., Ischia S. (edited by), *L'ipnosi nelle istituzioni. Ruolo e contributo,* Proceedings of the I Congresso Nazionale, Verona, 1985, Editions Istituto 'Bernheim', Verona, 1987.
- Guantieri G., Parietti P., Santini M., *L'ipnosi nell'informazione e nella formazione del medico e dello psicologo,* in Guantieri G., Ischia S. (edited by), *L'ipnosi nelle istituzioni. Ruolo e contributo,* Proceedings of the I Congresso Nazionale, Verona, 1985, Editions Istituto 'Bernheim', Verona, 1987.
- Guantieri G., *Hypnosis and the Therapeutic Relationship,* Proceedings of the 11th International Congress of Hypnosis and Psychosomatic Medicine, Leiden, Holland, 1988.
- Guantieri G., *L'ipnosi in ambito medico psicologico,* Proceedings of the Convegno Associazione Psicologi Bresciani, June 1988, Brescia.
- Guantieri G., *Prefazione* a David Waxman, *John Hartland, Medical and Dental Hypnosis,* (3rd edition), Publisher Bailliére Tindall, London, 1988.

- Guantieri G., *Ipnosi e terapia del dolore,* in *Newsletter* magazine, Year II, n. 2, 1989.
- Guantieri G., Angelozzi A., *Note sull'origine e l'evoluzione del Centro Studi 'Bernheim',* in *Newsletter* magazine, Year II, n. 1, 1989.
- Guantieri G., *L'emozione in prospettiva psicosomatica,* in *Prospettive in Psicologia* magazine, n. 1, 1990.
- Guantieri G., *L'approccio ipnotico al paziente psicosomatico,* Proceedings of the 5th European Congress of Hypnosis in Psychotherapy and Psychosomatic Medicine, Costanza, Germany, 1990.
- Guantieri G., *L'ipnosi come terapia,* in *Prospettive in Psicologia* magazine, n. 2, 1990.
- Guantieri G., *L'emozione in prospettiva psicosomatica,* in *Newsletter* magazine, Year IV, n. 1, 1991.
- Guantieri G., *L'ipnosi tra psicoterapia e psicopatologia,* Proceedings of the IX Congresso Nazionale di Ipnosi Clinica e Sperimentale A.M.I.S.I., Monastier (Treviso), 1991.
- Guantieri G., Gasparini D., Lafisca S., *Possibilità di applicazioni forensi dell'ipnosi alla luce del nuovo Codice di Procedura Penale,* in *Newsletter* magazine, Year II, n. 2, 1989.
- Guantieri G., De Benedetti L., *Learning of Hypnosis: Correlations and Personalities,* Proceedings of the 5th European Congress of Hypnosis in Psychotherapy and Psychosomatic Medicine, Costanza, Germany, 1990.
- Guantieri G., *L'ipnosi contro il dolore,* in *Il Polso* magazine, n. 16, 1991.
- Guantieri G., *Ipnosi e relazione interpersonale,* Proceedings of the Congresso *La gravidanza alle soglie del 2000: benessere e sicurezza,* Publisher S.G.E., 1991.
- Guerra G., Guantieri G., *Contributo alla conoscenza e all'impiego del rilassamento in varie situazioni esistenziali,* in *Giornale di Medicina Militare* magazine, n. 6, 1981.
- Guerra G., Guantieri G., Simonelli F., Sarao G., Tagliaro F., Luisetto G., *Livelli plasmatici di beta-endorfina e analgesia ipnotica,* IX Congresso Internazionale di Ipnosi e Medicina Psicosomatica, Glasgow, Scotland, in *Rivista Italiana di Ipnosi Clinica e Sperimentale* magazine, n. 2, 1982.
- Guerra G., Nano D., Quisi Q., *Ulcera peptica e medicina psicosomatica: un contributo clinico,* in *Rassegna di Studi Psichiatrici* magazine, n. 20, 1982.
- Guerra G., Tagliaro F., Cristofori P., Concari G., Melorio E., Luisetto G., *Livelli Plasmatici di betaendorfine negli stati ipnotici con suggestioni di dolore e di analgesia-anestesia,* in *Giornale di Medicina Militare* magazine, n. 2-3, 1982.
- Guerra G., Fazzari G., Ferrario M., Nano D., Quisi Q., Regazzini F., *Psicoterapia breve con tecniche ipnotiche presso servizi psichiatrici del territorio,* in *Rassegna di Studi Psichiatrici* magazine, n. 3, 1982.
- Guerra G., Nano D., Quisi Q., *Asma: la paura di perdere l'amore,* Proceedings of the XXXV Congresso S.I.P., Publisher Il Pensiero Scientifico, Rome, 1984.

- Guerra G., Nano D., Quisi Q., *Le Visualizzazioni Guidate: una tecnica per psicoterapia breve*, Proceedings of the XXXV Congresso S.I.P., Publisher Il Pensiero Scientifico, Rome, 1984.
- Guerra G., *Tecniche di induzione ipnotica, ipnotizzabilità e possibili applicazioni in ambito militare*, in *Giornale di Medicina Militare* magazine, 1984.
- Guerra G., Tagliaro F., Meneghini V., Poletti S., Cesa Bianchi G., *Livelli plasmatici di betaendorfine e ACTH in varie condizioni sperimentali di ansietà e di calma indotte in ipnosi*, in Guantieri G., Ischia S. (edited by), *L'ipnosi nelle istituzioni. Ruolo e contributo*, Proceedings of the I Congresso Nazionale, Verona, 1985, Editions Istituto 'Bernheim', Verona, 1987.
- Irone U., *La preparazione della gestante al parto mediante ipnosi*, in *Rassegna di Ipnosi Medica e Psicosomatica* magazine, n. 25, 1974.
- Irone U., *Ipnoterapia in un caso di nevrosi*, VII Congresso Internazionale di Ipnosi e Medicina Psicosomatica, Uppsala, Sweden, in *Rassegna di Ipnosi Medica e Psicosomatica* magazine, n. 31, 1976.
- Lanari A., Gramaccioni G.F., *Ipnosi e visualizzazioni guidate nel calciatore*, in Proceedings of the VI Congresso A.I.P.S., in *Movimento* magazine n. 3, 1986.
- Lanari A., Gramaccioni G.F., *Allenarsi con l'ipnosi*, in *Riza Psicosomatica* magazine, n. 78, 1987.
- Lanari A., Roncaroli P., *Ipnosi e visualizzazioni guidate nello sport*, Proceedings of the del Convegno *Tecniche di Intervento in Psicologia dello Sport*, Senigallia (Ancona), 1986, in *Equilibrio* magazine (Bulletin of C.M.P.S.), n. 1, 1987.
- Lanari A., *L'ipnosi: definizione e possibilità di impiego nello sport*, Proceedings of the Congresso Nazionale *Ricerca e Intervento in Psicologia dello Sport*, Verona, 1988.
- Lanari A., Gramaccioni G.F., *Ipnosi e visualizzazioni nello sport*, Proceedings of the XII Congresso Nazionale S.I.M.P., Milan, 1989.
- Lanari A., Gramaccioni, G.F., *Hypnosis and Ideomotor Training*, Proceedings of the 5th European Congress of Hypnosis in Psychotherapy and Psychosomatic Medicine, Costanza, Germany, 1990.
- Lanari A., Gramaccioni G.F., *Hypnosis and Mental Preparation for Sports Competitions*, Proceedings of the 5th European Congress of Hypnosis in Psychotherapy and Psychosomatic Medicine, Costanza, Germany, 1990.
- Lanari A., *L'ipnosi per partorire*, Proceedings of the XIII Congresso Nazionale S.I.M.P., Bologna, 1991.
- Lisanti S., Caldironi B., *Imprinting and Hypnosis in Psychotherapy*, in Guantieri G. (edited by), *Hypnosis in Psychotherapy and Psychosomatic Medicine*, Proceedings of the 3rd European Congress of Hypnosis, Abano Terme (Padua), Publisher Il Segno, Negrar, (Verona), 1985.
- Lodetti R., *Ipotesi interpretativa delle strutture mente-corpo*, Proceedings of the I Convegno Internazionale *Mente-corpo*, Milan, 1986, in *Riza Psicosomatica* magazine, Milan, 1987.

- Lodetti R., *Tre cervelli e tre "Io"*, *Ricerche strutturali*, Proceedings of the Proceedings of the XII Congresso Nazionale S.I.M.P., Milan, 1989.
- Lodetti R., *Il corpo umano: il modulo organizzatore nelle strutture fisiche e psichiche*, Publisher Dehoniane, Vol. I, Rome, 1990.
- Lodetti R., *Il corpo umano. Cibernetica degli apparati fisici per una nuova antropologia*, Publisher Dehoniane, Vol. II, Rome, 1991.
- Lodetti R., *Il corpo umano. Il modulo organizzatore nelle strutture organiche e psichiche*, Proceedings of the XIII Congresso Nazionale S.I.M.P., Bologna, 1991.
- Malesani P.G., *Self-Hypnosis and Abreaction: Exposition and a Case Discussion*, in Guantieri G. (edited by), *Hypnosis in Psychotherapy and Psychosomatic Medicine*, Proceedings of the 3rd European Congress of Hypnosis, Abano Terme (Padua), Publisher Il Segno, Negrar (Verona), 1985.
- Modenese M., Bonaldi T., *Modelli psicologici e terapia non farmacologica nell'ipertensione arteriosa essenziale*, in *Prospettive in Psicologia* magazine, n. 1, 1988.
- Modenese M., *La preparazione con l'ipnosi di un pesista olimpionico*, Proceedings of the Tavola Rotonda *L'ipnosi in ambito sportivo*, Verona, 1989.
- Modenese M., Castelli P., *Rilassamento e visualizzazioni in un gruppo di allievi I.S.E.F.*, Proceedings of the VIII Congresso Nazionale Associazione Italiana di Psicologia dello Sport, Senigallia (Ancona), 1990.
- Modenese M., *Visualizzazioni ed immagini mentali*, Proceedings of the Convegno Nazionale Società Italiana di Psicologia *Tecniche di intervento e implicazioni formative in psicologia dello sport*, Prato, 1991.
- Modenese M., Saltini P., *Neologismi ed induzione verbale di ipnosi*, Proceedings of the XIII Congresso Nazionale della Società Italiana di Medicina Psicosomatica, Bologna, 1991.
- Modenese M., Castelli P., *Ipnosi e psicoterapia*, Proceedings of the Convegno Associazione Psicologi Veronesi, Verona, 1991.
- Murgolo W., *Multidimensional Approach in the Treatment of two Cases of Psychogenic Impotentia*, in Guantieri G. (edited by), Hypnosis in *Psychotherapy and Psychosomatic Medicine*, Proceedings of the 3rd European Congress of Hypnosis, Abano Terme (Padua), Publisher Il Segno, Negrar (Verona), 1985.
- Muzi P.G., Monaco V., *Impiego terapeutico dell'ipnosi in un caso di oftalmoplegia intrinseca bilaterale di verosimile natura psicogena*, in *Medicina Psicosomatica* magazine, n. 15, 1970.
- Muzi P.G., *Suscettibilità e Refrattarietà all'ipnosi*, in *Rassegna di Ipnosi e Medicina Psicosomatica* magazine, n. 24, 1974.
- Muzi P.G., *Mente, corpo, identità tra fenomenologia e ontologia*, Proceedings of the convegno Internazionale *Mente-Corpo*, Milan, 1986.
- Muzi P.G., Angelozzi A., *How to do Trance with Words*, Proceedings of the 11th International Congress of Hypnosis and Psychosomatic Medicine, Leiden, Holland, 1988.

- Muzi P.G., *Suscettibilità e refrattarietà all'Ipnosi*, in *Newsletter* magazine, Year I, n. 1, 1988.
- Muzi P.G., Angelozzi A., *Che ci fa il mio cervello nel laboratorio di neurofisiologia?* Proceedings of the XII Congresso Nazionale S.I.M.P., Milan, 1989.
- Parietti P., *L'ipnosi quale ausilio alla psicoprofilassi ostetrica*, in *Medicina Psicosomatica* magazine, Anno 15, n.1, 1970.
- Parietti P., Minella E., *Psicoprofilassi ostetrica e metodiche ipnoterapiche*, Proceedings of the III Congresso Società Italiana Psicoprofilassi Ostetrica, Edizioni S.I.P.P.O., Milan, 1970.
- Parietti P., *Sulla preparazione psicologica del medico ipnologo*, in *Rassegna di Ipnosi Medica e Psicosomatica* magazine, n. 6, 1970.
- Parietti P., *Ipnoterapia nelle affezioni psicosomatiche*, in *Medicina Psicosomatica* magazine, n. 17, 1972.
- Parietti P., *L'ipnosi nella preparazione della gestante*, in *Rassegna di Ipnosi e Medicina Psicosomatica* magazine, n. 24, 1974.
- Parietti P., *La formazione dell'ipnoterapeuta*, in *Rassegna di Ipnosi e Medicina Psicosomatica* magazine, n. 25, 1974.
- Parietti P., *L'ipnosi alla luce delle teorie della comunicazione*, in *Rassegna di Ipnosi e Medicina Psicosomatica* magazine, n. 34, 1977.
- Parietti P., Guantieri G., *Ipnosi e psicoterapia*, in *Rassegna di Ipnosi e Medicina Psicosomatica* magazine, n. 34, 1977.
- Parietti P., Guantieri G., *Problems and Perspectives of Solution in the Teaching of Hypnosis*, in Pajntar M., Rosicar E., Lavric M. (edited by), *Hypnosis in Psychotherapy and Psychosomatic Medicine*, Proceedings of the II European Congress of Hypnosis, Dubrovnik, Croatia, University Press, Lubiana, Slovenia, 1980.
- Parietti P., *Il rilassamento ipnotico in psicosomatica*, in *Terapia in Psicosomatica*, Proceedings of the IX Congresso S.I.M.P., Turin, 1983.
- Parietti P., *Induzione e lettura del corporeo in ipnosi: una tecnica*, in Guantieri G. (edited by), *Il linguaggio del corpo in ipnosi*, Proceedings of the X Congresso Nazionale S.I.M.P., Publisher Il Segno, Negrar (Verona), 1985.
- Parietti P., Guantieri G., Santini M., *L'ipnosi nell'informazione e nella formazione del medico e dello psicologo*, in Guantieri G., Ischia S. (edited by), *L'ipnosi nelle istituzioni. Ruolo e contributo*, Proceedings of the I Congresso Nazionale, Verona, 1985, Editions Istituto 'Bernheim', Verona, 1987.
- Parietti P., *Esperienze di ipnosi in psicoterapia*, in *Prospettive in Psicologia* magazine, 1987.
- Parietti P., *Ipnosi in psicoterapia*, in Del Corno F., Lang M. (edited by), *Trattamento in Psicologia Clinica*, Publisher Franco Angeli, Milan, 1988.
- Parietti P., *L'aggressività del terapeuta quale difesa dall'impotenza*, Symposium *Dall'aggressività alla comunicazione terapeutica in campo ipnologico*, XI Congresso Nazionale S.I.M.P., Messina, 1987, in *Rassegna di Igiene Mentale* magazine, Year XI, 1989.

- Parietti P., Zenoni M.L., *Attività immaginativa ed ipnosi in medicina psicosomatica*, Proceedings of the XIII Congresso Nazionale S.I.M.P., Bologna, 1991.
- Pasetto A., Bartoloni A., Passerelli M., Ischia S., *Tecniche di sedazione psicologica in anestesia loco-regionale*, in *Acta Anaesthesiologica Italica* magazine, n. 29, 1978.
- Pasetto A., Seminara B., Guantieri G., Ischia S., Bartoloni A., *On a Case of Cholecistectomy under Hypnosis*, in Pajntar M., Roskar E., Lavric M. (edited by), *Hypnosis in Psychotherapy and Psychosomatic Medicine*, Proceedings of the 2nd European Congress of Hypnosis, Dubrovnik, Croatia, University Press, Lubiana, Slovenia, 1980.
- Pasetto A., Bartoloni A., Luzzani A., Passerelli M., Remondini P., Rigotti L., Antonello L., *Responsività ipnotica e valutazione del dolore*, in Guantieri G., Ischia S. (edited by), *L'ipnosi nelle istituzioni. Ruolo e contributo*, Proceedings of the I Congresso Nazionale, Verona, 1985, Editions Istituto 'Bernheim', Verona, 1987.
- Pasetto A., *Hypnotisability and Sensitivity to Pain*, Proceedings of the 5th European Congress of Hypnosis in Psychotherapy and Psychosomatic Medicine, Costanza, Germany, 1990.
- Pozzi U., *Il training psicosomatico: nuove acquisizioni*, Proceedings of the XII Congresso Nazionale S.I.M.P., Milan, 1989.
- Robazza C., *L'importanza dell'allenamento mentale nella preparazione sportiva*, in *Karate Oggi* magazine, n. 7, 1989.
- Robazza C., *L'ansia nella prestazione sportiva*, in *Karate Oggi* magazine, n. 8, 1989.
- Robazza C., *La preparazione mentale: tecniche di visualizzazione applicate al karate*, in *Karate Oggi* magazine, n. 12-13, 1990.
- Robazza C., *L'ipnosi nella preparazione mentale dell'atleta. Sperimentazione con soggetti praticanti karate*, VIII Congresso Nazionale di Psicologia dello Sport, Senigallia (Ancona), 1990, in *Movimento* magazine (Organo ufficiale dell'Associazione Italiana Psicologia dello Sport), n. 2, 1990.
- Robazza C., *L'ipnosi nello sport: ambiti di applicazione*, Proceedings of the XIII Congresso Nazionale S.I.M.P., Bologna, 1991.
- Robazza C., *Riduzione dell'ansia ed incremento delle capacità immaginative nello sport attraverso l'ipnosi*, Proceedings of the IX Congresso Nazionale di Ipnosi Clinica e Sperimentale A.M.I.S.I., Monastier (Treviso), 1991.
- Robazza C., *Preparazione mentale nel Karate attraverso l'ipnosi: sintesi di due ricerche*, in *Karate oggi* magazine, n. 24-25-26-27-28-32, 1991.
- Robazza C., Bortoli L., *Preparazione mentale attraverso ipnosi: un modello isomorfico*, Proceedings of the IX Congresso Nazionale di Psicologia dello Sport, Turin, 1992.
- Robazza C., *La preparazione mentale nel tiratore*, in *Quaderni di Tiro Sportivo* magazine, n. 3, 1992.

- Roncaroli P., Guantieri G., *Livelli di interazione nel rapporto interpersonale ipnotico,* Congresso Europeo di Ipnosi in Psicoterapia e Medicina Psicosomatica, Malmö, Sweden, in *Rassegna di Igiene Mentale* magazine, n. 4, 1979.
- Roncaroli P., Guantieri G., *Hypnosis as a Multidimensional Analysis in Psychotherapy,* in Pajntar M., Roskar E., Lavric M. (edited by), *Hypnosis in Psychotherapy and Psychosomatic Medicine,* Proceedings of the 2nd European Congress of Hypnosis, Dubrovnik, Croatia, University Press, Lubiana, Slovenia, 1980.
- Roncaroli P., Guantieri G., *Ipnosi e curva erotica femminile,* in *Rivista di Sessuologia Clinica* magazine, n. 5, 1980.
- Roncaroli P., *Double Semantic Hypnotic Induction in Psychotherapy and Psychosomatic Medicine,* in Guantieri G. (edited by), *Hypnosis in Psychotherapy and Psychosomatic Medicine,* Proceedings of the 3rd European Congress of Hypnosis, Abano Terme (Padua), Publisher Il Segno, Negrar (Verona), 1985.
- Roncaroli P., *Linguaggio delle mani in terapia ipnotica* in Guantieri G. (edited by), *Il linguaggio del corpo in ipnosi,* Proceedings of the X Congresso Nazionale S.I.M.P., Publisher Il Segno, Negrar (Verona), 1985.
- Roncaroli P., *Age Regression in hypnotic treatment and mental reversibility,* Proceedings of the X International Congress of Hypnosis and Psychosomatic Medicine, Toronto, Canada, 1985.
- Roncaroli P., *Applicazione dell'ipnosi in un Ospedale Generale di Zona,* in Guantieri G., Ischia S. (edited by), *L'ipnosi nelle istituzioni. Ruolo e contributo,* Proceedings of the I Congresso Nazionale, Verona, 1985, Editions Istituto 'Bernheim', Verona, 1987.
- Roncaroli P., *Subliminal Perception, Creativity and Hypnosis,* Proceedings of the IV European Congress of Hypnosis in Psychotherapy and Psychosomatic Medicine, Oxford, England, 1987.
- Roncaroli P., Lanari A., *Ipnosi e visualizzazioni guidate nello sport,* Proceedings of the Convegno *Tecniche di intervento in Psicologia dello Sport,* Senigallia (Ancona), 1986, in *Equilibrio* magazine (Bulletin of C.M.P.S.), n. 1, 1987.
- Roncaroli P., Angelozzi A., *Hypnotic Regression and Childish Structures of Thinking,* Proceedings of the XI International Congress of Hypnosis and Psychosomatic Medicine, Leiden, Holland, 1988.
- Roncaroli P., *Hypnosis in the therapy of High Risk Subjects,* Proceedings of the V European Congress of Hypnosis in Psychotherapy and Psychosomatic Medicine, Costanza, Germany, 1990.
- Roncaroli P., Campanella G., *Psico-oncologia ed ipnosi,* Proceedings of the XIII Congresso Nazionale S.I.M.P., Bologna, 1991.
- Roncaroli P., *Ipnosi e schema corporeo,* Proceedings of the IX Congresso Nazionale di Ipnosi Clinica e Sperimentale A.M.I.S.I., Monastier (Treviso), 1991.
- Santini M., Parietti P., Guantieri G., *L'ipnosi nell' informazione e nella formazione del medico e dello psicologo,* in Guantieri G., Ischia S. (edited by), *L'ipnosi nelle*

istituzioni. Ruolo e contributo, Proceedings of the I Congresso Nazionale, Verona, 1985, Editions Istituto 'Bernheim', Verona, 1987.
- Vannoni S., Castagna G., *Rieducazione funzionale e psicosomatica in ortopedia,* in Antonelli F., Lapiccirella V. (edited by), *Allucinogeni e Psicosomatosi,* Vol. III, Publisher Società Editrice Universitaria, Rome, 1972.
- Zanotti L., *L'ipnosi in ostetricia: studio retrospettivo di otto anni di attività in un reparto ospedaliero,* in Guantieri G., Ischia S. (edited by), *L'ipnosi nelle istituzioni. Ruolo e contributo,* Proceedings of the I Congresso Nazionale, Verona, 1985, Editions Istituto 'Bernheim', Verona, 1987.
- Zanotti L., *Preparazione al parto con ipnosi: nuovi orientamenti,* Publisher Il Segno, Negrar (Verona), 1990.
- Zanotti L., *Il parto in ipnosi: indagine su 100 gravide,* Publisher Il Segno, Negrar (Verona), 1990.
- Zanotti L., Esposito E., Andreotti M., *Preparazione al parto con l'ipnosi: riflessioni sui risultati di un questionario inviato alle gestanti dopo il parto nel decennio 1979/1989,* in *Newsletter* magazine, Year VI, n. 1, 1990.
- Zanotti L., *Giving Birth with Hypnosis: Ten Years of Experience in a Hospital Obstetrics Ward,* Proceedings of the V European Congress of Hypnosis in Psychotherapy and Psychosomatic Medicine, Costanza, Germany, 1990.
- Zanotti L., Esposito E., Andreotti M., *Esperienze di parti in ipnosi in un reparto ospedaliero,* Proceedings of the IX Congresso Nazionale di Ipnosi Clinica e Sperimentale A.M.I.S.I., Monastier (Treviso), 1991.
- Zenoni M.L., *La distensione immaginativa come tecnica integrativa in Medicina Psicosomatica,* Proceedings of the Proceedings of the Convegno Internazionale *Mente-Corpo,* in *Riza Psicomatica* magazine, 1987.
- Zenoni M.L., *Il tradursi dell'aggressività verbale e non verbale attraverso il linguaggio del corpo in campo ipnologico,* Congresso S.I.M.P., Messina, 1987, in *Rassegna di Igiene Mentale* magazine, Year I, 1989.
- Zenoni M.L., *Tre bocche più una: la distensione immaginativa come approccio, tecnica e terapia nell'approfondirsi della relazione terapeutica e sviluppo di vissuti corporei,* Proceedings of the II Convegno Internazionale *Mente-Corpo,* Milan, 1987.
- Zenoni M.L., Parietti P., *Attività immaginativa ed ipnosi in medicina psicosomatica,* Proceedings of the XIII Congresso Nazionale S.I.M.P., Bologna, 1991.
- Zenoni M.L., *L'ipnosi in un contesto relazionale sistemico: un caso,* Proceedings of the XIII Congresso Nazionale S.I.M.P., Bologna, 1991.

Reviews

- Angelozzi A., review: Erickson M.H., (edited by di Rossi E.L.), Opere, Vol. VI, *L'ipnoterapia Innovatrice,* Publisher Astrolabio, Rome, 1984, in *Newsletter,* Year I, n.1, 1988.
- Ferrari F., review: Bandler R., Grinder J., *I modelli della tecnica ipnotica di Milton H. Erickson,* Publisher Astrolabio, Rome, 1984, in *Newsletter,* Year II, n. 1, 1989.
- Ferrari F., review: Erickson M.H., Rossi E.L., Rossi S.L., *Tecniche di suggestione ipnotica,* Publisher Astrolabio, Rome, 1984, in *Newsletter* magazine, Year II, n. l, 1989.
- Ferrari F., review: Erickson M.H., Rossi E.L., *Ipnoterapia (Una ricerca clinica),* Publisher Astrolabio, Rome, 1982, in *Newsletter* magazine, Year II, n. 1, 1989.
- Ferrari F., review: Erickson M.H., Rossi E.L., *L'esperienza dell'ipnosi (Approcci terapeutici agli stati alterati), Publisher* Astrolabio, Rome, 1985, in *Newsletter* magazine, Year I, n. 2, 1988.
- Ferrari F., review: Hoffmann H.B., *Manuale di Training Autogeno,* Publisher Astrolabio, Rome, 1980, in *Newsletter* magazine, Year III, n. 3, 1989.
- Ferrari F., review: Edelstien M.G., *Trauma, Trançe e Trasformazione,* Publisher Astrolabio, Rome, 1987, in *Newsletter* magazine, Year III, n. 1, 1990.
- Ferrari F., review: Ferrucci P., *Crescere, teoria e pratica della psicosintesi,* Publisher Astrolabio, Rome, 1981, in *Newsletter* magazine, Year IV, n. 1, 1991.
- Ferrari F., review: Haley J., *Le strategie della psicoterapia,* Publisher Sansoni, Florence, 1977, in *Newsletter* magazine, Year IV, n. 2-3, 1991.
- Galvano O., review: Elizur A.J., Minuchin S., *Malattia mentale ed istituzioni,* Publisher Astrolabio, Rome, 1991, in *Newsletter* magazine, Year IV, n. 2-3, 1991.
- Grecchi V., review: Rossi E.L., *La psicobiologia della guarigione psicofisica,* Publisher Astrolabio, Rome, 1991, in *Newsletter* magazine, Year IV, n. 1, 1991.
- Guantieri G., review: Waxman D., *Hartland's, Medical and Dental Hypnosis, (3rd edition),* Publisher Bailliére Tindall, London, 1988, in *Newsletter* magazine, Year I, n. 1, 1988.
- Guantieri G., review: Hillgard E.R., Hillgard J.R., *Hypnosis in the Relief of Pain,* Publisher William Kaufmann, Los Altos, California, 1983, in *Newsletter* magazine, Year II, n. 1, 1989.
- Sambati M.A., review: Meier C.A., *Il sogno come terapia. Antica incubazione e moderna psicoterapia,* Publisher Edizioni Mediterranee, 1987, in *Newsletter* magazine, Year II, n.3, 1989.

Translations

- De Stavola W., translation: Volgpesi F.A., *Ipnosi umana e animale*, Publisher Piccin, Padua, 1972.
- De Stavola W., translation: Kline M.V., *Freud e l'ipnosi*, Publisher Piccin, Padua, 1976.

Congress Chronicles

- Benatti G., report: II Congresso Nazionale della Società Italiana di Medicina Psicosomatica (S.I.M.P.), Verona, 1969, in *Medicina Psicosomatica* magazine, n. 14, 1969.
- Benatti G., report: IX Congresso Nazionale della Società Italiana di Medicina Psicosomatica (S.I.M.P.), Florence, 1971, in *Neuropsichiatria* magazine, Year XXVI, n. 1, 1971.
- Benatti G., report: *Cenni orientativi alle lezioni del corso di aggiornamento in ipnologia medica*, presso il Centro Studi 'H. Bernheim', Verona, 1971.
- Benatti G., report: IV Congresso Nazionale della Società Italiana di Medicina Psicosomatica (S.I.M.P.), Messina, 1973, in *Medicina Psicosomatica* magazine, n. 18, 1973.
- Benatti G., report: Congresso Nazionale della Società Italiana di Psicoprofilassi Ostetrica, L'Aquila, 1973, in *Medicina Psicosomatica* magazine, n. 19, 1974.
- Benatti G., report: VI Congresso Internazionale di Ipnosi e Medicina Psicosomatica, Uppsala, Sweden, 1973, in *Medicina Psicosomatica* magazine, n. 19, 1974.
- Benatti G., report: IX Corso di Aggiornamento in ipnologia medica, Verona, 1975, in *Medicina Psicosomatica* magazine, n. 20, 1975.
- Benatti G., report: VI Congresso Nazionale della Società Italiana di Medicina Psicosomatica (S.I.M.P.), Milan, 1977, in *Medicina Psicosomatica* magazine, n. 23, 1978.
- Benatti G., report: VII Congresso Nazionale della Società Italiana di Medicina Psicosomatica (S.I.M.P.), Ancona, 1979, in *Medicina Psicosomatica* magazine, n. 24, 1979.
- Benatti G., report: VI Congresso Nazionale della Società Italiana di Medicina Psicosomatica (S.I.M.P.), Venezia, 1981, in *Medicina Psicosomatica* magazine, n. 26, 1981.
- Benatti G., report: IX Congresso Nazionale della Società Italiana di Medicina Psicosomatica (S.I.M.P.), Torino, 1983, in *Medicina Psicosomatica* magazine, n. 28, 1983.
- Benatti G., report: III Congresso Europeo di Ipnosi in Psicoterapia e Medicina Psicosomatica, Abano Terme (Padua), 1984, in *Rivista Italiana di Ipnosi Clinica e Sperimentale* magazine, n. 1, 1985.

- Benatti G., report: X Congresso Nazionale della Società Italiana di Medicina Psicosomatica (S.I.M.P.), Pescara, 1985, in *Medicina Psicosomatica* magazine, n. 30, 1985.
- Benatti G., report: XI Congresso Nazionale della Società Italiana di Medicina Psicosomatica (S.I.M.P.), Messina, 1987, in *Simp-News* magazine, n. 3, 1987.
- Benatti G., report: Convegno Internazionale di formazione e aggiornamento professionale *Mente-Corpo*: *La relazione terapeutica in Medicina Psicosomatica*, Milan, 1987, in *Simp-News* magazine, n. 4, 1988.
- Benatti G., report: XII Congresso Nazionale della Società Italiana di Medicina Psicosomatica (S.I.M.P.), Milan, 1989, in *Simp-News* magazine, n. 5, 1989.
- Benatti G., report: XIII Congresso Nazionale della Società Italiana di Medicina Psicosomatica (S.I.M.P.), Bologna, 1991, in *Newsletter* magazine, anno IV, n. 2-3, 1991.
- Modenese M., report: Tavola Rotonda *L'Ipnosi in Ambito Sportivo*, Verona, 18 novembre 1989, in *Newsletter* magazine, Year III, n. 18-20, 1990.
- Modenese M., report: Congresso *Cancro e Psiche*, Verona, 1989, in *Newsletter* magazine, Year II, n. 2, 1989.
- Zanotti L., considerations: Convegno *La gravidanza alle soglie del 2000: benessere e sicurezza*, Ravenna, 1991, in *Newsletter* magazine, Year IV, n. 2-3, 1991.

Disclosure Articles

- Guantieri G., *L'ipnosi nella terapia del dolore*, in *Riza Psicosomatica* magazine, Milan, January 1988.
- Parietti P., *Si rilassi... dalla psicoanalisi all'ipnosi, all'analisi immaginativa*, in *Riza Psicosomatica* magazine, n. 43, Milan, September 1984.
- Parietti P., *Ipnosi, una traccia*, in *Riza Scienze* magazine, n. 9, Milan, September 1985.
- Parietti P., *Un dolore sapiente*, in *Riza Psicosomatica* magazine, n. 67, Milan, September 1986.
- Parietti P., *L'ipnosi nella cura della cefalea*, in *Riza Psicosomatica* magazine, n. 67, Milan, September 1986.
- Parietti P., *L'ipnosi nella terapia del dolore*, in *Riza Psicosomatica* magazine, n. 68, Milan, October 1986.
- Parietti P., *Istinto o funzione di recupero, ipnosi e rilassamento*, in *Riza Psicosomatica* magazine, n. 71, Milan, January 1987.
- Parietti P., *Tenere le distanze: L'evoluzione del "toccare" nella relazione medico/paziente*, in *Riza Psicosomatica* magazine, n. 73, Milan, March 1987.
- Parietti P., *Dal sintomo alla scelta della terapia*, in *Riza Psicosomatica* magazine, n. 83, Milan, April 1987.

- Parietti P., *Le immagini del piacere e del dolore*, in *Riza Psicosomatica* magazine, n. 83, Milan, January 1988.
- Parietti P., *La terapia del grande fumatore... lei non fumerà più*, in *Riza Psicosomatica* magazine, n. 85, Milan, March 1988.

Thesis of Graduation

- Boldrin E., *Considerations on the evolution of hypnotherapy*, Degree Thesis in Psychology at the Faculty of Education of the University of Padua, Academic year 1986-87. Supervisor Prof. Paolo Santanastaso, Co-Supervisor Dr. Andrea Angelozzi.
- Cobello P., *Psychotherapeutic models in hypnosis*, Specialisation thesis in Psychiatry at the University of Verona, Institute of Psychiatry, Academic Year 1986-87, Supervisor: Prof. Antonio Balestrieri, Co-supervisor: prof. Lorenzo Burti.

Conferences and Interviews

- Guantieri G., Roncaroli P.: interview on *Swedish TV* about the situation of hypnosis in Italy, August 1988.
- Guantieri G., *Hypnosis as* a therapy, Anthropos Study Centre, October 1989.
- Guantieri G., *Hypnosis in sports, Channel 65 news*, November 1989.
- Guantieri G., *Hypnosis in Medicine* (edited by Baggio), in *Abitare a Verona* magazine, Year II, n. 9, November 1989.
- Guantieri G., *Psychosomatic medicine and clinical hypnosis* (edited by Della Bella), in *L'Arena*, 30 November 1989.
- Guantieri G., *Emotive storms*, Conference of the Italian Society of Psychosomatic Medicine (S.I.M.P., Brescia Section), November 1989.
- Guantieri G., *Hypnosis*, in *Elle* magazine, 1990.
- Guantieri G., *Emotions and Disease*, Anthropos Study Centre, 1990.
- Guantieri G., *That thing* (edited by Laura Zanoni), in *Verona* Magazine, January 1991.
- Guantieri G., *Hypnosis in Medicine* (edited by Claudio Capitini), *Telearena*, January 1991.
- Guantieri G., *Hypnosis: a foundation and a perspective*, Know, research and information group, Verona, January 1991.
- Guantieri G., *Psychosomatic medicine and hypnosis* (edited by Claudio Capitini), *RadioAdige*, February 1991.R

Bibliography of the studies of the 'Bernheim' institute published in *Acta Hypnologica*

Editions of the Italian Institute of Clinical Hypnosis and Psychotherapy 'H. Bernheim', School of Research and Training, San Martino B.A., (Verona), in the period 1997-2010.

- Alquati E., *Un po' di storia ..., di nuovo..., di antico. Some History..., Something New..., Something Old,* Year IV, n. 3, September 2000.
- Alquati E., *Ipnosi e medicine non convenzionali. Hypnosis and Non-conventional Medicines,* Year VI, n. 2-3, May-September 2002.
- Alquati E., *Mesmer: le 27 proposizioni tra Magnetismo e Immaginazione. Mesmer: the 27 propositions between Magnetism and Imagination,* Year VII, n. 2-3, May-September 2003.
- Andreoli V., *Ipnosi e neuroscienze. Hypnosis and Neurosciences,* Year VIII, n. 1-2, January-May 2004.
- Arena M., *Il linguaggio ipnotico nella comunicazione psicoterapeutica. The Hypnotic Language in Psychotherapeutic Communication,* Year I, n. 3, September 1997.
- Barbieri C., Locatelli F., Roncaroli P., *L'aggressività come disturbo della relazione terapeutica in caso di patologia neoplastica. Aggressiveness as a Disorder of the Therapeutic Relationship in Case of Neoplastic Pathology,* Year VIII, n. 1-2, January-May 2004.
- Barbieri C., Roncaroli P., *Consenso formale, confusione di ruoli e condivisione di esperienza di malattia: riflessioni in margine ad un caso di trapianto di midollo osseo in minore. Formal Consent, Role Confusion and Sharing of Illness Experience: Side Reflections on a Case of Bone Marrow Graft into a Minor,* Year VII, n. 1, January 2003.
- Benatti G., *Un omaggio a G. Guantieri. L'ipnosi nella storia dell'Istituto 'H. Bernheim'. 30 anni di studi e di ricerche. A Homage to G. Guantieri. Hypnosis in the History of 'H. Bernheim' Institute. 30 Years of Studies and Research,* Year I, n. 1, January 1997.
- Benatti G., *L'ipnosi: un possibile strumento nella realtà diagnostica. Hypnosis: a Possible Instrument in Diagnostic Practice,* Year I, n. 2, May 1997.
- Benatti G., *Una tecnica ipnotica per la scontentezza. A Hypnotic Technique for Discontent,* Year III, n. 1, January 1999.
- Benatti G., *La relazione ipnotica nei disturbi psicosomatici. The Hypnotic Relationship in Psychosomatic Disorders,* Year V, n. 1-2, January-May 2001.
- Bottoli A., *Ipnosi e ostetricia. Hypnosis and Obstetrics,* Year VI, n. 2-3, May-September 2002.
- Bottoli A., Brugnoli A., *Etica del dolore e della sofferenza alle soglie del terzo millennio. Ethics of Sorrow and Pain, on the Brink of the Third Millennium,* Year IV, n. 3, September 2000.

- Bottoli A., Brugnoli A., Schilirò G., *Linee guida per i corsi propedeutici di ipnosi clinica. Guidelines for Clinical Hypnosis Propaedeutic Courses,* Year II, n. 2-3, May-September 1998.
- Brugnoli A. (Review): Crosa G., *Il training autogeno di Schultz. Schultz's Self-Training,* Year II, n. 2-3, May-September 1998.
- Brugnoli A., *A Walter De Stavola. Dedicated to Walter De Stavola,* Year V, n. 1-2, January-May 2001.
- Brugnoli A., *Ipnosi e dolore: nuove vie dell'ipnoterapia del dolore cronico. Hypnosis and Pain: new Ways of the Hypnotherapy of Chronic Pain,* Year VI, n. 2-3, May-September 2002.
- Brugnoli A., *Autoipnosi e sindrome del burn-out professionale. Self-hypnosis and Occupational Burn-out Syndrome,* Year IV, n. 1, January 2000.
- Brugnoli A., *Stati di coscienza modificati ed ipnotici e possibile attivazione di fenomeni cosiddetti paranormali. Modified and Hypnotic States of Conscience and Possible Activation of So-called Paranormal Phenomena,* Year V, n. 3, September 2001.
- Brugnoli A., *Neurofisiologia di realtà percepita e realtà rappresentata: quale relazione tra "Working memory" e visualizzazione mentale in ipnosi. Neurophysiology of Perceived and Represented Reality: as Relationship between "Working memory" and mental visualisation in hypnosis,* Year V, n. 3, September 2001.
- Brugnoli A., Brugnoli M.P., *In ricordo del Dr. Alberto Piccoli. In Dr. Alberto Piccoli's memory,* Year VIII, n. 1-2, January-May 2004.
- Brugnoli A., *Gualtiero Guantieri: un medico coraggioso, un intuitivo geniale, un amico leale,* Year XII, n. 3, September 2008 and Year XIII, n. 1, January 2009.
- Brugnoli M.P., *Rilassamento ed ipnosi in età evolutiva. Relaxation and Hypnosis in the Age of Development,* Year VI, n. 1, January 2002.
- Brugnoli M.P., *Il "mental training" nello sport: ricerca sull'efficacia del mental training legata alla prestazione di forza con l'esecuzione del test di Bosco. Mental Training in Sports: a Research on the Effectiveness of Mental Training Linked to Strength Performance with Giving Bosco's Test,* Year VII, n. 2-3, May-September 2003.
- Brugnoli M.P., *Tecniche di rilassamento ed ipnosi nel controllo della sofferenza del Paziente Terminale. Relaxation Techniques and Hypnosis in the Control of the Terminal Patient's Pain,* Year VIII, n. 1-2, January-May 2004.
- Brugnoli M.P., (Review): *Brugnoli A., Tecniche di rilassamento e ipnosi clinica in terapia del dolore e cure palliative,* Year XIII, n. 3, September 2009 and Year XIV, n. 1, January 2010.
- Cacciacarne R., *Ipnosi nella pratica ambulatoriale: un modello efficace di approccio terapeutico,* Year XII, n. 3, September 2008 and Year XIII, n. 1, January 2009.
- Cacciacarne R., *Verso il sé integrato "A due mani ed una voce" con uso sinergico di parole guidate e manipolazioni cranio-sacrali,* Year XIII, n. 3, September 2009 and Year XIV, n. 1, January 2010.
- Caldironi B., *Commemorazione di Werther Ferioli. Werther Ferioli's Commemoration,* Year II, n. 2, January 1998.

- Caldironi B., *Parafrenia e parapsicologia. Paraphrenia and Parapsychology,* Year II, n. 2, January 1998.
- Carletti C., *Ulysses,* Year VII, n. 1, January 2003.
- Carletti C., *Testo poetico, ipnosi e fiaba terapeutica: una proposta sinergica. Poetic Text, Hypnosis and Therapeutic Tale: a Synergic Proposal,* Year VII, n. 2-3, May-September 2003.
- Carletti C., *L'arco e la tela,* Year XI, n. 3, September 2007.
- Carletti C., *Dafne e Atalanta: la corsa insostenibile,* Year XI, n. 3, September 2007.
- Carletti C., *S. Anna, la Vergine e il Bambino: l'ansia del tempo femminile,* Year XI, n. 3, September 2007.
- Carletti C., *L'aspra bufera,* Year XIII, n. 3, September 2009 and Year XIV, n. 1, January 2010.
- Carletti C., Piazza C., *Ipnosi e poesia: un uso del ritmo e della metafora in un'esperienza di formazione di gruppo. Hypnosis and Poetry. A use of Rhythm and Metaphor in a Group Training Experience,* Year X, n. 2-3, May-September 2006.
- De' Lutti P. (Review): Oberhuber W., *Ipnosi, terapia come comunicazione. Hypnosis Therapy as Communication,* Year IV, n. 2, May 2000.
- De Stavola W., *Considerazioni neurofisiologiche in tema di attraversate a nuoto su lunghe distanze. Neurophysiological Reflections about Swims across Long Distances,* Year V, n. 1-2, January-May 2001.
- Donadi P., *Parto e ipnosi. Childbirth and Hypnosis,* Year IV, n. 2, May 2000.
- Faretta E., Parietti P., *La psicoterapia ipnotica e l'EMDR nel disturbo di panico. Hypnotic Psychotherapy and EMDR in Panic Trouble,* Year VII, n. 1, January 2003.
- Ferioli W., *Induzione ipnotica: la gita in pullman. An Hypnotic Induction: The Trip By Coach,* Year II, n. 2, January 1998.
- Ferioli W., *Introduzione all'impiego dell'ipnosi in pediatria. Introduction to the Employment of Hypnosis in Pediatrics,* Year II, n. 2-3, May-September 1998.
- Ferrari F. (Review): Milton Erickson, *A scuola di ipnosi. In the School of Hypnosis,* Year I, n. 1, January 1997.
- Ferrari F. (Review): Michele Ritterman, *L'ipnosi nella terapia della famiglia. Hypnosis in Family Therapy,* Year I, n. 2, May 1997.
- Ferrari F. (Review): Del Castello E., Loriedo C., *Tecniche dirette ed indirette in ipnosi e psicoterapia. Direct and Indirect Techniques in Hypnosis and Psychotherapy,* Year I, n. 3 September 1997.
- Ferrari F. (Review): Caldironi B., *Seminari di psicoterapia immaginativa. Seminars of Imaginative Psychotherapy,* Year II, n. 1, January 1998.
- Ferrari F. (Review): Mosconi G., *Teoretica e pratica della psicoterapia ipnotica. Theoretics and Practice of Hypnotic Psychotherapy,* Year II, n. 2-3, May-September 1998.

- Ferrari F. (Review): Bandier R., Grinder J., *I modelli della tecnica ipnotica di Milton Erickson. Patterns of the Hypnotic Techniques of Milton H. Erickson*, Year III, n. 2-3, May-September 1999.
- Ferrari F. (Review): Erickson M, Rossi E.L., *Ipnoterapia. Hypnotherapy*, Year III, n. 2-3, May-September 1999.
- Ferrari F. (Review): Erickson M., Rossi E.L., *L'esperienza dell'ipnosi. The Experience of Hypnosis*, Year III, n. 2-3, May-September 1999.
- Ferrari F. (Review): Erickson M., Rossi E.L., Rossi S., *Tecniche di suggestione ipnotica*, Year III, n. 2-3, May-September 1999.
- Finco G., Polati E., Bartoloni A., Bonfante P., Bianchin E., Perini A., *Ipnosi in ospedale: problematiche e prospettive. Hypnosis at the Hospital: Problems and Perspectives*, Year I, n. 3 September 1997.
- Galili E., *Il mito dell'eroe sotto l'ombra del terrore. The Hero's Myth under the Shadow of Terror*, Year VIII, n. 3, September 2004.
- Galvano O., *Modificazione della coscienza nelle relazioni familiari. The Conscience Change in Family Relationships*, Year I, n. 2, May 1997.
- Gasparini D., *In tema di consenso esplicito e presunto. About Explicit and Assumed Consent*, Year I, n. 3, September 1997.
- Gasparini D., Piazza C., *Aspetti legali nella professione di psicoterapeuta. Legal Aspects of the Psychotherapist's Profession*, Year I, n. 1, January 1997.
- Gocci G., *L'ipnosi: storia, teoria e pratica. Hypnosis: History, Theory and Practice*, Year III, n. 2-3, May-September 1999.
- Gocci G., *Giovani e nuove droghe: un fenomeno sociale. Young People and New Drugs: a Social Phenomenon*, Year V, n. 1-2, January-May 2001.
- Gocci G., *Saturno e la depressione. Saturn and the Depression*, Year VIII, n. 3, September 2004.
- Gocci G., *Buddismo, cristianesimo ed individuazione. Buddhism, Christianity and Individuation*, Year IX, n. 1-2, January-May 2005.
- Gocci G., *I gruppi di individuazione (L'officina dell'immaginario). Individuation Groups (The workshop of imagery)*, Year IX, n. 1-2, January-May 2005.
- Gocci G., *L'anima perduta. The Missing Soul*, Year IX, n. 1-2, January-May 2005.
- Gocci G., *Psicologia al femminile. Womanly Psychology*, Year IX, n. 1-2, January-May 2005.
- Gocci G., *Un vomito che non voleva cessare. An Unremitting Vomit*, Year IX, n. 1-2, January-May 2005.
- Gocci G., Piazza C., *Corpo, sogno ed immagine in ipnosi senza trance. Body, Dream and Image in Hypnosis without Trance*, Year III, n. 1, January 1999.
- Gocci G., Piazza C., *Ipnosi moderna e comunicazione. Modern Hypnosis and Communication*, Year IV, n. 1, January 2000.
- Gocci G., Ranieri R., *Una ricerca sulla personalità del tossicodipendente con il test Myers-Briggs Type Indicator. A Search on the Drug Addict's Personality with the Myers-Briggs Type Indicator*, Year IV, n. 2, May 2000.

- Grecchi V., *Confronto e sviluppo delle idee e delle metodologie di due grandi maestri e innovatori: G. Guantieri e M. Erickson*, Year XII, n. 3, September 2008 and Year XIII, n. 1, January 2009.
- Grecchi V., *Ipnosi Ericksoniana, Tecniche Direttive, EMDR e Mindfulness*, Year XIII, n. 2, May 2009.
- Guantieri G., *Fondamenti e prospettive dell'ipnologia. Hypnology Foundations and Perspectives*, Year II, n. 2-3, May-September 1998.
- Guantieri G., *Schema di tecnica induttiva ipnotica. Outline of a Hypnotic Inductive Technique*, Year II, n. 2-3, May-September 1998.
- Guerra G., *"Ipnosi e sofferenza umana". Riflessioni e dati preliminari per un contributo alla ricerca sul coinvolgimento dei familiari e partners nell'utilizzo di tecniche ipnotiche. "Hypnosis and Human Pain". Reflections and Preliminary Data for a Contribute to the Research into the Relatives and Partners Involvement when Hypnotic Techniques are Used*, Year I, n. 1, January 1997.
- Handel D., *Hypnosis in advanced illness: Finding hope in the forest of pain and suffering (first part). L'ipnosi applicata a malattie in stato avanzato: come trovare la speranza nella foresta del dolore e della sofferenza (prima parte)*, Year XIII, n. 2, May 2009.
- Handel D., *Hypnosis in advanced illness: Finding hope in the forest of pain and suffering (second part). L'ipnosi applicata a malattie in stato avanzato: come trovare la speranza nella foresta del dolore e della sofferenza (seconda parte)*, Year XIII, n. 3, September 2009 and Year XIV, n. 1, January 2010.
- La Porta G., *Jung nella letteratura e nell'arte. Jung in Literature and Art*, Year IX, n. 3, September 2005 and Year X, n. 1, January 2006.
- Lodetti R., *L'anima neurofisiologica. The Neurophysiologic Soul*, Year VI, n. 1, January 2002.
- Lodetti R., *L'anima umana tra droga e ipnosi. The Human Soul between Drug and Hypnosis*, Year VII, n. 2-3, May-September 2003.
- Lora M., *Tra sogno e musica. Between Dream and Music*, Year III, n. 2-3, May-September 1999.
- Malesani P.G., *Gualtiero Guantieri: il Maestro Ipnologo*, Year XII, n. 3, September 2008 and Year XIII, n. 1, January 2009.
- Malesani P.G., *Ipnosi sciamanica tra bene e male. Terapia e manipolazione*, Year XV, n. 1, May 2 *comunicazione* 011.
- Martinelli G., *Ipnosi e odontoiatria. Hypnosis and Dentistry*, Year VI, n. 2-3, May-September 2002.
- Modenese M., *Congresso Europeo di Ipnosi. Gozo (Malta) Ottobre 2005: Presentazione in Assemblea Plenaria. Presentation in Plenary Assembly*, Year X, n. 2-3, May-September 2006.
- Modenese M., *Il trattamento con l'ipnosi della sindrome dell'arto fantasma. Alcune valutazioni psicodinamiche sul comportamento del soggetto. The Treatment through Hypnosis of Ghost-Limb Syndrome. Some Psychodynamic Remarks on the Subject's Behaviour*, Year II, n. 1, January 1998.

- Modenese M., *Sogno e ipnosi. Dream and Hypnosis,* Year III, n. 2-3, May-September 1999.
- Modenese M., *Ipnosi e psicoterapia. Hypnosis and Psychotherapy,* Year VI, n. 2-3, May-September 2002.
- Modenese M., *Ipnosi immaginativa in psicoterapia: tra mentale e corporeo. Imaginative Hypnosis in Psychotherapy, between Mind and Body,* Year X, n. 2-3, May-September 2006.
- Modenese M., *Formazione e Ipnologia,* Anno XII, n. 3, September 2008 and Year XIII, n. 1, January 2009.
- Montanari M., *Basi neurofisiologiche dell'ipnosi. Hypnosis Neurophysiological Bases,* Year II, n. 2-3, May-September 1998.
- Muzi P.G., Angelozzi A., *Costruire la trançe. Mezzi linguistici e modelli esplicativi. Building up Trance. Linguistic Means and Illustrative Models,* Year I, n. 2, May 1997.
- Norsa A., *Un'applicazione delle visualizzazioni guidate di Caldironi-Widmann con operatori sanitari. An Application of Caldironi's-Widmann's Guided Visualisations with Health Operators,* Year IV, n. 1, January 2000.
- Norsa A. (Review): Caldironi B., *Semi di luce. Seeds of light,* Year IV, n. 2, May 2000.
- Norsa A., *Ipnosi terapia nella depressione. Hypnosis Therapy in Depression,* Year VIII, n. 3, September 2004.
- Norsa A., Bilone F., Robotti C.A., *Ipnosi e cancro: una ricerca condotta presso l'Ospedale Civile Maggiore di Verona. Hypnosis and Cancer: a Research Carried Out at the Main Civilian Hospital in Verona,* Year V, n. 3, September 2001.
- Oliverio A., *Presentazione di Psicoterapia e Neuroscienze,* Year XII, n. 1-2 January-May 2 0 0 8 .
- Piazza C., *L'ipnosi come strumento di formazione per l'operatore socio-sanitario; un'esperienza con operatori psichiatrici. Hypnosis as a Training Instrument for the Socio-sanitary Operator; an Experience with Psychiatric Operators,* Year II, n. 1, January 1998.
- Piazza C., *Commemorazione di Luciano De Benedetti. Luciano De Benedetti's Commemoration,* Year III, n. 2-3, May-September 1999.
- Piazza C., *Considerazioni su pratica sportiva e disabilità, alla luce della psicoterapia ipnotica di Milton Erickson. Considerations about Sports Practice and Disability, in the Light of Milton Erickson's Hypnotic Psychotherapy,* Year III, n. 2-3, May-September 1999.
- Piazza C., *Esperienze di ipnosi senza trançe in gruppo. Group Hypnotic Experiences without Trance,* Year III, n. 2-3, May-September 1999.
- Piazza C., *Aspetti di rilievo nella formazione del personale impiegato nel trattamento di soggetti con problemi psichiatrici: la relazione ipnotica come strumento. Relevant Aspects of Training Psychiatric Operators,* Year III, n. 2-3, May-September 1999.
- Piazza C., *Dalla frammentazione specialistica alla comunicazione unificante; l'ipnosi nell'ottica psicosomatica. From the Fragmentation of the Specialisation to the Unifying*

- *Communication: Hypnosis from a Psychosomatic Point of View,* Year IV, n. 1, January 2000.
- Piazza C., *Due induzioni ipnotiche: il tappeto volante e Siddharta. Two Hypnotic Inductions: The Flying Carpet and Siddharta,* Year IV, n. 2, May 2000.
- Piazza C., *La relazione ipnotica nel tossicodipendente. The Hypnotic Relationship in the Drug Addict,* Year IV, n. 2, May 2000.
- Piazza C., *L'ipnosi e l'acqua: veicoli psicosomatici del linguaggio corporeo. Hypnosis and Water: Psychosomatic Means of the Body Language,* Year V, n. 1-2, January-May 2001.
- Piazza C., *Ipnosi e psicosomatica. Hypnosis and Psychosomatics,* Year VI, n. 2-3, May-September 2002.
- Piazza C., *Consapevolezza e guarigione. Awareness and Recovery,* Year VII, n. 2-3, May-September 2003.
- Piazza C., *Le depressioni. Esperienze cliniche e di vita. Depressions. Clinical and Life Experiences,* Year VIII, n. 3, September 2004.
- Piazza C., *Inconscio e approccio olistico,* Year XI, n. 1-2, January-May 2007.
- Piazza C., *Disturbo psichiatrico e comunicazione alterata,* Year XI, n. 1-2, January-May 2007.
- Piazza C., *Psicoterapia immaginativa nell'ansia prestazionale,* Year XI, n. 1-2, January-May 2007.
- Piazza C., *L'ansia normaloide,* Year XI, n. 1-2, January-May 2007.
- Piazza C., *Per una semeiotica dell'inconscio,* Year XI, n. 1-2, January-May 2007.
- Piazza C., Editorial and Review of the Conference Proceedings: *"Ipnosi Guntieriana e i suoi Sviluppi nel Tempo", San Martino B.A. (Verona), 15 Novembre 2008,* Year XII, n. 3, September 2008 and Year XIII, n. 1, January 2009.
- Piazza C., *Ipnosi in Progress,* Year XIII, n. 3, September 2008 and Year XIV, n. 1, January 2009.
- Piazza C., *Editoriale,* Year XIV, n. 2, May 2009.
- Piazza C., *Il dolore esistenziale, terra di confine tra corpo, mente e spirito; tecniche immaginative e di rilassamento in gruppo per l'approccio al dolore e alla malattia,* Year XIII, n. 2, May 2009.
- Piazza C., *Editoriale,* Year XIII, n. 3, September 2009 and Year XIV, n. 1, January 2010.
- Piazza C., Busani P. (Review): Jeffrey Zeig, *L'induzione: l'applicazione pratica dell'ipnosi ericksoniana. The Induction: Practical Application of Ericksonian.* Year I, n. 1, January 1997.
- Piazza C., Busani P. (Review): Camillo Loriedo, *Linguaggio diretto ed indiretto in ipnosi. Direct and Indirect Language in Hypnosis,* Year I, n. 3 September 1997.
- Piazza C., Carletti C., *Un'esperienza integrata tra analisi immaginativa Junghiana e psicoterapia ipnotica Ericksoniana. An Integration Experience between Jungian Imaginative Analysis and Ericksonian Hypnotic Psychotherapy,* Year X, n. 2-3, May-September 2006.

- Piazza C., Carletti C., *Editoriali. Editorials,* Year X, n. 2-3, May-September 2006.
- Piazza C., Modenese M., *Esperienze di trançe ipnotica in attività di gruppo a mediazione corporea. Experiences of Hypnotic Trance Bodily Mediated Group Activities,* Year VI, n. 1, January 2002.
- Regaldo G., *Tecniche di induzione rapida,* Year XII, n. 1-2 January-May 2008.
- Regaldo G., *Ipnosi in ostetricia,* Year XII, n. 1-2 January-May 2008.
- Roncaroli P., *Le emozioni primarie: loro importanza nelle fasi acute e croniche della malattia oncoematologica. Primary Emotions: their Importance in the Chronic and Acute Phases of the Oncohaematologic Illness,* Year V, n. 1-2, January-May 2001.
- Roncaroli P., *Ipnosi e gruppi nell'istituzione. Hypnosis and Groups in the Institution,* Year VI, n. 2-3, May-September 2002.
- Roncaroli P., Vallero E., Verri A., *Analisi di gruppo su base ipnotica in patologia oro-alimentare. Group Analysis on a Hypnotic Basis in Food Disorders,* Year II, n. 1, January 1998.
- Schilirò G., Bottoli A., Brugnoli A., *Nuovi modelli di studio dell'ipnotizzabilità mediante reti neurali artificiali. Suscettibilità e refrattarietà all'ipnosi. New Models to Study Hypnotizability through Artificial Neuro-networks,* Year III, n. 1, January 1999.
- Zenoni M.L., *L'ipnosi come processo olistico per operatori e utenti. Hypnosis as a Holistic Process for Operators and Users,* Year VI, n. 1, January 2002.

Index

02	**Introduction**
	Roots and fruits of Guantierian Hypnological Epistemology, by Consuelo Candida Casula
08	**In Memoriam**
	Dedicated to Gualtiero Guanteri, by Giuseppe de Benedittis
10	**Notations**
10	Preface
12	Considerations and memories, by hypnologists who were acquainted with Gualtiero Guantieri
12	- Directors of national and international institutes of hypnology
19	- Executives and Members of the 'Bernheim' Institute
33	Memories of Gualtiero Guantieri at various conventions and congresses
33	- XX Congress of the Italian Society of Psychosomatic Medicine (SIMP), dedicated to Gualtiero Guantieri. Anxiety in the clinic and in today's society, *Verona, 21-23 October 2005*
35	- *Conference of the 'Bernheim' Institute:* Guantierian Hypnology and its developments over time, *San Martino B.A. (Verona), November 15, 2008*
37	- *The 10th National Congress of the Italian Society of Hypnosis.* The languages of hypnosis: A bridge between mind and body, between past and future and between imagination and reality *Verona, 21-23 October 2016.*
38	Gualtiero Guantieri reconsidered in current hypnology by Andrea Angelozzi: Forty years later "Hypnosis: a foundation and a perspective"
43	Gualtiero Guantieri and his hypnology in virtual encyclopaedias
45	**Chapter 1**
	Gualtiero Guantieri: biographical notes
45	Origins
47	Childhood, adolescence and youth
48	The student
49	The Man
54	The family
57	The doctor, the hypnologist, the psychotherapist
61	The professor
63	The scientist
69	Old age and death
73	**Chapter 2**
	The 'H. Bernheim' Institute of Clinical Hypnosis and Psychotherapy

94	**Chapter 3**
	Epistemological foundations of Guantierian Hypnology
95	The need for a philosophical foundation of hypnology
98	The humanist and holistic conception of the person
98	- What vision of man?
99	- Theorising of the Self
101	- Hypnosis, spirituality and transcendence
103	The historicist and anthropological consideration of hypnological Phenomena
104	The multidisciplinary approach to the study of hypnosis
107	Psychosomatic inspiration
107	The need for a competent hypnological community
111	- The hypnologist between omnipotence and impotence
114	The future prospects of hypnological science
115	Conclusive comments
116	**Chapter 4**
	The Guantierian definition of hypnosis
120	**Chapter 5**
	Self-hypnosis and relaxation techniques
120	Self-hypnosis as a singular hypnotic modality
121	Differences between hypnosis and self-hypnosis
124	**Chapter 6**
	The Guantierian hypnotic induction method
124	The pre-inductive phase
125	The induction phase
127	The intensification of hypnosis
128	The de-hypnotisation phase
130	**Chapter 7**
	Compendium of Guantieri's 'L'ipnosi' (Hypnosis)
130	**Development of hypnosis studies**
130	- The pre-scientific phase
134	- The scientific phase
135	- The current state of hypnosis studies
138	**The Phenomenology of hypnosis**
138	- Hypnosis as a state and as an interpersonal relationship
139	- Expressions of hypnosis
141	- The effects of hypnosis
143	**The nature of hypnosis and some hypnotic phenomena**
143	- Neurophysiological interpretations of hypnosis
145	- Socio-psychological interpretations of hypnosis

146	- Psychoanalytic interpretations of hypnosis
148	- Dynamics of some hypnotic phenomena
149	**The induction of hypnosis**
149	- Hypnotisability
150	- Means of hypnotic induction
151	- Modes of hypnotic inductions and de-hypnotisation
153	- Hypnosis as a means of experimental investigation
154	- Hypnosis as a means of clinical investigation
155	**Hypnosis as a therapeutic means**
155	- Hypnotherapy for somatic disorders
157	- Hypnotherapy in psychosomatic disorders
162	- Principles of hypnotherapy in psychosomatic disorders
164	- Practical applications of hypnotherapy in psychosomatic medicine
166	- Hypnotherapy for mental disorders
167	**Other practical applications of hypnosis in medicine**
167	- The use of hypnosis in obstetrics
168	- The use of hypnosis in surgery
168	- The use of hypnosis in dentistry
170	**Appendix – Animal hypnosis**
171	**Supplement**
	Holistic conception of the person in neonatology, psychomotricity and neuroscience
171	**Introduction**
173	**Neonatology**
175	**Psychomotricity**
178	**Neuroscience**
179	**Conclusions**
182	**General Bibliography**
198	**Bibliography of the studies of the 'Bernheim' institute in the period 1988-1993**
198	**Original Works**
220	**Reviews**
221	**Translations**
221	**Congress Chronicles**
222	**Disclosure Articles**
223	**Thesis of Graduation**
223	**Conferences and Interviews**
224	**Bibliography of the studies of the 'Bernheim' institute published in Acta Hypnologica**

Pier Giorgio Malesani

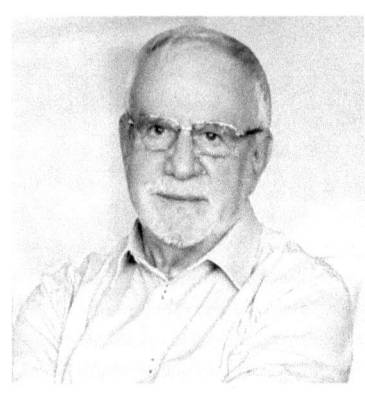

Pier Giorgio Malesani, (b. 1943) is a Psychologist, Psychotherapist, Hypnologist. He was a Founding Member and Past President of CISERPP (Italian Centre for Studies and Research in Psychology and Psychomotricity) of Verona and is Director of the 'H. Bernheim' Italian Institute for Clinical Hypnosis and Psychotherapy in Verona.

He graduated in Psychology at the University of Padua, in 1980, and acquired specialised theoretical-practical training in Hypnology and Relaxation Techniques at the same 'Bernheim' Institute between 1981 and 1984.

Since 1984, he has been a lecturer at the Advanced Professional School of Psychomotor Training at CISERPP in Verona and at the Two-year Theoretical-Practical Specialisation Course in Relaxation Techniques, organised by the same Centre.

Massimo Guantieri

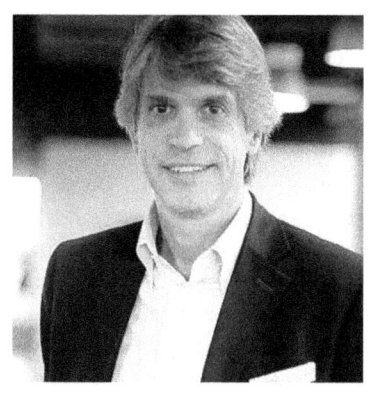

Massimo Guantieri (b.1965) is a husband and father. With over 25 years of experience in Education and Training, he is a seasoned educator, a dedicated professional trainer, and a compassionate observer of humanity. As a Senior Executive he worked and lived amidst diverse cultural and interdisciplinary contexts, from India and China to Vietnam, Europe, and South America, gaining profound insights into the essence of human existence: an interconnectedness with others, active engagement in life and the imperative to support fellow human beings.

He has a degree in Economics and Business, as well as an MBA in Communication and Relational Psychology and further specialisation in NLP, Enneagram, Communication, and Situational Leadership.

He actively participates in and teaches at national and international seminars, workshops and MBA courses.

Since 2016, Massimo has served as a Board Director of the 'H. Bernheim' Italian Institute of Clinical Hypnosis and Psychotherapy.

Beyond his professional endeavours, Massimo actively supports various volunteering associations, be it bringing smiles to hospital wards as a Clown Doctor in hospitals, aiding the homeless in Italy, or providing comfort to those in their final days at an end-of-life hospice in India.

Carlo Piazza

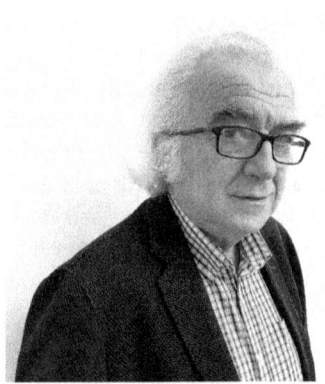

Carlo Piazza, born in 1956, a Basaglia-inspired psychiatrist, Jungian-trained psychodynamic psychotherapist with a Master's degree in Cognitive-Behavioural Psychotherapy, Guantierian and Ericksonian hyp-notherapist, specialist in Psychiatry, Pain Therapy and in Criminology and Forensic Psychopathology and expert witness for the Verona Tribunal since 1990, was a student of Gualtiero Guantieri in the years 1982-1988, gaining three diplomas (basic, advanced and analgesic hypnosis) in parallel with his own psychiatric training; he worked for 40 years in various public services in the Veneto region and directed in the latter part of his career first the Psychiatric Service of San Bonifacio (VR) and then the R.E.M.S. (Residenza per Esecuzione Misure di Sicurezza) regional facility in Nogara (VR), both in Aulss 9 Scaligera, before partially retiring in December 2019.

Since then he has been carrying out his clinical, hypnotherapeutic and psychotherapeutic professional activity at his private practice in San Martino Buon Albergo (VR). He is currently President of the Bernheim Institute and Honorary President Didactic and Supervisor of the School of Psychosynthetic Psychotherapy and Ericksonian Hypnosis in Vicenza and Trento, created in San Martino Buon Albergo (VR) from the Institute and of which he was co-founder in 2001. He has published 135 publications in book form, scientific articles, editorials, and has participated in books as author, co-author and with introductions, prefaces and afterwords.

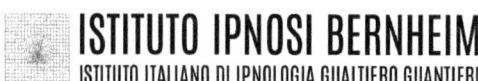
ISTITUTO IPNOSI BERNHEIM
ISTITUTO ITALIANO DI IPNOLOGIA GUALTIERO GUANTIERI

Contact

istitutobernheim@gmail.com
giomalesa@libero.it
massimo.guantieri65@gmail.com
carlo.piazza56@gmail.com